Physician's Guide to
Cancer Care Complications

FUNDAMENTALS OF CANCER MANAGEMENT

Series Editors

Norman M. Bleehen
Addenbrooke's Hospital
Cambridge, England

Eli Glatstein
National Cancer Institute
Bethesda, Maryland

1. Radiation Therapy Planning, *edited by Norman M. Bleehen, Eli Glatstein, and John L. Haybittle*

2. Physician's Guide to Cancer Care Complications: Prevention and Management, *edited by John Laszlo*

Other Volumes in Preparation

Physician's Guide to Cancer Care Complications

Prevention and Management

edited by
JOHN LASZLO

American Cancer Society
New York, New York

Marcel Dekker, Inc.   New York and Basel

Library of Congress Cataloging-in-Publication Data

Main entry under title:

Physician's guide to cancer care complications.

Includes bibliographies and index.
1. Cancer—Treatment—Complications and sequelae.
2. Cancer—Complications and sequelae. I. Laszlo,
John. [DNLM: 1. Neoplasms—complications.
2. Neoplasms—therapy. QZ 266 P5783]
RC270.8P48 1986   616.99'406   85-29361
ISBN 0-8247-7547-3

MARCEL DEKKER, INC.
270 Madison Avenue, New York, New York 10016

Current printing (last digit):
10 9 8 7 6 5 4 3 2 1

PRINTED IN THE UNITED STATES OF AMERICA

This book is dedicated to my father, the late Dr. Daniel Laszlo, and my stepmother, Dr. Herta Spencer. They taught many young physicians the principles of caring for patients with cancer at a time when this field was not popular, and they imbued me with the importance of these issues and of teaching them to the next generation. I am grateful both for the many skills that I learned from my clinical mentors at Duke, particularly Dr. R. Wayne Rundles and Dr. Eugene A. Stead, Jr., and to my co-worker physicians, nurses, and other health professionals from whom I have been so privileged to learn. Particular thanks go to the contributing authors for their enthusiastic support of this book, and to my data technician, Ms. Connie Fennema, who kept my efforts organized and purposeful.

Preface

We try to teach young physicians that just because a patient has cancer we
should not omit care that can extend or improve upon the quality of life;
however, we must not automatically initiate "standard" and expensive treatments if these are meddlesome and likely to cause more harm than good.
Nevertheless, errors of omission or commission are made easily even by experienced oncologists, and we try to learn from each patient and build a sound
knowledge base over the course of a lifetime of practice and therapeutic trials.
This book recognizes that we have some very potent therapeutic tools at our
disposal, thanks to advances made in the last half-century in surgery, chemotherapy, and radiation therapy. Our purpose, however, is to identify the many
potential hazards that go with usage of these therapies, some of which can be
anticipated clearly and therefore eliminated, minimized, or otherwise prepared
for in the context of an effective therapeutic alliance. We address the issues
of identifying the unique needs of the patient and family, and suggest means
with which to satisfy these needs in the hospital, clinic, and home.

The physician is required to orchestrate the care of the patient, but the
implementation of total care is largely the function of a multidisciplinary
group that often includes nurses, social workers, chaplains, recreation therapists,
technicians, other health professionals, and volunteers. The contributions of
our expert authors are partly technical and partly experiential. Although the
technical fields are changing rapidly, we trust that the wisdom regarding how
to approach such changes will endure and continue to serve us, as we serve
our patients with compassion.

John Laszlo

Contents

Preface   v
Contributors   xiii

1. INTRODUCTION   1
    John Laszlo

    References   4

2. GOALS OF PATIENT VERSUS GOALS OF PHYSICIAN   5
    Patricia Cotanch and John Laszlo

    I. Introduction   5
    II. Sensitivity to Goal Disparity   6
        References   13

3. MINIMIZING THE ECONOMIC HARDSHIPS OF DIAGNOSIS
    AND TREATMENT   15
    Harold R. Silberman

    I.   Cancer Costs and Today's Climate of Cost Containment   15
    II. Financing the Treatment of Curable Cancer   18
    III. Prevention of Cancer: The Real Economy   19
    IV. Saving Money While Still Making the Correct Diagnosis   20
    V.   Advanced Disease: Perhaps We Are Overdoing It   24

     VI. Very Late Disease and Terminal Care Can Tax All Concerned   29
     VII. Unproven Methods to Remedy Cancer: A Financial Shame   31
     VIII. Conclusions   32
           References   33

4. PREVENTING COMPLICATIONS OF SURGERY:
    EMPHASIS ON NUTRITIONAL FACTORS   37
    John P. Grant

      I. Introduction   37
     II. Preoperative Assessment   38
    III. Other Preoperative Concerns   54
     IV. Recognition and Minimization of Operative Risks   55
      V. Prevention of Postoperative Complications   57
     VI. Conclusions   58
          References   58

5. CHEMOTHERAPY   61
    John Laszlo, Virgil S. Lucas, and Diane Stevenson

      I.   Overview   61
     II.   Nausea, Vomiting, and Nutritional Depletion:
           Major Complications of Cancer Chemotherapy   63
    III.   Bone Marrow Toxicity   75
     IV.   Infections   87
      V.   Drug Extravasation and Vein Care   96
     VI.   Alopecia   106
    VII.   Cardiotoxicity   107
   VIII.   Pulmonary Toxicity   110
     IX.   Allergic Reactions   114
      X.   Skin Toxicity   116
     XI.   Gastrointestinal and Liver Toxicity   120
    XII.   Toxicity to the Urinary Tract   125
   XIII.   Endocrine   128
    XIV.   Late Complications, Including Secondary Malignancies   129
     XV.   Neurotoxicity of Chemotherapy   132
    XVI.   Ocular Side Effects   132
   XVII.   Reduction of Risk to Personnel Handling Antineoplastic
           Agents   133
           References   136

6. RADIATION THERAPY: ACUTE AND LATE MORBIDITY   147
    Gustavo S. Montana

      I. Introduction   147

    II. Head and Neck   148
   III. Thorax   159
   IV. Abdomen 165
    V. Pelvis 169
   VI. Gonads 172
  VII. Extremities 172
 VIII. Hematopoietic 174
   IX. Carcinogenesis 174
       Acknowledgment 175
       References 175

7. ANTICIPATION AND PREVENTION OF NEUROLOGICAL COMPLICATIONS OF CANCER AND CANCER THERAPY 179
S. Clifford Schold, Jr.

    I. Introduction 179
   II. Anticipation and Recognition of Direct Effects of Cancer on the Nervous System 179
   III. Nonmetastatic Effects of Cancer on the Nervous System 185
   IV. Neurotoxicity of Cancer Treatment 187
    V. Conclusion 194
       References 194

8. DEPRESSION AND OTHER PSYCHIATRIC DISORDERS ASSOCIATED WITH CANCER 197
Allan Maltbie and Patricia Cotanch

    I. Introduction 197
   II. Depression 197
   III. Association of Depression to Cancer 199
   IV. Suicide Among Cancer Patients 200
    V. Special Diagnostic Problems in Cancer Patients 201
   VI. Normal Expected Reactions to Cancer or Other Serious Illnesses 202
  VII. Differential Diagnosis 204
       References 214

9. SPECIAL CONSIDERATIONS FOR CHILDREN 219
William H. Schultz, Marilyn J. Hockenberry, and John M. Falletta

    I. Introduction 219
   II. Parent-Child Communication 220
   III. Implications of Informed Consent: Parents Speaking for Children 221

IV.   Therapeutic Orphans   223
V.   Problem of Undertreatment   223
VI.   Problem of Overtreatment   224
VII. Psychological Adaptation to Childhood Cancer   231
      References   233

10. COMPREHENSIVE CANCER CARE: SPECIAL PROBLEMS
    OF THE ELDERLY   237
    Harvey J. Cohen and Louis C. DeMaria, Jr.

    I.   Introduction   237
    II.   Diagnostic and Therapeutic Maneuvers and Their Implications
          in the Treatment of Elderly Cancer Patients   249
    III. Selected Needs and Problems of Elderly Cancer Patients   256
    IV.   Psychological Needs   263
    V.   Social Needs   267
    VI.   Closing Statements   268
          References   268

11. SUPPORT SERVICES FOR HOSPITALIZED PATIENTS   277
    Beverly K. Rosen, Louise Bost, and Paul W. Aitken

    I.   Family Support: A Hidden Ally (or Antagonist?) in
          Cancer Care   277
    II.   The Oncology Patient: Using Recreation Therapy
          to Alleviate Social Isolation and Depersonalization   289
    III. Religious Beliefs: A Help or a Hindrance?   299
          References   305

12. CARE OF THE DYING PATIENT   309
    Paula Balber

    I.   Introduction   309
    II.   Discussing Prognosis   309
    III. Reactions of Patients and Families: Useful Approaches   311
    IV.   Hospice   313
    V.   Conclusion   324
          References   325
          Appendix: Hospice Medicare Benefits   327

Index   333

Contributors

Paul W. Aitken, A.B., B.D., Th. M. Director, Chaplains Service, Duke University Medical Center, Durham, North Carolina

Paula Balber, R.N., M.A. Nurse, Triangle Hospice, Durham, North Carolina

Louise Bost, M.S. Director, Oncology Recreation Therapy Program, Duke University Medical Center, Durham, North Carolina

Harvey J. Cohen, M.D. Professor, Department of Medicine, Chief, Division of Geriatrics, and Director, Center for the Study of Aging and Human Development, Duke University Medical Center, and Director, Geriatric Research Education and Clinical Center (GRECC), Veterans Administration Medical Center, Durham, North Carolina

Patricia Cotanch, R.N., Ph.D. Associate Professor of Nursing, and Assistant Professor of Psychiatry, Duke University School of Nursing, Durham, North Carolina

Louis C. DeMaria, Jr., M.D. Assistant Professor, Department of Community and Family Medicine and Division of Geriatrics, Duke University Medical Center, Durham, North Carolina

John M. Falletta, M.D. Professor, Department of Pediatrics, and Chief, Division of Pediatric Hematology/Oncology, Duke University Medical Center, Durham, North Carolina

John P. Grant, M.D.   Associate Professor, Department of Surgery, Duke University Medical Center, Durham, North Carolina; and Chief of Surgery, Durham Veterans Administration Medical Center, Durham, North Carolina

Marilyn J. Hockenberry, R.N., M.S.N., P.N.P.   Pediatric Nurse Practitioner, Duke University Medical Center, Durham, North Carolina

John Laszlo, M.D. [*]   Professor, Department of Medicine, Duke University Medical Center, Durham, North Carolina

Virgil S. Lucas, B. Pharm.   Clinical Research Scientist, Department of Immunology/ Oncology, Burroughs Wellcome Company, Research Triangle Park, North Carolina

Allan A. Maltbie, M.D.   Associate Professor, Department of Psychiatry, Duke University Medical Center, Durham, North Carolina

Gustavo S. Montana, M.D.   Professor, Department of Radiology, Duke University Medical Center, Durham, North Carolina

Beverly K. Rosen, M.S.W., A.C.S.W.   Former Director, Oncology Social Work Program, Duke University Medical Center, Durham, North Carolina

S. Clifford Schold, Jr., M.D.   Associate Professor of Neurology, Department of Medicine, Duke University Medical Center, Durham, North Carolina

William H. Schultz, P.A.-C.   Clinical Associate, Department of Pediatrics, Duke University Medical Center, Durham, North Carolina

Harold R. Silberman, M.D.   Professor, Department of Medicine and Associate Clinical Professor, Department of Psychiatry, Duke University Medical Center, Durham, North Carolina

Diane Stevenson, R.N.   Chemotherapy Nurse Clinician, Division of Hematology/ Oncology, Duke University Medical Center, Durham, North Carolina

---

Current Affiliation: Vice President for Research, American Cancer Society, New York, New York

1
Introduction

John Laszlo[*]
Duke University Medical Center, Durham, North Carolina

Contrary to some impressions which the public may have, the fields of medicine and medical research do not always progress in smooth and orderly steps. They are subject to the same sorts of chaotic events as are the thought processes of its practitioners, the unanticipated finding, or the application of a discovery from one scientific field to another. Furthermore, medicine has always been susceptible to fads regarding what is and what is not scientifically acceptable, and it is being influenced increasingly by what the public thinks it wants.

Evolution of the discipline of clinical oncology is an important example of these influences; venereal diseases would be another, more limited, case. So many centuries of benign neglect of the patient with advanced cancer were generally consistent with the stigma associated with this disease. Surgeons dominated the field of oncology because their methods were potentially curative for patients who had localized disease. When radiotherapists began to show that palliation was possible even for patients with advanced disease, they —together with other physicians interested in medical oncology—began to take an interest in patients with advanced cancer. The development of chemotherapy in the past quarter century has caused great optimism among the medical community that cancer may be curable if only the right drugs can be found for the common tumors. Indeed the field of medical oncology has grown so rapidly that there is considerable concern that we will soon have an excess of specialists. Surgical, medical, and radiation oncologists have all

---

Current Affiliation: American Cancer Society, New York, New York

developed new approaches to diagnosis and to treatment which lead to greater curability in some types of cancer, and longer survival if not cure in still others; unfortunately there is too large a group of patients whose survival is not enhanced by our skills. The fields of oncology nursing, social work, and recreational therapy are fast becoming established at larger institutions as those voids in provision of care are being filled by those who have special training.

The public is far better informed (sometimes misinformed) about cancer and much more willing to question the doctor about treatment alternatives. They are concerned about the cost of being treated, and this includes the medical, social, and financial costs. With respect to finances, doctors are often unaware of the enormous economic burdens that we inflict with unnecessarily elaborate and even unproductive workups and therapy. Rehabilitation programs have been developed for the patient who has lost a body part, in response to the needs that these patients face. It is easy to recognize the concerns of an amputee who wants to return to a job; it is more difficult to understand the psychological disruption suffered by a patient who has undergone a mastectomy or faced the consequences of chemotherapy. The failure of our system of medical care (with exceptions, of course) to adequately provide for terminally ill patients— to palliate, to maintain the family structure, and not to deplete the last dollar in the process—has led to the dissemination of programs that provide hospice types of home care throughout the United States. The remarkable rapidity of public acceptance of this health concept may be unprecedented in this nation, and it should cause us to examine the limitations of some of our other cancer programs.

In evaluating the clinical programs of the Duke Comprehensive Cancer Center we have been struck repeatedly with the need to develop better means of responding to the diverse human concerns of patients; at the same time we strive to provide cures or significantly prolong their lives. The means of delivering first-rate supportive care for patients with chronic diseases such as cancer are still not well developed, as our daily experiences with patients reminds us. There has been sporadic, inspired, and major progress in use of blood products, diagnosis and treatment of infections, venous access, and antiemetics. Still, there has been little systematic research in supportive care, and the measurement tools available for assessing the needs and concerns of patients are often inadequate for the task.

Attention to the human needs of patients (i.e., pain control, nausea and vomiting, psychological problems) has taken on a relatively new and large part of the oncology literature. However, the subject of how to *anticipate* and *prevent* some of the complications of cancer and its potent treatments has not been systematically addressed. Although there clearly is an overlap with treatment of established complications or of conventional rehabilitation methods, the emphasis of this book differs in a significant fashion. Let us discuss openly that many of the things we do to treat patients have risks—some mild, some life threatening, some rare or common. We contend that many of the complications of cancer and particularly of its treatments are predictable and often quite preventable. Indeed the standard of practice should dictate that all reasonable preventive steps are taken and also that the patient is advised when there is a significant risk that treatment will produce disability. To the extent that prevention is preferable to treatment or rehabilitation, then clearly our patients would be grateful for progress along these lines.

This is a time of great change in expectations: patients want to be permanently cured of cancer and they certainly expect to be kept free from suffering during treatment if cure is not possible. It was not long ago that doctors had no tools to do more than manage the simpler ills and for alleviating some of the pain and suffering, if not all of the anguish, of chronic illness. Though not wanting to return to those days, we should not now substitute more advanced technical skills at the expense of practicing those older arts of medicine, though there are admittedly powerful forces pushing young doctors in such directions. One semiderogatory term that one sometimes hears from patients is that their doctors are overly "aggressive." And yet there need not be a conflict between technology and wisdom if one is aggressive in evaluating the total situation and dealing not only with the possible, but also with the most desirable choices, as seen from the viewpoint of the patient. Since there are often numerous choices to be made, the issue of minimizing the harm would seem to be a natural part of the decision-making process. We hope that by informing the reader about the potential complications of the various treatment options (versus the admittedly grim natural history of the disease itself), many problems can be avoided and the entire process of setting goals will become transparent to all of the participants. The subject matter dealt with in this book is quite diverse, from the imparting of highly technical knowledge to sharing our thoughts on philosophy, care of the young or elderly, and economics. Indeed, we do not guarantee that we will always be consistent in approaching controversial topics from different points of view. Nonetheless, the unifying theme of the book is that a gentle and thoughtful approach, one capable of being modified in accordance with changing circumstances, is most compatible with the highest professional calling that we can offer to the people we serve.

Most of the contributors for this book are drawn from the members of the Duke Comprehensive Cancer Center. They were encouraged to develop a "state-of-the-art" representation on the subject of prevention of complications, not an encyclopedia of cancer treatment, nor a recital of what various specialists do. The challenge was to effectively integrate overlapping fields of endeavor and to refer to other sources of information when pertinent. We might begin that process by referring to a selection of recent books which can be used to supplement some sections of our book (Rosenbaum and

Rosenbaum, 1980; Zimmerman, 1981; Cassileth and Cassileth, 1982; DeVita, Hellman, and Rosenberg, 1982; Holland and Frei, 1982; Higby, 1983; Laszlo, 1983; Wiernik, 1983; Perry and Yarbro, 1984).

REFERENCES

Cassileth, B. R., and Cassileth, P. A. (1982). *Clinical Care of the Terminal Cancer Patient,* Lea & Febiger, Philadelphia.

DeVita, V. T., Jr., Hellman, S., and Rosenberg, S. (1982). *Cancer: Principles and Practice of Oncology,* J. P. Lippincott Company, Philadelphia.

Higby, D. J. (1983). *Supportive Care in Cancer Therapy,* Martinus Nijhoff Publishers, Boston.

Holland, J. F., and Frei, E., III. (1982). *Cancer Medicine,* Lea & Febiger, Philadelphia.

Laszlo, J. (1983). *Antiemetics and Cancer Chemotherapy,* Williams & Wilkins, Baltimore.

Perry, M. C., and Yarbro, J. W. (1984). *Toxicity of Chemotherapy,* Grune & Stratton, Orlando, Fla.

Rosenbaum, E. H., and Rosenbaum, I. R. (1980). *A Comprehensive Guide for Cancer Patients and Their Families,* Bull Publishing Company, Palo Alto, Calif.

Wiernik, P. H. (1983). *Supportive Care of the Cancer Patient,* Futura Publishing Company, Mt. Kisco, New York.

Zimmerman, J. M. (1981). *Hospice: Complete Care for the Terminally Ill,* Urban & Schwarzenberg, Baltimore.

2

Goals of Patient Versus Goals of Physician

Patricia Cotanch
Duke University School of Nursing, Durham, North Carolina

John Laszlo*
Duke University Medical Center, Durham, North Carolina

I. INTRODUCTION

Fortunately, the practice of "protecting" patients from learning about their diagnosis of cancer is rapidly disappearing, at least in the United States. The advent of mandatory informed consents for protocol studies which are used in all oncology training programs, a well-informed lay public, and the popularity of being an assertive patient have all influenced the mores of the health professional. Indeed, the horrors of Solzhenitsyn's Cancer Ward where the patient describes himself as "a grain of sand" are hopefully relegated to the past. However, it is possible that the pendulum has swung too far in the other direction in the arena of "supportive care for cancer patients," which, while arguing for openness of communication, creates a demon that insists on deluging patients with facts about major complications that have only the slightest possibility of ever occurring in their specific case.

Emphasis is often placed on the physician to meet the objective of divulging a set body of information about the disease and treatment, rather than on a continuing interactive communication between patient and provider. The reader may recall classroom experiences where the teacher was frantically intent to cover certain information (teaching) and the students in turn were frantically taking notes but were totally confused. In that kind of setting the teachers were too busy "teaching" and not concerned with their primary purpose of assisting the students to learn.

Current Affiliation: American Cancer Society, New York, New York

The purpose of this chapter is to present information about how a direct approach to the patients' concerns can successfully be achieved. Although such an approach may be time consuming initially, it is so simple and effective that it is a wonder more doctors have not mastered this communication skill. Indeed, the failure to communicate increases the likelihood of noncompliance with therapy, among other problems, which in turn evokes feelings that further erode the patient-provider relationship, and this has psychological, medical, and legal ramifications.

The chapter presents pragmatic approaches that can be used to ward off crisis points that cancer patients frequently face. Information is presented based on the continuum of disease progression leading from cure, control, or, unfortunately, death. Strategies are presented that when employed or suggested can have a high probability of avoiding or delaying complications. Special attention is given to increasing sensitivity regarding potential disparity between the goals of the patients and provider. It is hoped that the disparity once recognized can be avoided by development of a successful therapeutic alliance.

II. SENSITIVITY TO GOAL DISPARITY

At first even the well-adjusted patient may have a lingering doubt about the accuracy of diagnostic tests, namely, "is it really cancer?" If there is no reasonable doubt then we explain the facts and treatment options—including no specific treatment or the option of delaying treatment. Discussion of the pros and cons of each option must include the necessary factual exposition and time for questions, and all questions will not necessarily be voiced at this first meeting. We can anticipate spoken or unspoken questions about unconventional treatments, the possibility of cure, life expectancy, a second opinion, causes of the cancer and whether it is contagious. If other key individuals (spouse, offspring, parent) are included in the conferences, the perceptive physician can quickly grasp the family dynamics—strengths, weaknesses, and concerns—and tailor the presentation to cover all the essentials. It is impossible to anticipate every possible concern without a thorough discussion, and time will not generally permit a full discussion with a succession of concerned family members or friends. If drug program A is unlikely to cause alopecia, that may be particularly reassuring news to this patient: if alopecia is likely, then advanced warning and advice about short- and long-term solutions will undoubtedly be appreciated.

A major goal at this point is to provide as much information as the patient wishes to have. Sometimes patients make it clear they are not ready to deal with the issues, and yet from the very beginning a major goal is to encourage the patient to have input into treatment decisions. It is important that the patient will be interacting with a competent and caring team who will be there to help. Specific instructions about whom to call with further questions (or in case of emergencies) will be quite reassuring, since afterwards there is bound to be concern that not all pertinent questions were properly anticipated or asked. In the long run it is more important for the patient to feel this kind of confidence than it is to cover every possible contingency in an overly encyclopedic presentation.

Often mere willingness to discuss the possibility that a recommended treatment might cause side effects instills confidence in the candor of the physician: it sets the stage for future honest communication, and facilitates acceptance of other complications, even those rarer ones that were perhaps not discussed. Indeed, in arguing for openness of communication we do not feel it is necessary to deluge each patient with every rare complication that might conceivably occur—the point can easily be made that beyond the more common complications there are others that are rare, unpredictable, and potentially very serious and even life threatening (so after all is the untreated disease). This type of climate creates a kind of trust that will go a long way towards defusing problems which are bound to arise at home between visits to the doctor. If there is reason to believe that key pieces of information will be needed by the patient or family at a later time, then the entire discussion can be recorded and given to the patient to keep. In the educational process it is useful to anticipate common concerns about pain or financial costs, and to reassure the patient that those problems will be addressed should they arise. These issues of communication with patients have been thoroughly discussed by Rosenbaum and Rosenbaum (1980).

Concerns and attendant behaviors associated with cancer can arbitrarily be divided into those which occur around the time of diagnosis, those which occur when there is evidence of tumor recurrence or progression, and those which occur during the terminal phase of illness. However, events preceding the time of diagnosis are also worthy of consideration: perhaps the patient had life experiences which caused awareness of the risk of cancer, such as high family incidence or carcinogen exposure, and chose some type of coping strategy from among a wide range of options; there may have been purposeful attempts at cancer detection, deliberate avoidance of known carcinogens, lack of interest, or denial. The past history can sometimes help to explain the surprise, guilt, anger, or denial which accompanies news that the diagnosis is cancer. Further, a person who has a long history of exposure to asbestos or cigarettes is conditioned to deal with lung cancer differently from someone who has not had that history, and if the spouse has been complaining for years about the exposure then the family dynamics could be adversely affected throughout the course of the illness.

When a diagnosis of cancer is first established, the options are finite, although still numerous. As the disease progresses and death becomes imminent the available choices become further constricted. It is often at this point that patients are referred to large centers to be cared for by specialists. By then the limited available options make it progressively more difficult for individuals to exert control over circumstances which affect their lives and welfare. Thus, from a clinical vantage point it seems clear that for patients who are not cured, the disease moves through a continuum during which the options for both patient and care provider diminish. During the course of the illness the health team periodically redirects its goals: these are initially curative in intent and are later geared towards palliation; although they generally parallel those of the patient, the specific concerns of the two parties may at times be so different as to become conflicting.

In a study of 26 veterans with advanced cancer, considerable disparity existed between patient and staff (doctors and nurses) perceptions (Nehemkis, Gerber, and Charter, 1984). Interestingly, oncology specialists tended to overestimate the importance of pain to the patient and to underestimate the value of simple daily activities such as being able to perform household chores and the sense of loss from disruption of leisure activities. In a more circumscribed study of patients' and physicians' perceptions as related to the consent form for participation in an investigational protocol (Penman et al., 1984), marked differences did exist. For example, 91% of patients thought that their physician wanted them to accept, whereas physicians thought that most of their patients were truly expressing their own preferences and only one-third were passive in their acceptance.

The disparity between the goals of the patient and provider may be in part related to a frequent clinical observation that with progressive illness the patient develops a shorter time frame for his/her concerns: this contrasts with the patient who is less ill (or the normal mature individual or health professional) and has a long-range perspective. A short-term outlook is not unique to terminally ill cancer patients, but occurs also in patients with other chronic illnesses who feel threatened or assaulted by dangerous or toxic procedures or by therapeutic interventions. We might say parenthetically that not much is known about the time frame changes that go on in family and "significant others." We have schematized our concept of these general issues and their effects on patient and staff in Table 1, without intending to specify the priority or to suggest that this is an exhaustive list of factors relevant to any given clinical situation.

Although other patients with advancing chronic illness experience a narrowing of options and time frame, cancer and cancer-related treatment seems to have an especially noticeable impact on patients and family. Unfortunately, all cancer treatments cause some degree of damage to the patient and they are often accompanied by physical and emotional discomfort. Some studies have compared the toxicity and psychological effects of treatments

Table 1   Issues Which Affect the Patient and Health Team at Various Times During the Illness

Diagnosis questions, concerns, and fears	Progression	Terminal
Patient		
Correct diagnosis?	Side effects of Rx	
Life expectancy?	Alternative therapy	
Best doctor and hospital?		Need for hospitalization
Causes of this cancer?		vs. home care
Contagious?		(Hospice)
Curable?		
Dying	Dying	Lack of communication
Family	Making family plans	Abandonment
Pain	Pain	Pain control
	Weight loss	Ambulation
Sexuality and	Nausea and vomiting	Bowel and bladder
body image	Venipunctures	Fear of unknown
Expenses	Expenses	
Business		
Activities of		
daily living		
Physicians and staff		
Accurate diagnosis	Family support	Emotional support
Extent of disease	Home needs	to patient and family
Co-morbid conditions	Planning salvage Rx	
Informing patient and	Palliation of	Palliation
family	symptoms	
	Prevention and treat-	
	ment of debility	
Developing therapeutic	Vein infiltration	
options	Malnutrition	
Surgery	Infection, bleeding,	
Radiation	fractures	
Chemotherapy		
Immunotherapy		
Hormones		

Note: This is a partial and schematic simplification to illustrate differences in perspective. The dotted lines are intended to symbolize the progressive constriction of available options.

(Meyerowitz, Sparks, and Spears, 1979; Todres, and Wojtivk, 1979; Cooper et al., 1979; Maguire, Tait, and Brooke, 1980; Silberfarb et al., 1983). While none of these was a large-scale, controlled investigation, all reports indicate that the treatment (mainly chemotherapy) may cause significant psychological morbidity that is directly related to the severity of side effects.

Silberfarb et al. (1983) found a greater incidence of depression and fatigue among patients on one arm of a randomized clinical trial than on the other, even though there was no difference in tumor response between the drug regimens. Perhaps the matter hinges upon the discrepancy between what is important to the patient and what is important to the physician at any given time. A solid therapeutic relationship cannot develop if the patient is distraught about losing her/his hair while the physician is mainly concerned with tumor measurements from the latest CAT scan reading. When this type of variance happens in the face of advancing disease, with its implications in terms of narrower treatment options and truncating time frame, as suggested in Table 1, it is understandably upsetting to physician, patient, and family. This triad may reach an impasse if the physician offers the "only" acceptable treatment option and the patient and/or family decide not to accept the treatment. An extreme example of this occurs when the doctor has a potentially curative but toxic treatment, such as with aggressive chemotherapy for testicular cancer, but the patient prefers to ask about nutritional or serum remedies or is adamant about not spending his life savings on expensive or uncomfortable treatments. Such impasses can be partly avoided if the patient/provider relationship is seen as an interactive process, with both parties making the effort to redirect goals and jointly choose among the treatment options.

If the patient's concerns are not adequately understood or his/her needs met, the result is likely to be unsatisfactory for the patient and frustrating for the health provider. From the point of view of the physician, the problem is usually identified as "noncompliance" a term that does not do justice to the situation and by its very nature suggests that the problem is an irremediable fault on the part of the patient. It is frequently and erroneously thought that education about a condition and compliance are directly related. Although educating the patient about the illness is important, it is not sufficient to guarantee compliance, nor do we recognize any specific factors which correlate closely with the ability of patients to follow the instructions of the health care team. In an extensive survey, Bissonett and Seller (1980) found that noncompliance with physician advice, either through error or by deliberate disregard, ranged from 20-70%. In one study (Itano, Tanahe, and Jum, unpublished manuscript) of 66 adults who were receiving chemotherapy in an outpatient clinic, 21% did not keep their scheduled appointments, complete lab work or receive chemotherapy as prescribed. Our own experience is that young males with testicular cancer may have rates of noncompliance, including delayed appointments and omission of treatments altogether, which are closer to 40 or 50%.

Given and Given (1984) argue for a climate of compliance in which patients with cancer undergoing long-term therapy have primary responsibility for implementing their therapeutic regimen and voluntarily choose behavior which coincides with the medical recommendations. Their view of compliance underlines the importance of provider-patient negotiation and ultimate agreement on objectives. Given the highly specialized nature of oncology and the use of complex technology, it is increasingly difficult for patients to take an active role in this way. Bissonette and Seller suggest that physicians can make several assumptions about the likelihood of a patient complying with their advice: (1) most patients will be passive and are unlikely to question the basis of the advice or to ask about the specifics of the program (often this passivity is encouraged by the behavior of the physician); (2) there will be a time-related diminution of compliance, even with short-term regimens; (3) patients whose therapeutic regimens involve major behavioral change will be especially difficult; (4) community values may be expected to reinforce the patient's noncompliance; and (5) the patient and physician will frequently not share the same expectations or goals, as mentioned above.

Some strategies for preventing noncompliance have been described elsewhere (Bissonnette and Seller, 1980; Given and Given, 1984; Richardson et al., 1983). The cornerstone of compliance strategies is to encourage active participation of patients in their treatment through the process of developing therapeutic alliance (Barofsky, 1978). Therefore, the intent is not simply to achieve compliance with a medical program, but also to provide the patient with the security and satisfaction needed to carry on with normal activities, without excessive preoccupation with health-related questions.

The constriction of options and time can potentially be balanced by the development of a therapeutic alliance. Indeed, if the patient and physician are committed to the development of such an alliance, then quality care and emotional rewards can be experienced even in the face of advancing disease and impending death.

Assumption of the role of "patient" almost always begins with a patient being directed as to what he/she is to do (comply). This is especially true for patients who seek treatment in large university-related medical centers, for patients may be intimidated by the reputation of the institution, advanced technology, and the presence of world renowned physicians. The patient arrives asking, "What can you do for me?" and "What do you want me to do?"

However, this initial relationship between provider (mainly physician) and patient needs to be viewed as the beginning of a continuum, not an *end* in itself. Almost all provider/patient relationships begin as unequal because of the difference in knowledge and experience, because of the site of interaction, and

Table 2 Social Control Continuum

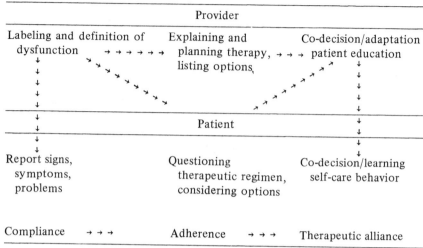

Provider		
Labeling and definition of dysfunction	Explaining and planning therapy, listing options	Co-decision/adaptation patient education
Patient		
Report signs, symptoms, problems	Questioning therapeutic regimen, considering options	Co-decision/learning self-care behavior
Compliance	Adherence	Therapeutic alliance

Note: Schematic representation of the interaction between a patient and a provider. It emphasizes that the interaction is reciprocal and that specific tasks or objectives can be identified that mark changes in the relationship. The goal of this process is development of self-care behaviors and movement along this continuum.
Source: Adapted from Barofsky (1978).

because one is ill and the other is not (Barofsky, 1978). (In this regard it is interesting to recall the admonition of Dr. E. A. Stead, Jr., who taught medical students that regardless of other demands and schedules, the sick never inconvenience the well.) Unfortunately, all too often the inequality remains and the relationship does not progress to more desirable forms of the therapeutic relationship. Barofsky has explained that in assuming the role of patient under the care of a provider, people are actually experiencing a type of socialization that can be depicted as a social control continuum (Table 2). Patients enter the process being told what to do: comply. Patient and provider may achieve adherence, which implies that both parties are communicating and are planning to conform to an external standard (i.e., explaining and understanding a medical or surgical clinical trial which requires that both parties read and sign an informed consent). Thus, adherence is the appropriate term when a patient and provider both expect and participate in a particular set of behaviors. Adherence requires some interaction between provider and patient and a concordance of expectations (Barofsky, Sugarbaker, and Mills, 1979). The term therapeutic alliance implies also that negotiations have occurred. However, for negotiation to occur, each party must have bargaining power—each exercising a degree of control.

The therapeutic alliance requires the patient to be an active participant in the decisions that are being made for him/herself, and therefore alliance demands a self-care responsibility from the patient. Development of such an alliance usually requires several reciprocal interactive sessions. If successfully achieved, a process of socialization is created between the patient and provider, which not only offers an opportunity for a rewarding interpersonal relationship but which may also be viewed as a developmental process for both. This approach may seem stilted or excessively formal but it is at least a useful exercise to consider carefully. Indeed in our experience, let us make the provocative suggestion that it is often those physicians who believe themselves to be most in touch with the goals of the patient who may be the ones least able to recognize the problems.

REFERENCES

Barofsky, I. (1978). Compliance, adherence, and the therapeutic alliance: Steps in the development of self-care, *Soc. Sci. Med., 12*:369-376.

Barofsky, I., Sugarbaker, P., and Mills, M. (1979). Compliance and quality of life assessment, in *New Directions in Patient Compliance* (S. Cohen, ed.), D. C. Heath & Company, Lexington Books, Lexington, Mass., pp. 59-75.

Bissonnette, R., and Seller, R. (1980). Medical noncompliance: A cultural perspective, *Man and Med., 5*:41-62.

Cooper, A., McArdle, C., Russell, A., and Smith, D. (1979). Psychiatric morbidity associated with adjuvant chemotherapy following mastectomy for breast cancer, *Brit. J. Surg., 66*:362.

Given, B. A., and Given, C. W. (1984). Creating a climate for complaince, *Cancer Nursing, April*:139-147.

Itano, J., Tanahe, P., and Jum, J. Compliance of cancer patients, unpublished manuscript.

Maguire, G., Tait, A., and Brooke, M. (1980). Psychiatric morbidity and physical toxicity associated with adjuvant chemotherapy after mastectomy, *Brit. Med. J., 281*:1179-1180.

Meyerowitz, B., Sparks, F., and Spears, I. (1979). Adjuvant chemotherapy for breast carcinoma: Psychological implications, *Cancer, 43*:1613-1618.

Nehemkis, A. M., Gerber, K. E., and Charter, R. A. (1984). The cancer ward: Patient perceptions—staff misperceptions, *Psychother. Psychosom., 41*:42-47.

Penman, D. T., Holland, J. C., Bahna, G. F., Morrow, G., Schmale, A. H., Derogatis, L. R., Carnrike, C. L., Jr., and Cherry, R. (1984). Informed consent for investigational chemotherapy: Patients' and physicians' perceptions, *J. Clin. Oncol., 2*:849-855.

Richardson, J. L., Johnson, C. A., Selser, J., Evans, L. A., Kishbaugh, C., and Levine, A. M. (1983). Compliance with chemotherapy: Theoretical basis and intervention design, *Progress in Cancer Control IV: Research in the Cancer Center*, Alan R. Liss, New York, pp. 379-390.

Rosenbaum, E. H., and Rosenbaum, I. R. (1980). *A Comprehensive Guide for Cancer Patients and Their Families*, Bull Publishing Company, Palo Alto, Calif.

Silberfarb, P., Holland, J., Anbar, D., Bahna, G., Maurer, H., Chahinian, A., and Comis, R. (1983). Psychological response of patients receiving two drug regimens for lung carcinoma, *Am. J. Psychiat., 140*:110-111.
Todres, R., and Wojtivk, R. (1979). The cancer patient's view of chemotherapy, *Cancer Nursing, 2*:283-286.

3

Minimizing the Economic Hardships of Diagnosis and Treatment

Harold R. Silberman
Duke University Medical Center, Durham, North Carolina

I. CANCER COSTS AND TODAY'S CLIMATE OF COST CONTAINMENT

By 1984, a generalized concern about rising costs of health care coupled with the concept of a potential to bankrupt the Medicare Trust Fund has led to the accusation that physicians have been fiscally irresponsible. Those of us who practice the art and science of medicine have been accused of "overdoing it" by one group, while other critics simultaneously claim that we are "underdoing it"!

Here, in this chapter, emphasis is placed upon containing costs where possible and reasonable within the context of the management of oncologic disease. First, one must ask what are the current costs? According to one economist, Thomas A. Hodgson (of the Office of Analysis and Epidemiology, National Center for Health Statistics, in the Department of Health and Human Services), we should consider three categories of costs (Hodgson, 1984): "direct costs, resulting from the use of resources; indirect costs, resulting from the loss of human resources including economic output that is forgone; and psychosocial costs, resulting from intangible impact such as pain and suffering." The last of these three divisions is discussed thoroughly in other sections of this book. As regards direct costs, even by adding up the expenditures for hospitalizations, outpatient clinical services, nursing home care, home health services, fees for primary physicians and specialists, as well as other health practitioners, drugs and drug sundries, rehabilitation charges, the costs of prostheses, appliances, etc., and the amount required for terminal care of patients, we arrive at only part of the figure. It is necessary to consider the other direct costs borne by patients and family members that arise because of transportation or living away from home while en route to/from health providers. If one takes all of that and other factors into consideration, a conservative estimate places the current cost of medical care for malignant neoplasms at more than $10 billion annually in the United States. By way of comparison, the country spends $42.8 billion on alcoholic beverages, $20.4 billion on tobacco for personal consumption, and $89 billion for gasoline and oil.

Major advances achieved in cancer chemotherapy and the development of high energy radiotherapy equipment now allow for the delivery of chemicals or x-irradiation sufficient to effect a cure or at least eradicate local disease. These improvements in two modalities have not come cheaply, but no one today is truly prepared to put a cap on the price of saving either many lives or even a few. Moreover, when diseases are not cured, the individuals with them still require much attention, many medications, and most supportive services. Indeed, one can make the case that curative regimens are cost-effective for any population with a specific neoplasm and an increase in cure rate could reduce the $10 billion figure cited above.

Only rough calculations can be made for the cost of curing certain malignancies. For pediatric acute lymphocytic leukemia, much of the medication can be given and most of the procedures can be accomplished without repeated hospitalizations. Although it may take 2.5-3 years to complete entire multimodal regimens, the total bill would be about $15,000. For adult care myelogenous leukemia, on the other hand, several hospitalizations are necessary and the first one, for induction of remission, can be lengthy (4-12 weeks) resulting in an estimated cost of $35,000 for each cured patient. Hodgkin's disease, stages III and IV, is treated principally in an outpatient clinic over 6-9 months at an estimated cost of $8,000. Disseminated testicular carcinoma requires a more rigorous drug combination and often patients require some hospital time to complete the usual four courses necessary to be successful; $10,000 would be a conservative estimate for effecting a single complete, enduring response.

Failure to cure is always more expensive. For example, if a youngster with acute lymphocytic leukemia does not remain in complete remission, several hospitalizations are required with an estimated cost of $40,000 (cf. $15,000 for permanent complete remission). When the patient with acute nonlymphocytic leukemia does not remain well, the sum of medical bills till time of death would total conservatively $65,000 (cf. $35,000 for permanent complete remssion). To care for a patient with Hodgkin's disease who is not cured by the initial approach, repetitive hospitalizations, radiotherapy, supportive care, and clinic visits come to an estimated $80,000, or ten times the price of a cure (Frei, 1984). Finally, studies of the use of services in the last year of life document that hospital expenses contribute greatly to the total and that the consumption of resources by cancer patients is especially intense during the last 2 months of life (Gibbs and Newman, 1982).

Unfortunately this kind of cost analysis does not address other major items such as dollar equivalents for time lost from work, costs for travel and the sometimes necessary lodging away from home, and perhaps most importantly, the loss of income by others created by having a spouse, parent, or other relative accompany the patient back and forth for outpatient treatment or to provide a variety of supportive measures in the hospital or in the home. It is clear that most illnesses can create a variety of burdens for patients and their families.

A recent review of the economics of lung cancer (Loeb et al., 1984) did incorporate estimates for both direct and indirect losses analyzing individual perspectives as well as social ramifications and also reflected the fiscal burdens for businesses, government, and private insurance companies. The sheer magnitude of this disease overshadows everything one can say about other malignancies. In 1984, the American Cancer Society estimated 121,000 lung cancer deaths in the United States (85,000 in men and 36,000 in women), with lung cancer accounting for 35% of all cancer deaths in men and 18% in women (Silverberg, 1984). In 1980, medical expenditures on all lung cancers in men totaled $1.003 billion with $595 million spent on care of women with the same diagnosis. Estimating the proportion of lung cancer attributable to smoking (males 76.5% and females 45.5%) suggests a total expenditure of $1.038 billion for cigarette-associated pulmonary neoplasia. If productivity losses are valued at $5.876 billion and a proportional share of the total morbidity course is $446 million, then the total reaches $7.36 billion. It is even more disturbing to express the sum in 1984 dollars—$10 billion!—and to realize that we are discussing a disease for which *there is prevention.*

Awareness of these tangible, though not necessarily perfectly accurate, economic data should motivate us to look for the potential to reduce expenses in any of several areas. Shortening hospitalizations, even by a couple of days, produces a dramatic effect for the economist but can also be a real gain for the afflicted individual and the family. By paying constant attention to every single detail in the treatment plan, excesses can be eliminated. After that, other important savings can also be achieved because the patient and family members often are quite aware of specific and sometimes unique problems. These are created by the date or time of a visit: the date selected to begin a hospitalization; the temporary events that restrict their resources in a given week or month; the need for certain items which could be supplied by cancer societies, support groups, or church organizations. It is therefore urgent that someone in the treatment team ask at many steps along the way, "Is there a way that all of this can be made more practical or economical for you at this time?" Of certain braver patients it is eventually reasonable to ask: "How much of your personal resources do you want to expend upon battling the late stages of your illness?" It goes without saying that patients often still find it easier to make their requests of or statements to nurses, social workers, or chemotherapy assistants than to physicians.

Then there is even the question of whether doctors charge more than a procedure or visit is *really* worth. Clearly physicians have little if any control over much in the final bill except their fees, but often they do control these. Fee structures are certainly variable and perhaps disparate, both as regards differences in reimbursement for cognitive and procedural tasks, as well as for similar tasks performed in different regions of the country. Because wide variations do exist in our prevailing fees and since there is yet no national solution to these apparent discrepancies, it is appropriate for each of us to consider a resource-cost analysis that shows which of our services are not overvalued.

II. FINANCING THE TREATMENT OF CURABLE CANCER

In designing a proper approach to the patient with a newly diagnosed neoplasm, there is the potential for conflict if one focuses primarily on cost containment of medical care without adequate consideration for complete therapy of those who can be cured and of the high priority that should be placed on continuing clinical cancer research. It is critically important that the two goals, cost containment and therapeutic gains in cancer, not come into conflict. The requirements to achieve a cure at the outset of disease must be met because, as already pointed out, those not cured will have recurrent and episodically progressive disease. Such individuals survive for months to years during which time there can be repetitive "consumption" of acute medical or surgical services, frequent outpatient care, and intermittent hospitalizations.

Thus, when approaching the individual with a potentially curable neoplasm many of the caveats discussed in later pages about exercising diagnostic and/or therapeutic restraint must be abrogated. In their place one may want to substitute a euphemism: *My best chance for curing this individual is now by the use of appropriate treatment up front.* A sensible design of catastrophic medical insurance must take that statement into account.

Several diseases fit this model including Hodgkin's disease; large cell lymphoma (so-called histiocytic lymphoma or reticulum cell sarcoma); testicular carcinoma; acute lymphocytic leukemia in children; rarely acute nonlymphocytic leukemia, particularly in adults; certain pediatric tumors (Wilm's, rhabdomyosarcoma, Ewing's, and perhaps osteosarcoma); and, in 90% of instances, trophoblastic disease. Note that these are neoplasms that often require a multimodal approach utilizing the techniques of surgery, radiotherapy, and chemotherapy.

Because of the potential for cure or at least very long lasting complete remissions, other considerations such as displacement of the patient from the home to a cancer center, with attendant travel expenses for family members, time lost from employment, and emotional costs of facing the facts early on, without delay, all must be relegated to receive secondary attention at most.

This posture can also be defended, in selected situations, when a truly novel, investigational approach is available and has been designed with the intent to be curative. Furthermore, discussions of economic impact should not obscure the cogent fact that dosages of cytotoxic drugs have been shown to be critical. Therefore, modifying regimens just to lower the cost and/or prevent toxicity can result in reduced efficacy (Frei and Canellos, 1980; Carpenter et al., 1983).

The designers of new systems for the support of medical care, whether they be at the federal level or in the insurance industry, must take all of these concepts into consideration. Otherwise we may lose our perspective and overspend limited resources transplanting baboon hearts and human "spare" or cadaveric parts before obtaining those cures that can be achieved in cancerous disease with current day methodology. Indeed, right now today, Medicare laws are severely restrictive in sponsoring what HCFA calls experimental therapy.

Anticipating a need for a cancer insurance policy is not a high priority for people today but must be encouraged in some form by both the public and the private sectors. There are data showing that when cost sharing is used in conjunction with a national health insurance for catastrophic coverage there is actually a decrease in the use of hospital services (Mitchell and Phelps, 1976). Certainly, there is a need for such catastrophic coverage in some situations where the principal diagnosis is a neoplasm. However, if oncologists (and other organized groups such as the American Society of Internal Medicine) are successful in an effort to achieve such an insurance arrangement, there will be a need to decide when a situation (and not just the diagnosis) merits this designation of catastrophic. In the past several decades physicians have not created a good track record in making exact determination of total disability and severity of illness. In part this has occurred because they have been too strong an advocate for their patients and in part because more subjective than objective criteria were used. Doctors must narrow the credibility gap by being both more accurate and more honest. Otherwise, much of the treatment given for the 60% of cancers which are incurable and for which the technology is still crude can be unnecessarily aggressive and economically unsound.

III. PREVENTION OF CANCER: THE REAL ECONOMY

Only by itemizing and categorizing (just as is required in preparing a household budget) can one begin to look at the potential sites where the exercise of restraint might reduce unnecessary expenses. Where might the economic hardships occur? All diseases have a beginning and so it is with cancer. Obviously the most specific way to eliminate costs of a problem is to prevent that problem. Specific examples of cancer prevention have been clearly defined. They include stopping or never starting a cigarette habit, which reduces the incidence of lung

cancer (by 80-90%) as well as head and neck cancers; carefully planned schedules of testing for occult blood in the stool combined with periodic proctosigmoidoscopy and/or double contrast barium enema to detect and then
resect early colonic neoplasms before they metastasize (Winawer, Miller, and
Sherlock, 1984); attention to use of the Papanicolaou smear, which reduces
the incidence of invasive cervical carcinoma; and, in the past two decades, more
intense application of techniques of self-examination combined with mammo-
graphy so that breast cancer can be resected when it is still stage I. Obviously,
prevention and screening by whatever approach are not free of costs. Moreover,
many projects still await the kind of studies which define the most cost-
effective approach to early detection (Eddy, personal communication, 1984).

IV. SAVING MONEY WHILE STILL MAKING THE
CORRECT DIAGNOSIS

For purposes of discussion, prevention and the technical approaches to ac-
complishing it are quite separate from the ways in which doctors "work up"
and stage the individual whose suspected malignancy is almost certain or already
proven. In the setting of established disease, it is appropriate to suggest that
physicians can learn to be prudent in the ordering of tests. Judging from the
response that followed a sounding board article in the New England Journal of
Medicine on this subject (Reuben, 1984), it is quite evident that the issue is
hotly contested and extensively debated. Excessive ordering of tests/studies is
often defended by the concept espoused by those who review charts for research purposes: "Later it will be nice to have lots of data when we analyze
these cases to write them up retrospectively; it is so frustrating to go through
charts and find that something is missing." In the past, a good deal of information has become available by serendipity. Now, it is necessary that such data
be sought through prospectively planned research protocols, and remember, not
all patients can or should participate in such clinical research. It then becomes
incumbent upon the practitioner to determine which diagnostic approaches are
mandatory; which ones are required to make a clinical decision and what is
needed to establish an unequivocal diagnosis. So many of us extrapolate from
cooperative group protocols designed for studying the treatment of groups of
patients having specific neoplasms to the management of that disease in a single individual who is not enrolled in the protocol. One result is a rigid pattern of
test ordering for research purposes when all that was necessary was a scaled-
down test-ordering process. The researchers who teach students, residents and
postgraduate fellows and those who have been their learners often come away
with a catechism of rigid order writing. As a result they stand accused of
"equating their ability to know with the need to know and letting their desire
to know predominate because they were once accustomed to being able to
know" (Reuben, 1984),

If we are to encourage the exercising of restraint, then there is the challenge of finding ways to change physician behavior. One such approach, which may be less traumatic than others, is the Peer Data Method (Kincaid, 1984) which focuses on the patterns of care that physicians exhibit, thus avoiding second-guessing them on their care of a specific patient. There is little reason to doubt that patterns of behavior, especially excesses, begin to change when internists submit to a monitoring process (Kincaid, 1984).

It is usually easier to prevent undesirable habits than change them and so it is in the training of doctors (Schroeder et al., 1984). Therefore, medical schools must continue to pursue those revisions in their teaching curricula that emphasize appropriate and economically sound approaches to the diagnosis of and continued evaluation of disease. Reasonable beginnings can be found regularly in the *Journal of the American Medical Association* under a section entitled "Toward Optimal Laboratory Use," and in the *Annals of Internal Medicine* under the sections devoted to diagnosis and treatment. Unfortunately, only rarely are such discussions in these or other journals devoted specifically to cancer per se (Safran, Desforges, and Tsichlis, 1977) indicating a need for more thought and publication in this area. Although older physicians have either resisted or misunderstood algorithms and decision trees, there is certainly a place for them in teaching medical students and in training house officers.

One appropriate place on which to focus is lung cancer, a disease of increasing frequency and such severity that it caused 117,000 deaths in 1983 or 25% of all cancer deaths in that year. An orderly, sensible approach to the diagnosis of this (or any) cancer is the ideal and results in an economy. Such a schema promoting efficiency in the workup of suspected lung cancer has been published (Koh and Prout, 1982). The authors begin by reminding us, with tongue in cheek, that for a "tumor whose doubling time is theoretically as short as 20 days, it is scientifically unsound to spend one or two doubling times evaluating the condition of the patient!" Proposed specific guidelines were offered to obviate inefficiency and to reach a treatment plan quickly. Their emphasis suggested that an efficient workup confirms the diagnosis and, at the same time, determines stage and operative status. For instance, guideline number five states: "A node biopsy should be the initial study if palpable adenopathy is found." Their tenth principle reads: "Routine radionuclide scans are not indicated in asymptomatic patients."

In contrast, consider the more frequent scenario detailed next. It is distressing because an undisciplined yet stereotyped approach eventually results in defining the correct histological diagnosis and extent of disease.

M.F., a 49-year-old twice-divorced truck driver, a "heavy drinker" with approximately a 55-pack-year cigarette habit (1 pack per day age 18-24; 2 per day age 24-34; 1 per day age 34-42; 3 per day age 42-49) was found to have left hilar and suprahilar masses with a left upper lung field density when a chest x-ray was obtained in a family medicine clinic to evaluate 2-3 months of cough and streak hemoptysis of two weeks duration. He was referred to a teaching university thoracic surgical service; was admitted directly to hospital in an ambulatory state; had a repeat chest x-ray; and had the following orders written on his chart: Chem. 6 and 12, AM sputum x 3 for cytology (and AFB/fungi), complete pulmonary function tests with arterial blood gases. On the third hospital day bronchoscopy defined a friable endobronchial mass in the left upper lobe, biopsy of which established the diagnosis, small cell undifferentiated carcinoma. Liver/bone scans plus a brain CT were ordered; and consults were directed to radiation as well as medical oncology. The latter arrived first and directed by the data accumulated found a small, but hard, clearly abnormal node at the base of the left sternocleidomastoid muscle. Apparently it had been missed by the surgical house officer. Feeling the need to know for sure the extent of disease, the oncologist aspirated the node and demonstrated small cell carcinoma. In the same hour he did bilateral posterior iliac aspirations/ biopsies, proving marrow involvement. Later the next day, when advised of all the findings (liver, bone, and brain scans were normal) this patient declined an offer to participate in a cooperative group protocol designed to further study a previously published six-drug regimen (Sierocki et al., 1980).

What went on with this case is *not* an isolated event. Without deciding ahead of time what was needed for sure or whether the patient would participate in a clinical research program, almost one of everything on the diagnostic menu was ordered. Worse than that, everything could have been accomplished in an outpatient setting eliminating the hospital charges for room and board. By the way, two of the three sputum cytologies (one returned later on the day of bronchoscopy) demonstrated malignant cells consistent with small cell undifferentiated carcinoma.

For too long some physicians have practiced by certain simplifying heuristics which can often be heard in hallways and conference rooms: "Costs should not be considered in decisions about individual patients;" "When in doubt, do it;" "An error of commission is to be preferred to an error of omission!" It is now time to substitute better heuristic commandments (Meeroff, 1984) such as: "Sequence paraclinical tests;" "Do not be redundant with paraclinical tests;" "Once the degree of reliability needed to make a decision is reached, tests should be stopped;" "There should be a reason for every datum gathered;" and, finally, "If the result of a paraclinical procedure will not change the course of treatment, the procedure should not be ordered."

Although this case study focused on the first trimester of an illness, many of the principles stressed can be carried over into the second and the early portions of the third trimesters of most neoplasms. There are specific though controversial examples that can be cited under the general heading of followup of patients who have undergone definitive treatment. The first is not my case but has been published several times as part of a classified advertisement (advertisement in New Engl. J. Med., 1984) for Centocor's CA 125, a radioimmunoassay based on monoclonal antibody technology, that has an 80% sensitivity for the detection of surgically demonstrable ovarian cancer. Their case in point was "a 46-year-old mother of three with stage IV endometrioid ovarian cancer" who "underwent cytoreductive surgery, an aggressive course of chemotherapy, and two second-look laparoscopies which revealed no recurrence. Therapy was discontinued. Within 8 months, her CA 125 levels had risen dramatically yet her CEA levels remained normal, and she had no symptoms of recurrence. But 7 months later a CT scan revealed a small pelvic mass. Despite subsequent palliative treatment, the disease progressed and the patient died." Their justified claim was that the CA 125 technique predicted the course of her disease 7 months before the earliest evidence of recurrence appeared. But was it necessary to know that far in advance when there was no reasonable curative treatment remaining?

Consider how some practitioners use yet another assay for the early serologic detection of tumor recurrence. Techniques to measure and quantitate carcinoembryonic antigen have been generally available for 10 years. When surgical plans include a second-look approach, with the intent of achieving cure by resecting small recurrences, then one cannot debate very forcefully the proposition that serial CEA determinations are warranted for those patients selected to participate in such a plan. However, all too often the use of the assay is typified by this example:

A 70-year-old retired farmer sought medical attention after 9 months of a change in his bowel habit toward increasing constipation, 3 months of bright-red rectal bleeding, and 2 weeks of vague lower abdominal discomfort. At laparotomy, a Duke's C poorly differentiated adenocarcinoma of the sigmoid was resected. During quarterly examinations by a surgical oncologist (but there are many instances in which the individual could be a medical oncologist), he underwent palpation of his abdomen, proctosigmoidoscopy, and CEAs were obtained. Forty-eight months postoperatively, the CEA, which had been 36 preoperatively and 6 one month postoperatively, had risen to 84 while the patient continued to feel relatively well. A liver-spleen scan and abdominal CT failed to define anatomic evidence of recurrent disease. Six months later his CEA had risen to 180; appetite had declined somewhat; and there were occasional somewhat vague discomforts in the epigastrium. Three months after that, the edge of his left hepatic lobe was palpable and tender. A repeat abdominal CT demonstrated low density areas in the left lobe certainly, and in the right lobe probably. Moreover there were tiny nodules in the right midlung field and at the left lung base. The patient was

informed of the findings; he declined needle aspiration of the hepatic lesion
for proof of recurrence; and agreed to a trial of single-agent chemotherapy
with 5-fluorouracil. After 3 months of administration of the drug, the CEA
had risen further; abdominal pain had increased; and the hepatic edge was
4 cm more below the xiphoid. At that point this man declined the offer of
experimental approaches in a very stoical manner and succumbed 6 months
later.

Could not the CEAs have been omitted and ordering of an abdominal CT been
deferred until the 57th postoperative month when he had both symptoms and a
palpable tender liver edge?

Perhaps one important generalization can be made about these examples
which involve very sensitive immunoassays for the detection of disease at a
time when treatment modalities lag far behind: unless it is going to help the
patient and the doctor, do not order something that is going to worry them
both before it is absolutely necessary to think about the issue. This is quite
contrary to the concept of justifying serial assays because such a test is safe,
noninvasive, relatively cheap, and provides some "peace of mind" for the patient,
their family, and the physician! It is hard to find the peace of mind in these
two cases and easy to find the extra costs.

V. ADVANCED DISEASE: PERHAPS WE ARE OVERDOING IT

There exists for the oncologist multiple pressures to do something about uncontrolled, progressive, and no longer curable malignancy. Relapse after an
aggressive primary chemotherapeutic regimen, recurrence despite an intense
adjuvant program, and periodic reports in the daily press about new approaches
to curing cancer lead naturally to the patient's (and family's) expectation that
something more can and should be done. Instead of careful explanations of current day limitations, this kind of pressure often leads to trying a multiple drug
program reported in the latest journal or sketchily reported in an abstract at a
national meeting. Infrequently are the results worth the effort or the price.
But the fact remains that the demand for medical resources is virtually limitless.
Use of those resources should require that there be a reasonable expectation,
i.e., that the patient's health will be benefited. An obvious corollary exists—
stop when there has been no realistic benefit. Such axioms are easily followed
when prescribing a palliative chemotherapy program if one remembers certain
rules: (1) find something to monitor/measure and keep careful serial records
of it; (2) include use of the performance status as well as some indicators of
the quality of life and remeasure both after application of the treatment; (3)
remember the caveat that if two courses of a combination of drugs do not
influence a solid tumor, then there is no reason to expect benefit from a third
and fourth cycle of those agents.

It may be painful to admit defeat, but it is sensible and usually more humane. Far too many patients with cancer continue to receive cytotoxic drugs that were never or are no longer effective right up to and including their final weeks of life.

This problem of meeting expectations is even more complex when the approach selected requires something other than prescribing oral and/or parenteral medications. How difficult it is to resist apparently marvelous technological advances in medicine is well demonstrated by the totally implantable infusaid pumps (Infusaid) currently delivering chemotherapeutic agents directly into hepatic metastases via their arterial blood supply (Ensminger et al., 1982). There is little reason to doubt that such an approach is usually beneficial in terms of transient relief of some symptoms, generally when the metastases have produced hepatomegaly (Balch et al., 1983). But it is also apparent that such symptomatic gains do not extrapolate into significant prolongation of life (Weiss et al., 1983). Two randomized trials are just now in progress comparing intra-arterial with either continuous intravenous infusion or intermittent intravenous injections of floxuridine (Kemeny et al., 1984; Stagg et al., 1984b).

Here, the clinician is faced with a dilemma: who gets this hardware and at what point in the course of their illness? When anecdotal experience and nonrandomized trials guide practice, there is less science and even less data collection/analysis. What is needed are steps three and seven of the seven-step description of the development, diffusion, and use of medical technologies employed in 1976 by the President's Biomedical Research Panel. Step three advised evaluation of the safety and efficacy of new technology through such means as controlled clinical trials. Step seven suggested skillful and balanced application of the new development to the population. It is not clear that either step has been fully applied yet to the delivery of intra-arterial chemotherapy of colonic hepatic metastases.

Various models of such an infusion pump cost about $2,000-4,000 and are not reuseable so that, with attendant surgery, the total cost to the patient, according to Medical Letter consultants, may be $10,000 or more (Med. Lett., 1984). Use of this type of equipment is not limited to a single drug (Stagg et al., 1984a); nor is the approach limited to the liver (Baker and Wheeler, 1982). Nevertheless, because of the eventual lack of an effective agent to infuse, the pump often becomes useless before the disease has finished running its course.

Remarkable advances in medical technology are considered to contribute quite significantly to the rising cost of medical care and to the increased percentage of the gross national product spent on health care. Indeed, Dr. William Schwartz, whose recently published book, *The Painful Prescription: Rationing Hospital Care,* which he coauthored with Henry Aaron of the Brookings

Institute, believes that the latest DRG/PRO cost-reducing efforts will show
only an "illusory short-term reduction in costs" *because* that illusion will become transparent when technological forces continue to increase the cost of
medical care. It is time to convince and encourage those who create or invent
that it is appropriate to submit their new technologies for some type of evaluation. Unfortunately, there are few arbiters bold enough and confident enough
to perform such a task. One is the American College of Physicians' small but
highly regarded program, the Clinical Efficacy Assessment Project (CEAP).
Another may be the recently proposed Medical Technology Assessment Con-
sortium intended to be under the auspices of the National Academy of Sciences
and the Institute of Medicine.

Savings should be effected in areas other than those that come under the
heading of specific therapy too, of course. Each might be small by comparison
with the items discussed up to this point but when multiplied many times over
the total could be significant. But where are the opportunities and what are
the means to accomplish such a postulate? There are several excellent well-
organized texts (Cassileth, and Cassileth, 1982; Higby, 1983) devoted to the
techniques of prescribing for common medical problems and medical complications in the cancer patient. Unfortunately, the modern physician knows mostly
about prescribing through pharmacies and very little about home remedies. For
example, Dr. Michael Levy's 45-page chapter in one of those texts (Cassileth
and Cassileth, 1982), entitled *Symptom Control Manual,* is superbly arranged
and is very specific as to what can be prescribed. However, there are virtually
no nonproprietary remedies and no one ever mentions traditional medications,
herbal approaches, or grandmother's measures! Perhaps few are truly available
but more than likely our abilities to be innovative about managing or easing
symptoms have atrophied. We should initially encourage and endorse such
alternate approaches as are available, inviting the patient and the family to
participate in this search for remedies that might be less expensive than a
physician's prescription.

Before embarking upon symptomatic measures, certain distinctions must be
made necessitating that specific questions be answered. Is the symptom a side
effect of chemotherapy? Does the patient have an urgent requirement for
aggressive supportive therapy to manage infection, hemorrhage, anemia, or
specific sites of tissue destruction (e.g., chemical cystitis, oral mucositis,
radiation-induced esophagitis, tumor associated spinal cord compression, tumor-
ous pericarditis)? There are singular differences between a child at the nadir of
granulocyte/platelet counts following a first attempt with chemotherapy during
remission-induction and an ambulatory, adult outpatient with a solid tumor
whose host defenses are only minimally impaired at the time fever develops.
All too often "in-house" treatment approaches for the former situation are
extended to the latter setting when an oral antibiotic with careful periodic

observation in clinic might suffice as a first approach. There is *no* reason to make the treatment *more desperate* than the clinical predicament and it is always much more costly to do so.

Next, after fever of infection, we should address an important question, Are there home remedies or simple ameliorating approaches for the large glossary of disturbances that occur in cancer patients? Unfortunately, the answer is not yet, and they may be a long way off since research in the field of primary care has only recently been re-emphasized (Mushlin, 1984) and is not likely to study symptom control in cancer victims first.

In the paragraphs that follow several challenging disturbances are addressed in alphabetical order and the author apologizes for his own and the failings of colleagues to provide more specific advice.

A. Anorexia

This universal complaint usually requires preparation of food out of sight and smell; presentation in small amounts; trial of alcoholic beverages to relax while stimulating appetite; and total freedom in selecting what and when to eat.

B. Cough

Codeine usually cannot be surpassed and it is less expensive than other agents such as dextromethorphan. Inhalation of the vapors while sipping hot tea, laced generously with honey, lemon, and whiskey, is sometimes effective in croup-like situations and can be tried when the etiology is interstitial lung problems from metastases. Sometimes careful (on an empty stomach) inhalation of aerosolized xylocaine can be helpful (Stewart and Coady, 1977).

C. Diarrhea

Relatively digestible and somewhat constipating foods such as rice, banana, applesauce, and toasted white bread should be eaten and along with amphogel might replace diphenoxylate and atropine, the ingredients of Lomotil. A liquid bismuth subsalicylate preparation such as Pepto-Bismol, very effective in traveler's diarrhea, deserves more emphasis when the gastrointestinal mucosa has been denuded by drugs rather than by bacteria. Fluid replacement can be accomplished by oral hydration approaches (Abramowicz, 1983).

D. Dysuria (Cystitis)

Marked dilution of urine by large fluid intake is clearly a preventive measure when certain drugs such as cyclophosphamide and its cogeners are administered, and it also diminishes burning once the chemical insult has occurred. Neutral or acid pHs are usually better tolerated than alkaline urines so advise drinking tomato juice (acetic acid) and eliminate orange juice (citric acid). Beyond that, it is worth remembering that a combination of methylene blue and hyoscyamine (Urised) is more expensive than phenazopyridine (Pyridium) (two 12.5¢ q.i.d. vs. one 6.6¢ tablet t.i.d.) (Medical Economics, 1984).

E. Dyspnea

Home oxygen more often makes psychological than physiological sense, but can nevertheless be an ally especially if one orders it to be used intermittently as before/after trips to the bathroom or in preparation for any exertion. Unfortunately, in order to have Medicare sponsor its use, a patient's PO_2 has to be below 55 mm Hg. Nothing allays the anxiety associated with dyspnea better than morphine, and instructing family members in its subcutaneous administration is made easier if the physician remembers that a half milligram error in one direction or the other is not really critical.

F. Nausea

Currently neither grandmothers nor physicians have much to offer. At least the latter have suppositories, phenothiazines, or trimethobenzamide (Tigan), which is only slightly less expensive than prochlorperazine. However, before writing a prescription for 50-100 tablets of an antiemetic, be certain that the act of swallowing the first few does not precipitate vomiting.

G. Pain and Psychological Suffering

This remains an area of considerable controversy with numerous prescription drugs—analgesics, tranquilizers, antidepressants, and sedatives—to relieve the two symptoms. There is no one correct position in the issue of someone else's pain, despondency, anxiety, and insomnia. At least be certain that the patient expresses his/her intentions—to live drug-free when possible and tolerable or to eliminate suffering above all. Finally, keep in mind relative prices for medications. A combination of oxycodone and Tylenol (Percocet-5 or Tylox) is two times as expensive when not ordered as a generic drug and five times as expensive as 5 mg of methadone; 60 mg of phenobarbitol costs 1/18 as much as 5 mg of Valium. Finally, dosage for all of these can be reduced or eliminated by loving massage.

H. Sore Mouth

Some patients advise rinsing and gargling with a glass of luke warm water with salt dissolved in it. That approach and/or coating the mouth thinly with Milk of Magnesia are certainly worth trying before prescribing viscous xylocaine.

I. Vomiting

No single symptom in the field of cancer is more vexing or leads to hospitalization as often as repeated emesis. The armamentarium for its management is
broad and covered thoroughly in Chapter 5.

Endorsement by the physician early on of certain principles such as oral
rather than parenteral routes, of prescribing less expensively whenever possible,
and reducing symptoms by a non-prescription approach will help with the
transition to a concept of Hospice later on (see Chapter 12).

An extreme example of cost control in the relief of symptoms can be
illustrated by the development of annoying thirst, perhaps in someone with
very late or terminal disease.   Frequent moistening of the lips and tongue
with ice chips is a simple and effective approach even though it does not correct the fluid deficit. This method is clearly far less expensive than I.V.
fluids in managing thirst when the concern is no longer that dehydration will
lead to hypovolemia and thence to renal failure with death by uremia. Again,
the use of ice chips and sips of fluid takes the focus away from the parenteral
route and reduces the dependency upon doctors or nurses.

Unfortunately, there is no single perfect manual to guide those who seek
practical and cheap solutions for annoying symptoms. One recently published
volume (Wilen and Wilen, 1984) reads very easily, offers reasonable suggestions,
and at least entertains while never advising dangerous methods.

VI. VERY LATE DISEASE AND TERMINAL CARE CAN TAX
ALL CONCERNED

Acute intercurrent illness does occur in the late stages of advanced cancer. It
may or may not herald the terminal state and should be treated, but managerial
decisions might well be different than those made when dealing with an otherwise healthy individual having the same problem. Clearly there is a time for
simple empirical therapy stripped of most, if not all, the extra trimmings that
accompany many outpatient or in-hospital treatment plans. Unfortunately, as
Dr. Feinstein so aptly stated it, "At every level of clinical practice today . . .
the use and evaluation of therapy is beset by controversy, discussion, and
doubt" (Feinstein, 1983). On the other hand, there should be no real doubt
about the goals of treatment in those with terminal cancer. They are preserve
locomotion and continence; protect the ability to think; relieve pain and suffering; and support dignity.

As it has been asked in geriatrics (Weksler, Durmaskin, and Kodner, 1983),
so should it be asked in the terminal stages of cancer: Why *must the physician
be captain of the health care team in the final stages of cancer?* This almost
heretical question could be the beginning of solving some of the ethical issues

facing us today and could help change the emphasis away from caring too much about documentation towards heightening the sensitivity about what the patient truly needs.

Regardless of who becomes these new team leaders, they will have to know when enough is enough. Consider the patient admitted to the hospital for an acute problem with expectation of quickly again being well enough for discharge home, but whose neoplasm takes a so-called turn for the worse. Continuation of active therapy is no longer warranted. Furthermore, by current day standards, such a patient no longer requires an expensive intermediary care bed. What is needed can be provided by the concepts of Hospice. To be prepared for that eventuality is currently the only available technique for conserving dollars in this final phase of illness. All too often the question of how to arrange for this kind of care has been postponed, creating unnecessary delays and extra attendant costs before finding a suitable structure, whether it be the home or a nursing home. Early attention to discharge planning is the key and has been strongly endorsed by all hospital utilization review committees. Indeed, Medicare's definitions of levels of care has mandated this type of fiscal responsibility and sometimes it is painful for all concerned (Lind, 1984).

Next, it is legitimate to ask what to do about the patient with advanced cancer whose intercurrent problem escalates and there is no simple stopping point. Often there is a clinical temptation to believe that just a little more information, such as a lung biopsy, and a few days of more intensive therapy with aggressive support will "get him/her over this complication." This description is not a fanciful thesis, rather it is a scenario played out frequently on intensive and critical care units leading to marginally useful results and extraordinary bills. Such expenditures on the terminally ill are not only very costly but also unreasonable and disproportionate to the dollars that this country could be devoting to clearly available solutions for several serious medical problems. Unfortunately, not everyone can or will agree with this proposition and for those who do, the solutions to the problems are waiting for a societal commitment to solving them (Bayer et al., 1983).

And then there is the agonizing final step in saving the very terminal hemorrhaging of dollars: turning off life support. Until all physicians get more comfortable with discontinuing mechanical ventilation and intravenous fluids that only support vital signs without sustaining meaningful life (and almost always initiated on an ICU), it is impossible to give specific advice in this area of the practice of medicine. Nevertheless, the issue is timely and currently, significant support is available for the physician (Bedell et al., 1983; Low, 1984; Wanzer et al., 1984; Uhlmann, McDonald, and Inui, 1984). A proliferation of ethicists and hospital ethics committees stand ready to advise families in making responsible decisions.

VII. UNPROVEN METHODS TO REMEDY CANCER: A FINANCIAL SHAME

This chapter, devoted to minimizing the economic burden borne by us all, would not be complete without some discussion of the waste created when patients resort to unproven methods of cancer management. Despite efforts at educating the public, legislative activities, and some progress which we, in the establishment, label medical advances, unconventional approaches may be gaining in popularity. One study of over 600 patients suggests that 54% of them were participating in a conventional program while simultaneously using an unorthodox form of therapy (Cassileth et al., 1984). It is difficult to obtain estimates for the charges incurred while pursuing such alternative approaches. Theoretically, the selling price of metabolic therapy, megavitamins, and "immune" therapy represent higher direct costs than those for dietary regimens, mental imagery as applied for antitumor effect, and spiritual or faith healing. However, for all of these there can be traveling expenses, especially to places outside the United States, professional fees, testing costs, and, of course, suggested donations, all of which influence the tally greatly. Even the preparation of unique diets, consisting of very specific and relatively rare foods, which must be prepared in a particular manner, can be quite expensive.

Prevention or modification of this behavior by patients is a formidable task. It requires that the physician be aware of the magnitude of the problem; the frequency with which both conventional and unconventional therapy is being "taken" simultaneously; and that those who initiate alternative therapy are as likely to do so when their disease shows distant spread as when there is localized tumor or no evidence of disease!

Our advice to the clinician and his team is as follows: (1) do not ever ignore the issue—it has not and will not go away; (2) keep up to date about some of the things being offered (American Cancer Society, 1982); (3) feel free to bring it up periodically during discussions with patients while making it clear that the patient can do likewise; (4) be prepared to provide factual data where possible (American Society of Clinical Oncology, 1983); and (5) offer some self-help alternatives that can be achieved without undue costs (Simonton, Matthews-Simonton, and Creighton, 1981) such as relaxation techniques, for which there is scientific support and the proposal that intense concentration to favorably direct effective drugs or x-irradiation, for which there is no substantial proof. Remember, there are varied reasons for the appeal of these alternative remedies. Some are life-style oriented; others are antimedicinal; a few are strictly based on religious beliefs; many focus on detoxifying the body; most incorporate an unproven but *apparently* sensible dietary revision; almost all promise patients an *active role* in their own health care; and finally, they may represent a last resort for the terminal patient who cannot give up.

VIII. CONCLUSIONS

The "overdoing it" in medicine may have cost everyone dearly and those in clinical cancer research even more so, since Medicare currently lists *"experimental therapy" as a "noncovered" service* (Medicare and Medicaid Guide). This term experimental, which conjures up the image of a procedure done to or with animals, or one done to humans that has little or no clinical scientific basis, has become a monetary obstacle to the delivery of best patient care. A more accurate operational term such as novel or new approach seems warranted since clinical investigation is a fundamental construct in modern medicine and represents an attempt to improve medical care or to extend the boundaries of clinical science. Moreover, a novel approach may equate to best care available to that patient. Even some standard modes of therapy should be carried out as one does a laboratory experiment in the sense that all effects, both beneficial and detrimental, must be measured, recorded, and evaluated. The anticipated or hoped for result obviously cannot be guaranteed with any certainty and therefore great care and judgment are required to decide when to begin what treatment and in which patient, whether to continue, and how to stop. Adhering to such principals and combining them with the caveat that not every individual can or should participate (speaking of patients as well as doctors) in clinical research should effect significant savings without abandoning the entire concept of chemotherapy trials.

Remembering to focus upon certain important clues, usually available from the sick and their relatives, will assist the physician further in budgeting critically restricted resources within a single family. It is no longer advisable to practice with the philosophy that *only* the doctor knows what is best for a patient and that costs should never be a consideration when caring for a given individual.

There are some pearls for more perfect practice that will affect part of the spiraling costs that are now the principal concerns of all third-party carriers: (1) to think about how to study a patient's problem is now (and always has been) an outpatient procedure; (2) to review data (slides, x-rays, operative notes, pathology reports, discharge summaries) is an office process; (3) when a patient (or the family) requests time in days to think things over, they must be informed that such consideration should be carried on out-of-hospital; and (4) when one can conclude that what is to be done to/for a patient could be accomplished in a clinic setting (if the individual lived near by and the M.D. was not too busy— or going on a lecture tour—and had time to review/study/counsel the person), then an advisor for a peer review organization would issue a "denial" should such a patient be admitted.

Finally, paying heed to one of my favorite quotations usually will keep physicians from overdoing it: "intellect distinguishes between the *possible* and the *impossible*; reason distinguishes between the *sensible* and the *senseless*; even the *possible* can be *senseless*" (Born 1968).

REFERENCES

Aaron, H. J., and Schwartz, W. B. (1984). *The Painful Prescription: Rationing Hospital Care*, Brookings Institute, Washington, D.C.

Abramowicz, M. (ed). (1983). Fluid replacement by oral hydration approaches, *Med. Lett. Drugs Ther., 25*:19-20.

Advertisement. (1984). Monitoring the course of ovarian carcinoma: A promising new approach, *New Engl. J. Med., 310*:6 (ad pages).

American Cancer Society. (1982). *Unproven Methods of Cancer Medicine*, American Cancer Society, New York.

American Society of Clinical Oncology, Subcommittee on Unorthodox Therapies. (1983). Effective cancer therapy: A guide for the layperson, *J. Clin. Oncol., 1*:154-163.

Baker, S. R., and Wheeler, R. H. (1982). Long-term intra-arterial chemotherapy infusion of ambulatory head and neck cancer patients, *J. Surg. Oncol., 21*: 125-131.

Balch, C. M., Urist, M. M., Soong, S., and McGregor, M. (1983). A prospective phase II clinical trial of continuous FUDR regional chemotherapy for colorectal metastases to the liver using a totally implantable drug infusion pump, *Ann. Surg., 198*:567-573.

Bayer, R., Callahan, D., Fletcher, J., Hodgson, T., Jennings, B., Momsees, D., Sieverts, S., and Veatch, R. (1983). The care of the terminally ill: Morality and economics, *New Engl. J. Med., 309*:1490-1494.

Bedell, S. E., Delbanco, T. L., Cooke, F., and Epstein, F. H. (1983). Survival after cardiopulmonary resuscitation in the hospital, *New Engl. J. Med., 309*: 569-576.

Born, M. (1968). *My Life and My Views*, Charles Scribner & Sons, New York.

Carpenter, J. P., Jr., Maddox, W. A., Laws, H. L., Wirtschafer, D. D., and Soong, S. J. (1983). Favorable factors in the adjuvant therapy of breast cancer, *Cancer, 50*:18-23.

Cassileth, B. R., and Cassileth, P. A. (1982). *Clinical Care of the Terminal Cancer Patient*, Lea & Febiger, Philadelphia.

Cassileth, B. R., Lusk, E. J., Strouse, T. B., and Bodenheimer, B. A. (1984). Untemporary unorthodox treatments in cancer medicine, *Ann. Intern. Med., 101*:105-112.

Ensminger, W., Niederhuber, J., Gyves, J., Thrall, J., Cozzi, E., and Doan, K. (1982). Effective control of liver metastases from colon cancer with an implanted system for hepatic arterial chemotherapy, *Proc. ASCO, 3*(Abstr. C-363):94.

Feinstein, A. R. (1983). An additional basic science for clinical medicine. I. The constraining fundamental paradigms, *Ann. Intern. Med., 99*:393-397.

Frei, E., III. (1984). Clinical therapeutic investigation in cancer research centers: Cost benefit considerations, *Minutes Annual Meeting of the Association of*

American Cancer Institutes, Memorial Sloan-Kettering Cancer Center, New York, pp. 5-14.

Frei, E., III, and Canellos, G. P. (1980). Dose: A critical factor in cancer chemotherapy, *Am. J. Med., 69*:585-594.

Gibbs, J., and Newman, J. (1982). Study of health services used and costs incurred during the last six months of a terminal illness, Contract No. HEW-100-79-0110, Blue Cross and Blue Shield Association, Chicago.

Higby, D. J. (1983). *Supportive Care in Cancer Therapy* (D. J. Higby, ed.), Martinus Nijhoff Publishers, Boston.

Hodgson, T. A. (1984). The economic burden of cancer, presented at the Fourth National Conference on Human Values, American Cancer Society, New York, March 15-17, 1984.

Kemeny, N., Daly, J., Oderman, P., Chun, H., Petroni, G., and Geller, N. (1984). Randomized study of intrahepatic vs. systemic infusion of fluorodeoxyuridine in patients with liver metastases from colorectal carcinoma, *Proc. ASCO, 3*(Abstr. C-551):141.

Kincaid, W. H. (1984). Changing physician behavior: The Peer Data Method, *Quality Rev. Bull., 10*:238-242.

Koh, H. K., and Prout, M. N. (1982). The efficient workup of suspected lung cancer, *Arch. Intern. Med., 142*:966-968.

Levy, M. (1982). Symptom control manual, in *Clinical Care of the Terminal Cancer Patient* (Cassileth, B. R., and Cassileth, P. A., eds.), Lea & Febiger, Philadelphia.

Lind, S. E. (1984). Transferring the terminally ill, *New Engl. J. Med., 311*: 1181-1182.

Loeb, L. A., Ernestler, V. L., Warner, K. E., Abbotts, J., and Laszlo J. (1984). Smoking and lung cancer: An overview, *Cancer Res., 40*:5940-5958.

Low, D. (1984). The death of Clarence Herbert: Withdrawing care is not murder, *Ann. Intern. Med., 101*:248-251.

Medical Economics (1984). *Annual of Pharmacists Reference (Redbook),* Medical Economics, Oradel, N.J.

Medicare and Medicaid Guide, Commerce Clearing House *1*: 1777-1788 (paragraph 405.422).

Meeroff, J. C. (1984). Ten heuristic commandments for clinical problem-solving, *V.A. Practitioner, 1*:58-59.

Mitchell, B., and Phelps, C. P. (1976). National health insurance: Some costs and effects of mandated employee coverage, *J. Pol. Econ., 3*:533-571.

Mushlin, A. I. (1984). New knowledge for primary care: A glimpse at general practice research in Great Britain, *Ann. Intern. Med., 100*:744-750.

News Item. (1984). An implanted infusion pump for chemotherapy of liver metastases, *Med. Lett., 26*:89-90.

Reuben, D. B. (1984). Learning diagnostic restraint, *New Engl. J. Med., 310*: 591-593.

Safran, C., Desforges, J., and Tsichlis, P. N. (1977). Decision analysis to evaluate lymphangiography in the management of patients with Hodgkin's disease, *New Engl. J. Med., 296*:1088-1092.

Schroeder, S. A., Myers, L. P., McPhee, S. J., Showstach, J. A., Simborg, D. W., Chapman, S. A., and Leong, J. A. (1984). The failure of physician education as a cost containment strategy, *JAMA, 252*:225-230.

Sierocki, J. S., Hilaris, B. S., Hopfan, S., Goldby, R. B., and Wittes, R. E. (1980). Small cell carcinoma of the lung—experience with a six drug regimen, *Cancer, 45*:417-422.

Silverberg, E. (1984). Cancer statistics, 1984, *CA Cancer J. Clin., 34*:7-23.

Simonton, O. C., Matthews-Simonton, S., and Creighton, J. L. (1981). *Getting Well Again,* Bantam Books, New York.

Stagg, R. J., Lewis, B. J., Friedman, M. A., Ignoffo, R. J., and Hohn, D. C. (1984a). Hepatic arterial chemotherapy for colorectal cancer metastatic to the liver, *Ann. Intern. Med., 100*:736-743.

Stagg, R., Friedman, M., Lewis, B., Ignoffo, R., Goodnight, J., Viele, C., and Hohn, D. (1984b). Current status of the NCOG randomized trial of continuous intra-arterial (IA) versus intravenous (IV) floxuridine (FUDR) in patients with colorectal carcinoma metastatic to the liver, *Proc. ASCO, 3*(Abstr. C-577):148.

Stewart, C., and Coady, T. (1977). Letter to editor: Suppression of intractable cough, *Brit. Med. J., 1*:1660.

Uhlmann, R. F., McDonald, W. J., and Inui, T. S. (1984). Epidemiology of no code orders in an academic hospital, *W. J. Med., 140*:114-116.

Wanzer, S. H., Adelstein, S. J., Cranford, R. E., Federman, D. D., Hook, E. D., Moertel, C. G., Safer, P., Ston, A. A., Taussig, H. B., and Van Eys, J. (1984). The physician's responsibility toward hopelessly ill patients, *New Engl. J. Med., 310*:955-959.

Weksler, M. E., Durmaskin, S. C., and Kodner, D. L. (1983). New goals for education in geriatric medicine, *Ann. Intern. Med., 99*:856-857.

Weiss, G. R., Garnick, M. B., Osteen, R. T., Steel, G. D., Jr., Wilson, R. E., Schade, D., Kaplan, W. D., Boxt, L. M., Kandarpa, K., Mayer, R. J., and Frei, E. T., III. (1983). Long-term hepatic arterial infusion of 5-fluorodeoxyuridine for liver metastases using an implantable infusion pump, *J. Clin. Oncol., 1*:337-344.

Wilen, J., and Wilen, L. (1984). *Chicken Soup and Other Folk Remedies,* Fawcett Columbine, New York.

Winawer, S. J., Miller, D. G., and Sherlock, P. (1984). Risk and screening for colorectal cancer, *Advances in Internal Medicine,* Vol. 29, Yearbook Medical Publishers, Chicago, pp. 471-496.

4

Preventing Complications of Surgery: Emphasis on Nutritional Factors

John P. Grant
Duke University Medical Center and Veterans Administration Medical Center, Durham, North Carolina

I. INTRODUCTION

The performance of operative procedures on patients harboring malignant diseases may be associated with greater morbidity and mortality than comparable procedures in non-cancer bearing patients. The presence of cancer can significantly alter fluid and electrolyte balance, blood volume and hemoglobin concentration, function of vital organs (lungs, heart, kidney, gastrointestinal tract), nutritional status, host immune status and resistance to infection, as well as the psychological state of the patient and the will to live. Therapeutic interventions such as radiation therapy, chemotherapy, or both, and the use of steroids and broad-spectrum antibiotics can further alter the response to and tolerance of surgery. Finally, the consequences of extirpative surgery must be considered as total or subtotal removal of organs such as the lung, gastrointestinal tract, pancreas, adrenal glands, or ovaries may have significant physiological effects, and removal of other organs such as extremities, breasts, testicles, uterus, and extensive tissue from the head and neck area may have a particularly significant psychological impact.

Prior to any surgical intervention, therefore, it is necessary to carefully review the total status of the patient with cancer. Recognition of risk factors and knowledge of the physiological and psychological processes that contribute to increased risk will allow for optimal preoperative preparation. When risks are recognized and minimized in this manner, the potential benefit of surgical intervention can be correctly weighed and the patient properly advised.

II. PREOPERATIVE ASSESSMENT

A. Psychological Aspects

Psychological stress that is experienced by a patient who has a newly diagnosed or suspected malignancy cannot be overemphasized (Ahned, 1981;
Kardinal and Porter, 1981). Thoughts of impending death, financial burdens,
and concerns for family can consume the patient's and family's energy thereby
distracting them from efforts needed to recover from surgery. What is of
"significant" concern versus what is fantasy often cannot be discerned by the
patient or family. The surgeon and nursing staff should make a special effort
and take time with the patient and family to be sure they understand, in
realistic terms, the nature of the disease and the need for surgical intervention.
At no time should the attitude of impatience or disinterest in the patient's
concerns be conveyed. As important as assuring that the patient and family
have available all the factual information necessary for an informed decision
concerning surgical intervention is that they not be misled. Where doubt
exists or questions remain as to the best approach to therapy, the surgeon
should identify the area of uncertainty or the gap of knowledge. As discussed
in an earlier chapter, when the patient and family have complete confidence
in their care team, and are fully informed and actively playing a role in
decision making, it is easier to encourage their efforts toward facing the
surgical procedure and participating in postoperative recovery. When questions
remain, the surgeon should not hesitate to call in other consultants. Post-
mastectomy patients can give insight to new patients with breast cancer,
patients with intestinal ostomies can help allay fears about intestinal resection
and patients with prostheses can discuss consequences of various forms of
extremity amputation. At other times a physical therapist, speech therapist
or rehabilitation expert can be of great value. Not to be overlooked is the
value of a second surgical opinion if the patient does not fully understand or
accept the need for surgery. Patients may be hesitant to request a second
opinion for fear of insulting or embarrassing their physician.

In addition to discussing the indications for and consequences of surgical
intervention, the patient must be made fully aware of the potential risks of
undergoing an operative procedure. Again, the physician must spend ample
time discussing the risks of bleeding, wound infection, cosmetic complications,
pain, and disability. With full disclosure, informed consent can be obtained
and the patient can become part of the care team. Occasionally a psychiatrist
can be helpful in dealing with hidden concerns of the patient.

B. Imbalance of Fluids, Electrolytes, and Blood

Often patients who have malignant diseases present to the surgeon with alterations in fluid, electrolyte, and blood balance. Obstructive lesions may lead to

sequestration of fluid within the gastrointestinal tract or tissue spaces, or to external loss by vomiting and diarrhea. Intra-abdominal lesions may lead to accumulation of ascitic fluid. Nausea, vomiting, and diarrhea are commonly associated with chemo- and radiotherapy. Decreased dietary intake can lead to progressive dehydration and malnutrition. Use of diuretics or the presence of fever may further contribute to fluid and electrolyte disturbances. Finally, total blood volume and red blood cell mass may be depleted because of external losses from the tumor.

A careful evaluation of fluid and electrolyte abnormalities, blood volume, and red blood cell concentration should be performed prior to surgical intervention. Detected abnormalities should be corrected at a rate dependent upon the chronicity of the disturbance, the urgency for surgical intervention, and the physiological status of the patient. Rapid correction of chronic fluid and electrolyte disturbances may lead to congestive heart failure or pulmonary edema, whereas a lethargic response in patients with acute losses can result in major organ dysfunction due to poor arterial perfusion.

Water represents 55-70% of the body weight. It moves freely between membranes to balance concentration gradients between various compartments. Total body water is regulated by antidiuretic hormone. The amount of body water determines osmolarity, which is defined as the concentration of ions and proteins in solution, and normally is approximately 300 mOsm/L. A formula useful in estimating osmolality is $Posm = 2 (Na + K) + BS/18 + BUN/2.8$. Two-thirds of the body water is intracellular fluid, which is that part of the body water from which sodium is excluded. Potassium is the primary ion in this cellular compartment. One-third of the body water is made up of extracellular fluid; one-fourth of this is plasma, and three-fourths is in interstitial spaces. The volume of extracellular fluid is controlled by total body sodium, which in turn is regulated by aldosterone. The final fluid space, which is really part of extracellular fluid, is third-space fluid. This fluid is not functionally available. Table 1 depicts the electrolyte content of the body water spaces.

When evaluating patients for fluid and electrolyte replacement, it is important to determine the presence and severity of any fluid and electrolyte disturbances, quantitate ongoing losses, and approximate daily maintenance requirements.

C. Determination of Fluid and Electrolyte Status

Body Water Excess

Clinical symptoms of excessive total body water depend on the degree of overload and the rate of accumulation. Mild to moderate overload that has occurred over a long period of time may result in few clinical symptoms. Generally,

Table 1   Composition of Body Fluids (mEq/L)

	Extracellular fluid		Intracellular fluid
	Plasma	Interstitial	
Cations			
Sodium	142	146	10
Potassium	5	4	150
Calcium	5	3	0
Magnesium	3	2	40
Totals	155	155	200
Anions			
Chloride	103	115	0
Bicarbonate	27	30	10
Protein	16	1	40
Sulfate	1	1	10
Phosphate	2	2	140
Organic acid	6	6	0
Totals	155	155	200

Source: After Bland (1963).

the serum sodium will be mildly depressed, there will be an increased urinary output and increased total body weight. No pitting edema will be present. As water excess becomes marked, or if it occurs over a short period of time, edema of the brain can occur with resulting nausea, vomiting, and convulsions. Serum sodium concentration will often be less than 120 mEq/L. Treatment includes restriction of water intake, administration of diuretics, and, in case of renal failure, dialysis. Only if convulsions occur with cerebral edema should 5% sodium chloride be administered. It should be remembered that the problem is not salt depletion, even though the serum sodium concentration is low, but rather it is water overload.

Water Depletion

Clinical features of water depletion are thirst and decreased sweating. When less than 1.5 L of water deficit is present, patients usually present with only mild symptoms of thirst. As depletion increases from 1.5-4.0 L, marked thirst develops, the mouth becomes dry, and the groin and axilla demonstrate no evidence of moisture. Serum sodium concentration increases, urinary volume falls and specific gravity increases. When greater than 4.0 L of body water is lost, the patient will express an intolerable thirst and hypernatremia and oliguria will be present. Body weight will be decreased. There may be a slight increase in hematocrit, the patient may become apathetic and perhaps stuporous and, if not corrected, hyperosmolar coma and death may follow. Note should be made that in water depletion skin turgor usually remains normal as does the serum hematocrit and blood pressure. Again, serum sodium concentration reflects total body water rather than total body sodium. Indeed, the amount of body water deficit can be estimated based on the measured serum sodium. Current body water in liters can be calculated by multiplying normal body water by the ratio of 140 divided by measured serum sodium. For the purpose of this formula, normal body water is assumed to be 60% of usual body weight in kilograms. The difference between normal body water and the current body water is equal to the body water deficit or excess.

Sodium Excess

The clinical symptoms of sodium excess are edema and weight gain. With marked sodium excess anasarca will be present. The treatment is specific: sodium restriction. Diuretics may be given to increase sodium loss if the free water and potassium losses are replaced. Rarely with sodium loading does serum concentration become elevated. As one adds more sodium to the body, more water is retained so an increase in body weight is evident but the serum concentration of sodium remains normal.

Sodium Depletion

Loss of salt from the body results in progressive loss of body water. Clinical symptoms result from changes in the extracellular fluid space. Loss of up to 450 mEq of sodium, equivalent to 3.0 L of extracellular fluid, is associated with loss of skin turgor, development of a furrowed, dry tongue, the neck veins become collapsed, there is an increased hematocrit due to hemoconcentration, urinary sodium falls below 40 mEq/L in response to aldactone secretion, and tachycardia develops. There is little or no thirst present and usually not much craving for salt. The serum sodium concentration remains normal. When more than 600 mEq of sodium are lost, representing more than 4.0 L of extracellular fluid, there is a marked increase in serum hematocrit and oliguria occurs which is pre-renal in nature. Hypotension, especially orthostatic, is often observed and the patient becomes apathetic and feels nauseated. There is some decrease in serum sodium concentration when salt depletion becomes extreme. If uncorrected, hypovolemic shock follows.

Potassium Excess

Increased concentrations of potassium result in abnormalities of cardiac conduction with tenting of T waves, a wide QRS complex, prolongation of the PR interval, and cardiac arrhythmias. There is generalized weakness and, with progressive potassium excess, reflexes are depressed. Paresthesias develop and respiratory paralysis finally ensues. The treatment of hyperkalemia is potassium restriction. Emergency therapies include administration of intravenous calcium which antagonizes the effects of potassium on the myocardium, sodium bicarbonate which shifts potassium intracellularly with alkalinization of the cells, 50% glucose and insulin which also shifts potassium intracellularly, and administration of Kayexalate orally or even hemodialysis.

Potassium Depletion

Changes in the electrocardiogram seen with potassium depletion include sagging ST waves, inverted T waves, a long QT interval, and decreased voltages. As potassium depletion progresses, generalized malaise and weakness develop along with gastrointestinal ileus. Cardiac arrhythmias are not uncommon and a pseudodiabetic glucosuria is often observed. Paradoxical aciduria may develop with metabolic alkalosis. In assessing for hypokalemia, it is important to remember that serum potassium concentration is a poor reflection of total body potassium. Since most potassium is within cells, major changes in total body potassium can occur, as in malnutrition, with only minor changes observable in the serum concentration. In addition, acid-base status must be considered in interpreting serum concentrations as acidosis results in passage of potassium out of the cell into the serum, and alkalosis results in the reverse. The average male, in a normal state of health, has 45 mEq/kg total body potassium and the female has 35 mEq/kg potassium. Use of Figure 1 facilitates calculation of total body potassium deficit or excess based on the state of nutrition and acid-base balance thereby allowing better estimation of initial potassium needs. Another useful laboratory value in determining total body potassium status is measurement of urinary potassium concentration. Normally, urinary concentration of potassium is equal to or greater than 40 mEq/L. Potassium overloading results in increased potassium excretion whereas potassium depletion is associated with decreased excretion. However, unlike sodium, there is a limit to the ability of the kidneys to conserve potassium, being unable to reduce losses below 15-25 mEq/day. The treatment of potassium depletion is intravenous or oral administration of potassium salts.

D. Other Electrolyte Abnormalities (Grant, 1980)

Progressive phosphorus depletion has been observed in patients receiving phosphate-binding antacids, with respiratory alkalosis, vomiting or other malabsorption syndromes, acute and chronic alcoholism, and with increased renal phosphate clearance such as in vitamin B_{12} deficiency, hyperparathyroidism, severe hypokalemia, and hypomagnesemia. Phosphate depletion is associated with progressive weakness, tremors, circumoral paresthesias, hyperventilation, loss of deep tendon reflexes, mental obtundity, and death. The red blood cell and platelet survival times are decreased and the oxyhemoglobin curve is

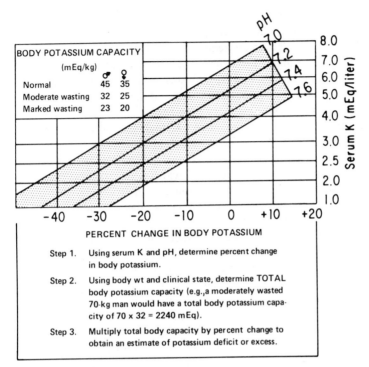

Figure 1 Calculation of body potassium stores with corrections for acid-base abnormalities. (From Condon, R. E., and Nyhus, L. M. (1972). *Manual of Surgical Therapeutics*, 2nd Edition, Little, Brown, Boston, p. 200. With permission.)

shifted to the left resulting in impaired oxygen delivery to tissues. Leukocyte chemotaxis and phagocytosis are also impaired. Clinical symptoms of phosphate depletion usually do not occur until the serum inorganic concentration is less than 1.0 mg/dl.

Hyperphosphatemia is usually the result of renal failure. Other causes include neoplastic diseases treated with cytotoxic agents, oral phosphate administration, and administration of phosphate-containing enemas. Metastatic calcifications may occur in soft tissues and organs due to the formation of colloidal complexes with calcium. Treatment consists of withholding all phosphate salts and oral administration of phosphate-binding antacids such as aluminum hydroxide, which decreases gastrointestinal tract absorption of phosphate.

Depletion of body magnesium can occur with various malabsorption syndromes, administration of certain drugs such as cisplatin and amphotericin B, intestinal or biliary tract fistulas, with prolonged vomiting or nasogastric suction, chronic alcoholism, pancreatitis, parathyroid diseases, and diabetes, especially if high doses of insulin are required. Clinical symptoms of hypomagnesemia rarely occur unless the serum concentration falls below 1.0 mEq/L. The symptoms include positive Trousseau's and Chvostek's signs and perhaps overt tetany with carpopedal spasm. Muscle fasciculations, tremors, and generalized muscle spasticity have been observed and ataxia, vertigo, and muscular weakness are common. Mental changes include psychotic behavior, generalized apathy, depression, and irritability. A renal diuresis of potassium may occur and a distal renal tubular acidosis has been reported. Digitalis toxicity has been reported which is reversible with administration of magnesium. Treatment of magnesium deficiency is by replacement, giving up to 40 mEq of magnesium sulfate per day depending on the severity of the clinical situation.

Hypermagnesemia is most often seen in patients with renal failure, diabetic acidosis, aldosterone deficiency, hyperparathyroidism, and those in whom magnesium-containing laxatives and enemas are given excessively. The symptoms of hypermagnesemia include alteration in neuromuscular transmission as reflected by hypotension, nausea, vomiting, weakness, lethargy, hyporeflexia, and respiratory depression. As the syndrome progresses, coma and cardiac arrest can occur. There are various degrees of AV block observed in the electrocardiogram with QT prolongation and a prolonged PR interval. Treatment consists of withholding all magnesium. Cardiac and pulmonary support may be necessary. Dialysis has been effective in reducing serum magnesium concentrations in acute settings.

Zinc deficiency is common in patients with malignancy, malabsorption, chronic liver diseases, and those who have undergone long-term corticosteroid therapy. Major stress or sepsis has been associated with an acute depletion syndrome. Clinical symptoms include diarrhea and mental depression with development of a paranasal, paraoral, scrotal, and generalized dermatitis. There may be a change in taste and smell acuity with occasional perverted taste and smell, anorexia, and subsequent weight loss. Zinc is an important trace element in wound healing. Deficiency has been associated with impaired formation of mature collagen. Zinc replacement can be accomplished by intravenous administration of zinc sulfate, giving between 100-200 mg of zinc a day.

Once the nature and severity of fluid and electrolyte deficits has been determined, approximately one-half of the estimated deficit should be replaced over 8-10 hours at which time the patient should again be assessed for deficits and new estimates made. Over the next 8 hours, half of the new estimate should be replaced and so on, until all deficits have been replaced. Likewise, patients with excess fluid or electrolytes should have their excesses drawn off over similar periods of time.

Blood Volume Alterations

Acute loss of blood as with gastrointestinal hemorrhage is associated with a rapid decrease in blood volume, tachycardia, hypotension, decreased urinary output, and, if severe, vascular collapse. Serum hematocrit may not change unless blood losses are replaced solely with crystalloid solutions. Measured or estimated losses should be rapidly replaced with either packed red blood cells and crystalloid or with whole blood. To avoid potential complications of macroaggregate transfusion with blood products, a microfilter should be used whenever more than 2 units of blood per square meter body surface area per 24 hours are to be given, especially if the blood is over 7 days old. As storage of blood at $4°C$ damages platelets and greatly reduces their survival, massive transfusion may be associated with dilutional thrombocytopenia. If 10 or more units of blood are transfused rapidly, or if bleeding persists, a platelet count should be obtained and platelet transfusions given to maintain the platelet count above $50,000/mm^3$. Bleeding due to deficiency of plasma clotting factors with massive blood transfusions is a rare problem and the use of fresh frozen plasma is seldom indicated. If only packed red blood cells are used, however, hypofibrinogenemia can occur.

With chronic blood loss, the body adapts by increasing plasma volume. Serum hematocrit and hemoglobin concentrations fall. Blood volume is normal and signs of vascular collapse are not present. Due to the fall in hemoglobin concentration, however, oxygen transport properties of the blood progressively deteriorate increasing morbidity and mortality during anesthesia and surgery. It is therefore preferable that time be taken preoperatively to replenish the red blood cell mass until serum hemoglobin concentration is greater than 10 gm/dl, or hematocrit greater than 30%. As the plasma volume is already increased, it is most appropriate to replenish these patients with packed red blood cells. As one replenishes the red blood cell volume, the patient will diurese excess fluid and the hematocrit and hemoglobin concentration will progressively rise (approximately one gram percent hemoglobin concentration or three percent hematocrit per unit of packed red blood cells transfused). Only 2-3 units of blood should be administered over a 24-hour period to allow for shifts in plasma volume. Acute replenishment of red blood cells in patients who have compromised cardiac or pulmonary function, especially if administered as whole blood, may well result in volume overload, congestive heart failure, and respiratory distress.

Determination of Ongoing Fluid and Electrolyte Losses

In preparation for a surgical procedure, it is also necessary to keep up with ongoing measurable losses. Nasogastric drainage, biliary tube drainage, diarrhea, and excessive urinary or fistula losses should be replaced on an every-4-hour basis. Table 2 depicts the typical electrolyte composition of various drainage fluids which can help select replacement solutions. When volume losses are excessive, however, a sample of the drainage fluid should

Table 2 Approximate Electrolyte Concentrations of Various Body Fluids (mEq/L)

Source	Volume/day		Na	K	Cl	HCO$_3$
Gastric	2000 to 2500	pH < 4	60	10	90	-
		pH > 4	100	10	100	-
Pancreas	1000		140	5	75	90
Bile	1500		140	5	100	35
Small bowel	3500		100	15	100	25
Diarrhea	1000 to 4000		60	30	45	45
Urine	1500		40	40	20	-
Sweat			50	5	55	-

be sent for electrolyte determination so more exact replacement can be accomplished.

Provision of Maintenance Fluid and Electrolytes

As imbalances are corrected and ongoing losses replaced, daily maintenance fluid and electrolytes must also be provided. Fluid requirements can be estimated based either on body surface area, giving 1500 ml/M^2 body surface area, or based on weight, giving 100 ml/kg for the first 10 kg of body weight, 50 ml/kg for the next 10 kg, and 20 ml/kg for each kg above. Using body weight, fluid requirements can be overestimated in an obese patient and underestimated in the thin patient, whereas calculations based on body surface area are less influenced by unusual body weights. Normally 60-100 mEq of sodium and 40-60 mEq of potassium are required per day. Generally calcium, magnesium and phosphorus are not supplemented when hypocaloric intravenous fluids are administered as release of intracellular fluid in the catabolic state is adequate to meet daily requirements.

It is important to remember that daily supplementation of B vitamins is essential in patients maintained on intravenous fluids. There are minimal body reserves and deficiencies can develop rapidly, especially during stress. Deficiency of vitamin B$_1$ (thiamine) can result in beriberi, Wernicke's encephalopathy, and congestive heart failure. Vitamin B$_2$ (riboflavin) deficiency can result in cheilosis which is a dry cracking about the lips, as well a magenta tongue. Deficiency of vitamin B$_3$ (pantothenic acid) probably causes malaise, headache, nausea and vomiting, and easy fatigability, although the syndrome remains to be well documented. Deficiency of vitamin B$_5$ (niacin) results in a well-defined syndrome of pellegra, with dermatitis, glossitis and diarrhea. Headaches and loss of memory have been reported. Deficiency of vitamin B$_6$ (pyridoxine) can result in irritability, depression and stomatitis with acneiform rash on the forehead and seborrhea of the nasolabial folds. Vitamin B_7 (biotin) deficiency has recently been shown to result in a fine, scaly desquamation of the skin. Deficiency of vitamin B_9 (folic acid) can result in diarrhea and a megaloblastic anemia with glossitis. Deficiency of vitamin B_{12} (cyanocobalamine) can result in a megaloblastic anemia with glossitis and peripheral paresthesias and dorsolateral column involvement. Deficiency of vitamin C (ascorbic acid) can result in scurvy with joint pain, petechial hemorrhages, and ecchymosis with swollen gums.

Deficiencies of the fat-soluble vitamins A, D, E, and K are less common due to larger body stores but can occur after prolonged poor dietary intake or during intravenous nutritional support. Deficiency of vitamin A can result in night blindness with xeropthalmia, Bitot's spots, phrynoderma, and keratomalacia. Vitamin D deficiency can result in osteomalacia and tetany. Vitamin E deficiency can give anemia with increased platelet aggregability and membrane instability. Deficiency of vitamin K can result in an abnormal prothrombin time and bleeding tendencies.

Finally, patients who are markedly malnourished or those who have been supported for a prolonged period of time on fat-free intravenous infusions have a high probability of developing essential fatty acid deficiency. Clinical symptoms of essential fatty acid deficiency include mild diarrhea, coarsening of the hair with hair loss, impaired wound healing, increased susceptibility to infection, and a characteristic desquamating skin rash usually about the nose, mouth, and eyes, but spreading diffusely over the body as the deficiency progresses. Biological changes include thrombocytopenia, altered platelet aggregation, increased capillary permeability, red blood cell fragility and subsequent anemia, and decreased prostaglandin synthesis. Fatty acid supplementation can be accomplished by administering 10 or 20% fat emulsion solutions intravenously or by administering safflower oil or corn oil by mouth, giving 15 ml/day.

Optimization of fluid, electrolyte, and vitamin balance and normalization of red cell mass can reduce morbidity and mortality associated with surgical intervention. This effort should take high priority when patients are evaluated and only after the clinical status is normalized should elective surgery be entertained. Even in emergent situations, attention should be directed toward normalization of these parameters, delaying surgery as long as safely possible.

E. Paraneoplastic Syndromes

Up to 75% of patients who have cancer present with or will develop at least one paraneoplastic syndrome during the course of their illness. The paraneoplastic syndromes include characteristic cutaneous, neurological, hematological, and renal manifestations, as well as a variety of endocrine disorders that are due to ectopic hormone production. In addition to their importance in signaling the initial diagnosis of malignancy, the paraneoplastic syndromes must be considered in preoperative planning, especially those syndromes that are associated with ectopic hormone production. Nearly all neoplasms, regardless of histological type, produce ectopic proteins. Some neoplasms also metabolize these proteins to biologically active substances which result in clinical syndromes. Examples of biologically active ectopic hormone production include corticotropin, parathormone, erythropoietin, growth hormone, chorionic gonadotropin, aldosterone, insulin and insulin-like factors, antidiuretic hormone, and calcitonin. Thus, clinical presentations include clinical features of Cushing's syndrome, hypercalcemia, hypoglycemia, and marked sodium retention. These syndromes must be appreciated and appropriate action must be taken to counteract the effects of the ectopic hormone production in order to avoid serious intraoperative complications. Of the nonendocrine paraneoplastic syndromes, thrombotic thrombocytopenic purpura, nonbacterial thrombotic endocarditis, disseminated intravascular coagulation, anemia, and leukemoid reactions also may play a significant role in morbidity and mortality encountered in the operating room. Nephrotic syndrome and renal disease secondary to hyperuricemia, hypercalcemia, amyloid, or paraproteins also adversely affect clinical outcome and require preoperative assessment and treatment.

F. Malnutrition

Marked malnutrition and wasting is a frequent and important systemic effect of cancer. Although it tends to be a late manifestation, it is not unusual for significant weight loss to be the presenting symptom of malignancy. The Eastern Cooperative Oncology Group (ECOG) examined the frequency of weight loss at the time of entry into chemotherapy protocols in 3047 cancer patients having 12 different kinds of tumors. The incidence of weight loss ranged from 31% in favorable histology non-Hodgkin's lymphomas to 87% in patients with measurable gastric carcinomas (DeWys et al., 1980).

The etiology of cancer cachexia is multifactorial. One factor is altered ingestion of food substrates due to either obstruction of the gastrointestinal tract or anorexia. In turn, the anorexia may be due to secretory products of the tumor, mental depression, or toxic effects of therapy such as mucositis with radiation of the head and neck or nausea and vomiting associated with chemotherapy. Another factor is alteration in food assimilation. Rapid transit, diarrhea, and malabsorption are common due either to the presence of the tumor in the gastrointestinal tract or to therapeutic measures. Radiation therapy to the head and neck area may produce loss of salivation and difficulty swallowing while irradiation to the abdomen may result in endarteritis, fibrosis or ulceration of the bowel with loss of motility and absorptive function. Intestinal fistula may result in shunting of food substrates either to the skin or bypassing segments of bowel producing a short bowel syndrome. Finally, there may be alteration in utilization of absorbed substrates. Several authors have demonstrated a significant increase in the basal metabolic rate of patients harboring malignant diseases compared to age- and sex-matched non-cancer patients (Bozzetti, Pagnoni, and DelVecchio, 1980; Waterhouse, 1974). This heightened energy expenditure can result in rapid deterioration when energy intake is minimal. In addition to increased basal metabolic rate, there are alterations in substrate utilization (Buzby and Steinberg, 1981). Carbohydrate tolerance is abnormal with a higher incidence of a diabetic-type state in patients with malignant disease. There is increased resistance to the effects of insulin in both hepatic tissue and peripheral muscle and there is increased gluconeogenesis from alanine and lactate with increased activity of the Cori cycle. Protein metabolism is altered by increased protein turnover and decreased protein synthesis. There may also be some nitrogen trapping by the tumor. Fatty acid oxidation is impaired similar to that observed in severe stress with infrequent development of starvation ketosis in spite of inadequate caloric intake.

Consequences of malnutrition were reported by Warren (1932) in 400 autopsy reports on cancer patients. He found that cachexia accounted for at least 22% of cancer deaths and felt that the estimate was conservative as cachexia was implicated as an ancillary contributor to death in many other patients. Progressive protein calorie malnutrition in the non-cancer patient has been shown to produce progressive dysfunction of skeletal and respiratory muscle, altered gastrointestinal tract motility and absorption, impaired renal function with decreased glomerular filtration rate, decreased myocardial contractility with reduced tolerance to myocardial stress, altered immuno-competence with impaired cellular and humoral immunity, impaired liver function with decreased drug metabolism and protein synthesis, and impaired wound healing with delayed mature collagen deposition, decreased wound tensile strength, and increased incidence of wound infections (Grant, 1983). Although not as well documented, similar dysfunction most certainly occurs in the malnourished cancer patient. DeWys et al. (1980) noted median survival was significantly shorter in patients with malignancies who had lost weight compared to those who had not. Copeland et al. (1975) have noted a correlation between weight gain and tumor regression among chemotherapy patients, with those failing to gain weight during nutritional support generally being those with intractable disease. Nixon et al. (1980) have related anthropometric and biochemical abnormalities to survival in a study of hospitalized cancer patients, with a majority of patients who died within the first 70 days of cancer treatment having creatinine-height ratios and triceps skinfold thickness values less than 60% of standard and serum albumin concentrations of 3.5 g/dl or less. Harvey et al. (1981) have developed a prognostic indicator formula which relates complications in cancer patients to serum albumin concentrations and the presence or absence of cancer.

Although there are several studies that document impaired survival in cancer patients who are severely malnourished, and indeed chemotherapy or radiation therapy and even surgical therapy must often be interrupted or altered due to severe malnutrition, there are little data suggesting improved patient survival associated with institution of nutritional support (Brennan, 1981). Studies have documented improved tolerance to chemotherapy and radiation therapy, improved tolerance to surgical intervention, improved sense of well-being of the patient, significant weight gain and improvement of blood protein concentrations, and even in some cases improved tumor response when aggressive nutritional support is part of the care plan. *Although results of a well-controlled, randomized, prospective clinical study remain to be obtained, it makes little sense to initiate aggressive chemotherapy, radiation therapy, surgical therapy, or combination therapy while permitting the patient to starve to death.* Patients admitted with a diagnosis of cancer who require surgical intervention should therefore undergo a screening nutritional assessment to determine the presence and significance of malnutrition. *Those who suffer from moderate or severe malnutrition and who have an otherwise reasonable chance for successful therapeutic intervention should be given aggressive nutritional support, whether via the enteral or parenteral route.* The support should begin at least 7-10 days prior to surgical intervention, allowing for replenishment of fluids, electrolytes, minerals, trace elements, and vitamins and then continued following the operative procedure until restoration of adequate oral intake. A cooperative study is ongoing at the time of this publication in the Veterans Administration system whereby 7-10 days of preoperative intravenous nutritional support are being evaluated for reduction of morbidity and mortality with major abdominal or thoracic surgery.* Approximately one-half of these patients will be undergoing operative procedures for malignant processes. Half will be randomized to preoperative feeding and the other half will undergo early surgical intervention. Hopefully results of this study and others to come will determine the clinical effectiveness of preoperative nutritional intervention in improving patient survival.

When nutritional support is necessary, the gastrointestinal tract should be preferentially used when feasible and safe. Some patients will respond to simple dietary manipulations. In most, however, anorexia is severe enough that voluntary intake will be inadequate regardless of dietary selection. These patients are best treated by placement of a nasogastric or nasojejunal tube for direct instillation of nutrients into the gastrointestinal tract. These nutrients may be administered either by continuous drip or by intermittent infusion. Selected patients appear to do better with nighttime infusions, allowing voluntary oral intake during the daytime. If the gastrointestinal tract is unavailable or if attempts at enteral feeding result in severe intolerance with cramping, bloating, and diarrhea, nutrients can be given intravenously in the form of total

*Principal Investigator Dr. Gordon Buzby, Philadelphia VA Hospital, Cooperative Study #221.

parenteral nutrition. Typical intravenous nutrition regimens for cancer patients include a mixture of 20-30% dextrose and 3.5-5.0% amino acids supplemented with vitamins, minerals, and electrolytes. Essential fatty acids are provided as 0.5-1.0 L of a 10 or 20% fat emulsion each week. Usual caloric and protein requirements during enteral and parenteral nutrition range between 35 and 45 kcal/kg/d and 1.5-2.0 g protein/kg/d. If possible, the cancer patient should undergo indirect calorimetry to better define his actual caloric needs as the effects of the tumor on metabolic rate are hard to estimate. The exact combination of fat and carbohydrate for nonprotein caloric support, which is optimal for the cancer patient, remains to be determined.

A wide variety of complications have been reported during enteral nutritional support but most are avoidable with close supervision. Appropriate monitoring of serum chemistries is essential during initiation of nutritional support and routinely during continued support. In particular, potassium, phosphorus, and magnesium must be monitored as these electrolytes are concentrated in the intracellular fluid space. With onset of anabolism, a significant increase in requirements may be seen due to decreased mobilization from cells and synthesis of new lean body mass. Glucose tolerance must be monitored by routine blood checks as well as glucose measurements of the urine. Insulin is not infrequently needed to maintain normal glucose concentrations. To avoid antibody formation to exogenous insulin, only recombinant human insulin should be given. Use of more than 100 units insulin per day is seldom indicated. If glucose intolerance cannot be controlled, the amount of carbohydrate infused should be reduced. Severe glucosuria with marked diuresis can rapidly lead to a syndrome of hyperglycemic, hyperosmotic, nonketotic, acidosis which, if not promptly treated by interruption of carbohydrate infusion, rehydration, and correction of acidosis, can lead to coma and death. Aspiration is not an infrequent complication of tube feeding. Patients should be monitored to assure complete gastric emptying and the head of the bed should be elevated 45° during feeding if possible. If gastric residuals are observed, the feeding tube should be advanced into the distal duodenum or proximal jejunum under either fluoro- or endoscopic guidance or by spontaneous passage thereby reducing the risks of regurgitation. Finally, patients can suffer diarrhea and malabsorption if the tube feeding is administered too rapidly, if it has too high osmolality, if bacterial overgrowth of the feeding solution occurs, if lactose or fat intolerance is present, or if hypertonic drugs are administered via the catheter as a bolus.

Similarly, many complications of intravenous nutritional support have been reported. Those associated with placement of a subclavian catheter include pneumothorax, hemomediastinum, brachial plexus injury, arterial injury, and injury to the thoracic duct. The incidence of these complications is minimal (usually less than 1.0%) if the individual placing the catheter is experienced with the technique. Long-term catheter maintenance has been associated with thrombosis of the subclavian vein and/or superior vena cava in 10-15% of patients. It is felt that thrombosis has been reduced by use of silastic or polyurethane catheters instead of polyvinylchloride catheters, but the evidence is not conclusive. Low-dose Coumadin therapy has proved efficacious as prophylaxis. One thousand units of heparin added to each liter of feeding solution has reduced catheter clogging and has perhaps also reduced the incidence of subclavian vein and superior vena cava thrombosis. When thrombosis is detected clinically by either swelling of the arm or neck and face, or both, the catheter should be removed and the patient should be heparinized. Although not proven helpful, most continue anticoagulation for 2-6 months with Coumadin. If continued intravenous support is required, a new catheter can be placed in the opposite subclavian vein or, in exceptional cases, in the groin. If a subsequent venogram shows resolution of the thrombosis, the subclavian vein can again be utilized. Usually, however, the vein remains obliterated or severely narrowed with development of collateral vessels and is no longer useful for venous access. Patients with cancer may be at a higher risk due to a hypercoagulable state induced by the tumor or perhaps due to AT-3 deficiency or vitamin E deficiency.

The risk of catheter sepsis is ever present and requires strict maintenance of the catheter exit site and adherence to aseptic techniques of catheter care. Studies have shown a marked reduction of catheter-related complications when catheters are placed and maintained by a designated team of professionals (Nehme, 1980). With the team approach, catheter-related complications are usually less than 5%, compared to complication rates as high as 15-25% without a team. It therefore behooves the surgeon who employs intravenous nutritional support to have a nutritional support team guided by a well-designed protocol for catheter placement and maintenance as well as solution administration.

As for enteral support, patients receiving total parenteral nutrition also can develop fluid, electrolyte, trace element, and essential fatty acid abnormalities; therefore, blood chemistries must be monitored carefully, especially during the first week after initiation of support. Hyperglycemia and glucosuria are more common with intravenous feeding than enteral feedings and administration of insulin is often necessary. The same precautions in the use of insulin as with enteral feeding must be observed.

G. Drug Therapy

Patients with malignant diseases often present with other chronic illnesses for which they receive prescription drugs. These drugs should be carefully reviewed to determine their appropriateness and, if indicated, should be continued in the preoperative and postoperative period. Diuretics and digitalis for cardiac function, thyroid supplementation, oral hypoglycemics and insulin for control of diabetes, antihypertensives, antihistamines, bronchodilators, and expectorants for pulmonary function are examples of these drugs. Consultation with the anesthesiologist should be obtained to assist in the management of drugs which may interfere or interact with anesthetics during surgery.

Some patients receive steroids as part of their therapy while others may have metastatic disease to the adrenals. The possibility of adrenal insufficiency must therefore be considered in all cancer patients. If insufficiency is suspected or documented, preoperative steroid supplementation should be given to avoid an acute adrenal crisis. An initial dosage of 100 mg of cortisone acetate given intramuscularly at bedtime and repeated on call to the operating room, supplemented as necessary during surgery with Solu-Medrol, followed by divided doses of 75-100 mg Solu-Medrol a day intravenously with gradual tapering over the next 3-7 days to maintenance support is one recommended regimen. It must also be recognized that steroid therapy can significantly alter a patient's response to catastrophic events such as a perforated viscus or major sepsis. Clinical findings during such times may be minimal. Awareness that steorids are being administered may help avoid a mistaken diagnosis. When pharmacological doses of steroids are given during operative procedures, in addition to masking clinical findings of acute crises, alterations in glucose metabolism are common with resultant hyperglycemia and glucosuria. Due to the catabolic effects of steroids, wound healing is impaired as well, which may lead to subsequent dehiscence or wound infections. Special attention should be given to tissue handling during the operative procedure to minimize trauma, dead space, hematoma formation, and contamination. Spontaneous intestinal performation and gastrointestinal bleeding due to ulceration during steroid administration also can occur.

Patients receiving chemotherapeutic agents just prior to surgery present particular risks and therefore timing of surgical intervention must be carefully considered. Wound healing will be impaired and infection resistance diminished. Some drugs have specific toxic side effects on myocardial, pulmonary, and renal function and may therefore impair the patients ability to tolerate surgical procedures as well as the postoperative period of stress. Patients who have received prior bleomycin therapy represent a greatly increased risk for surgery and anesthesia (Goldinger and Schweiger, 1979). To improve the risk it appears useful to reduce the administered oxygen concentration during and immediately after surgery and to pay close attention to replace fluid with colloid solutions to prevent pulmonary edema.

III. OTHER PREOPERATIVE CONCERNS

A. Preoperative Irradiation

Preoperative irradiation of the operative area impairs wound healing and may
lead to wound separation, fascial dehiscence or fasciitis, breakdown of intestinal anastomoses, fistula formation, or subsequent stricture formation of
the gastrointestinal tract. If the operative procedure is done within 4-6 weeks
following radiation therapy severe radiation fibrosis is seldom encountered.
If an anastomosis is done in edematous or inflamed irradiated bowel, it may
be wise to initiate postoperative intravenous feeding and delay oral intake
for 10-14 days to allow complete healing. However, if the radiation therapy
has been given years prior to the planned surgical intervention, significant
radiation enteritis and intestinal adhesions might be anticipated which can
increase morbidity and mortality. There is no proven method to decrease the
incidence of radiation injury to the surgical field or other tissues.

B. Antibiotic Preparation

Appropriate antibiotic preparation prior to surgical procedures is extremely
important. The use of prophylactic antibiotics, both in sterilization of the
gastrointestinal tract and as a systemic drug just prior to surgical intervention,
has been shown to be beneficial in patients undergoing various operative
procedures where there is an appreciable risk of infection (Polk and Lopez-
Mayor, 1969). For example, routine use of antibiotics in surgery of the
stomach for peptic ulcer disease is of little value, whereas antibiotics are of
great value in surgery for gastric cancer due to bacterial overgrowth in the
stomach when achlorhydria is present as part of the malignant process. In
all cancer procedures, consideration should be given to the possibility of
anaerobic as well as aerobic infections. In particular, whenever pelvic surgery
is done or the bowel is traversed, antibiotics effective against both aerobic
and anaerobic organisms should be given. When given prophylactically, antibiotics should be administered when the patient is called to the operating
room. This will assure establishment of adequate tissue levels. There is no
need to give antibiotics any earlier and they are of doubtful usefulness as
prophylaxis when first given during the operation. Maximal clinical benefit
of prophylactic antibiotics is obtained with fewer side effects when only
two or three doses are given postoperatively. (Prophylactic use of antibiotics in the leukemic patient is discussed in Chapter 5.) Extended use of
antibiotics as therapeutic treatment of known infections is dictated by each
clinical setting. If an appropriate bowel preparation is impossible in patients
with colonic malignancy due to tight obstruction, it is preferable to stage
the operative procedure with a diverting colostomy and simultaneous or

delayed resection of the tumor to allow restoration of an oral diet and recovery of nutritional status. Following subsequent bowel preparation, the
patient can be taken back to the operating room for reanastomosis of the
diverted colon.

C. Skin Preparation

Attention should also be directed toward effective skin preparation to minimize
skin-born contamination of the operative field. The patient should be instructed to thoroughly scrub the skin in the operative field the night before
surgery using a bactericidal soap, both to defat the skin and to reduce skin
bacteria. The patient should be isolated from other patients with infections
and all personnel should take special precautions not to transmit infection
from one patient to another.

D. Biliary Obstruction

Biliary obstruction is associated with impaired absorption of fat and fat-soluble
products. This may well lead to vitamin K deficiency. From 5 to 10 mg
vitamin K should be given orally or intramuscularly in these patients two days
prior to surgical intervention, regardless of the prothrombin time. This will
assure adequate vitamin K supplementation, which may need to be continued
postoperatively.

IV. RECOGNITION AND MINIMIZATION OF OPERATIVE RISKS

Avoidance of surgical complications requires careful attention to detail in the
operating room. As for other patients, the intensity of intraoperative monitoring needed must be determined during the initial pre-anesthesia evaluation.
Patients at high risk should be carefully monitored with arterial catheters,
urinary drainage tubes, and Swann-Ganz catheters. Selected patients may occasionally benefit from an overnight admission to the intensive care unit for
stabilization and monitoring. Ample blood should be available in anticipation
of potential complications and one should be aware of the necessity for repeat-
ing antibiotic doses in cases lasting more than 6-8 hours. Many patients with
cancer suffer a degree of immunoincompetence because of steroid administration, malnutrition, and radiation therapy or chemotherapy. A decreased white
blood count and lymphocyte dysfunction may render the cancer patient
further susceptible to operative infections. Special attention should therefore
be given to skin preparation to assure as thorough skin cleaning as possible.
A full 5-minute cleansing with a defatting soap followed by application of antimicrobial solution is recommended. The use of povidone iodide-impregnated

plastic drapes may be of value in selected patients. It is important to perform a wide skin preparation in anticipation of potential complications or need to extend the wound beyond the initial incision. An upper abdomen or lower chest procedure should be prepared and draped in anticipation of possible need to enter the adjacent cavity. Extremity and head and neck incisions should anticipate extension if unsuspected extension of disease is identified. For the same reason, when an incision is placed it should be so oriented as to allow extension if further exposure is required during the operative procedure. Ongoing studies by Moylan (1982) have found use of disposable gowns and drapes to significantly reduce clean wound infections due to decreased porosity and reduced penetration of bacteria through the gown.

When incisions are placed for *biopsy*, careful thought should be given to their location and orientation, taking into consideration the incision required for the definitive operative procedure if the biopsy proves to be malignant. An inappropriately placed biopsy incision can render cosmetic results unsatisfactory and at times compromise the surgical margins of subsequent procedures. When biopsies are taken as a preliminary procedure to a resection, care should be taken not to spill viable tumor cells within the operative field during the biopsy procedure. The area should be packed off and the capsule should be closed when possible following the biopsy with sutures or clips and the area irrigated with distilled water prior to reexposure of the operative field.

Once the extent of disease has been documented by the exploration, a decision must be made as to whether to proceed with an extirpative or palliative procedure. This requires sound clinical judgment and familiarity with the natural history of the disease and the risks of the operative procedure. For example, the effect of metastatic liver disease on estimated median survival, if identified during an operative procedure such as for an intestinal neoplasm, has been characteized by Jaffe et al. (1968). Heroic measures taken to remove the primary disease may not be justifiable in view of the prolonged recovery period and severely shortened expected life survival. Another example is patients explored for small bowel obstruction who are found to have extensive carcinomatosis. In this case, a palliative procedure such as anastomosis of the proximal small bowel to the transverse colon or even a drainage gastrostomy may be optimal therapy rather than an attempt to dissect adhesions or resect an extensive segment of bowel.

When a decision is made to extirpate a tumor, the procedure should be performed with minimal manipulation and with early ligation of venous and lymphatic channels. Once the tumor has been excised, irrigation of the operative field should again be performed in a very thorough fashion to remove viable tumor cells. At this point, consideration should be given to marking any residual tumor or the tumor bed with metallic clips to allow radiographic localization, especially if radiotherapy is to be administered later. On the other hand, the placement of metallic clips within the abdomen renders performance of subsequent computerized tomography more difficult due to artifact formation and should be avoided if close monitoring by computerized tomography is needed.

A final consideration to be given during the operative management of patients with malignant processes is the establishment of an appropriate feeding access if a prolonged period of poor oral intake is expected. If anorexia has been present preoperatively but there is no contraindication to use of the gastrointestinal tract in the postoperative period, a feeding gastrostomy or jejunostomy should be included as part of the routine operative procedure if the abdomen is exposed. If the gastrointestinal tract will not be available for an extended period of time following surgery or if aggressive chemotherapy or radiation therapy will be initiated postoperatively resulting in anorexia and nausea, consideration should be given toward establishment of long-term vascular access via a silastic catheter inserted into the superior vena cava. Establishment of either vascular or enteral access will make postoperative care simpler for the physician, providing an easy access for fluid and electrolytes, antibiotic and chemotherapy administration, and, for the patient as well, reduce the necessity of multiple needle punctures.

V. PREVENTION OF POSTOPERATIVE COMPLICATIONS

Following surgery, fluid and electrolyte supplementation must be carefully monitored and adjusted to avoid volume overload and subsequent congestive heart failure, pulmonary failure, or intravascular dehydration, resulting in renal failure or impaired cardiac output. A technique for estimation of third-space fluid losses into the operative area suggested by Filston and Izant (1978) that works well for pediatric and adult patients is the provision of 25% more fluid above maintenance for each quarter of the abdomen entered during an intraabdominal operative procedure. After the first 24 hours, the volume status should be reassessed and the rate of infusion altered to assure 1200-1500 cc of urinary output a day. Careful measurement of extra fluid losses, such as from nasogastric or drainage tubes, should be made and replaced to avoid fluid and electrolyte derangements. Blood replacement in the operating room and in the immediate postoperative period must be carefully reviewed to assure its adequacy to maintain the hemoglobin concentration above 10 or the hematocrit above 30%. The use of packed red blood cells or whole blood will depend upon components required.

If nutritional support was provided preoperatively because of significant malnutrition, it should be restarted 24-36 hours following surgery and continued until an adequate oral diet or tube feeding is established. If the patient had borderline preoperative malnutrition, consideration should be given to institution of postoperative nutritional support if an oral diet is not recovered within five days following surgery. If the patient was otherwise healthy preoperatively, he can be followed for up to 7-10 days without nutritional support. However, if an extended period of time before adequate oral intake is expected or if complications occur, nutritional intervention should be undertaken.

Early ambulation is an important parameter in reduction of postoperative morbidity and mortality. Ambulation reduces stasis in the lower extremities decreasing the incidence of venous thrombosis and pulmonary embolization. Early ambulation allows for better diaphragmatic movement with fuller expansion of the lungs and reduction in atelectasis and pneumonia. Ambulation also improves the patient's general attitude, encouraging him that recovery is expected, helping him to be optimistic. As soon as feasible, drainage tubes should be removed—especially those which restrict the patient's ability to ambulate. Nasogastric tubes left in an inappropriate length of time contribute to morbidity with an increasing incidence of nasopharyngeal irritation, gastroesophageal erosions with bleeding, and aspiration of saliva or regurgitation of gastric juice with aspiration. Indwelling Foley catheters significantly increase risks for subsequent urinary tract infections and intravenous lines increase risks for thrombophlebitis. Pain medication should be appropriate to allow patient mobility, but not so generous as to result in respiratory or mental depression, decreasing mobility. Antibiotics administered preoperatively prophylactically should be continued no longer than 48-72 hours postoperatively to avoid development of antibiotic resistant infections. When antibiotic therapy is delivered as a therapeutic venture, it should be continued for 7-10 days to assure eradication of bacteria from even poorly perfused tissues.

VI. CONCLUSIONS

With careful attention to preoperative assessment and preparation of patients, and attention to special techniques in the operating room and to postoperative care, the potentially increased surgical risk of the cancer patient can be converted to an acceptably low incidence of actual morbidity and mortality.

REFERENCES

Ahned, P. (ed.) (1981). *Living and Dying with Cancer,* Elsevier, New York.
Bland, J. H. (1963). *Clinical Metabolism of Body Water and Electrolytes,*
    W. B. Saunders, Philadelphia.
Bozzetti, F., Pagnoni, A. M., and Del Vecchio, M. (1980). Excessive caloric
    expenditure as a cause of malnutrition in patients with cancer. *Surg.*
    Gynecol. Obstet., 150:229.

Brennan, M. F. (1981). Total parenteral nutrition in the cancer patient, *New Engl. J. Med., 305*:375.

Buzby, G. P., and Steinberg, J. J. (1981). Nutrition in cancer patients, *Surg. Clin. North Am., 61*:691.

Copeland, E. M., III, MacFadyen, B. V., Lanzotti, V. J., and Dudrick, S. J. (1975). Intravenous hyperalimentation as an adjunct to cancer chemotherapy, *Am. J. Surg., 129*:167.

DeWys, W. D., Begg, C., Lavin, P. T., Band, P. R., Bennett, J. M., Bertino, J. R., Cohen, M. H., Douglas, H. O., Jr., Engstrom, P. F., Ezdinli, E. Z., Horton, J., Johnson, G. J., Moertel, C. G., Oken, M. M., Perlia, C., Rosenbaum, C., Silverstein, M. N., Skeel, R. T., Sponzo, R. W., and Tormey, D. C. (1980). Prognostic effect of weight loss prior to chemotherapy in cancer patients, *Am. J. Med., 69*:491.

Filston, H. C., and Izant, R., Jr. (1978). *The Surgical Neonate,* Appleton-Century-Crofts, New York, p. 8.

Goldinger, P. L., and Schweizer, O. (1979). The hazards of anesthesia and surgery in bleomycin-treated patients, *Semin. Oncol., 6*:121-124.

Grant, J. P. (1980). *Handbook of TPN,* W. P. Saunders, Philadelphia, pp. 125-154.

Grant, J. (1983). Clinical impact of protein malnutrition on organ mass and function, in *Amino Acids. Metabolism and Medical Applications* (G. L. Blackburn, J. P. Grant, and V. R. Young, eds.), John Wright PSG, Boston, pp. 347-358.

Harvey, K. B., Moldawer, L. L., Bistrian, B. R., and Blackburn, G. L. (1981). Biological measures for the formulation of a hospital prognostic index, *Am. J. Clin. Nutr., 34*:2013.

Jaffe, B. M., Donegan, W. L., Watson, F., and Spratt, J. S., Jr. (1968). Factors influencing survival in patients with untreated hepatic metastases, *Surg. Gynecol. Obstet., 127*:1.

Kardinal, C. G., and Porter, G. H. (1981). The psychologic care of the cancer patient, *Compr. Ther., 7*:65.

Moylan, J. A. (1982). Clinical evaluation of gown-and-drape barrier performance, *Bull. Am. Coll. Surg., May.*

Nehme, A. E. (1980). Nutritional support of the hospitalized patient: The team concept, *JAMA, 243*:1906.

Nixon, D. W., Heymsfield, S. B., Cohen, A. E., Kutner, M. H., Ansley, J., Lawson, D. H., and Rudman, D. (1980). Protein-calorie undernutrition in hospitalized cancer patients, *Am. J. Med., 68*:683.

Polk, H. C., Jr., and Lopez-Mayor, J. F. (1969). Postoperative wound infection: A prospective study of determinant factors and prevention, *Surgery, 66*:97.

Warren, S. (1932). The immediate cause of death in cancer, *Am. J. Med. Sci., 184*:610.

Waterhouse, C. (1974). How tumors affect host metabolism, *Ann. NY Acad. Sci., 230*:86.

5

Chemotherapy

John Laszlo* and Diane Stevenson
Duke University Medical Center, Durham, North Carolina

Virgil S. Lucas
Burroughs Wellcome Company, Research Triangle Park, North Carolina

I. OVERVIEW

It has been about a quarter century since the goal of curing the first patients of a disseminated malignancy was realized when single agent chemotherapy was used for women with choriocarcinoma. Since that time, a massive international cancer research effort has resulted in the development of more aggressive and innovative programs for all types of patients. Now the possibility of cure exists for patients who have disseminated testicular cancer, diffuse histiocytic lymphoma, Hodgkin's disease, acute lymphocytic leukemia, and a number of childhood cancers. Furthermore, the use of combination chemotherapy as an adjuvant to surgical removal of primary tumors is beneficial in diseases such as breast cancer and seemingly also in osteosarcoma. Unfortunately, even aggressive use of multiagent chemotherapy or additive radiation therapy has not yet cured the more common disseminated malignancies such as those originating from breast, gastrointestinal tract, or lung, although remissions may be achieved with variable degrees of frequency and length.

Successful treatment depends upon not only the antitumor effectiveness of drugs, but also the ability of physicians to develop strategies for preventing or managing the potential consequences of marrow suppression and life-threatening thrombocytopenia and granulocytopenia, as well as to prevent serious toxicity to vital organs (liver, kidneys, heart). Major advances in platelet transfusion, in the recognition and treatment of opportunistic infections, and in strategies for preventing unique organ toxicities from drugs such as

---

*Current Affiliation: American Cancer Society, New York, New York

cisplatin, bleomycin, and doxorubicin have made it possible to make major advances in the treatment of cancer. We are just beginning to consider means of preventing the late complications of curative chemotherapy, such as developmental abnormalities in treated children and in chemotherapy-induced second malignancies.

Complications that may be produced by different chemotherapeutic drugs range from minor to life threatening and, although some are far more common than others, no organ system is exempt. Toxic effects may be considered to be local or mechanical, as with drug infiltration or fluid overload, specific and/or unique as on peripheral nerves, kidney or heart, or more systemic because of excessive toxicity to rapidly dividing normal cells, such as marrow or G.I. epithelium. Depending upon the changes produced, the patient may even be unaware of the complication; more often, however, it will effect the quality of life for some period of time. Some of these complications are predictable and preventable, some are predictable and not preventable if aggressive treatment is being pursued, and in some instances these complications are so sporadic as to be unpredictable.

Apprehension, or even unfounded fear of potential complications, can at times be so debilitating as to cause the patient to decline or postpone chemotherapy. When such probems exist they are frustrating also to family and physician; fortunately, they too can often be prevented by appropriate care (see Chapter 2).

It is vitally important for the physician to make clear to the patient why this particular course of treatment is being chosen. While the possible reasons or options are many, and beyond the scope of this book, there does need to be a reasonableness of fit with the patients' hopes and expectations. Is it reasonable for a practitioner to use very aggressive and toxic programs of combination chemotherapy for metastatic colon or non-small cell lung cancer which have never been shown to prolong survival? We would argue strongly that this type of treatment would be inappropriate whereas other approaches are most consistent with the interests of the patient, and certainly will prevent unnecessary complications which encroach seriously on good quality time at home. This is not to say that experimental programs (not just minor variations on a theme) would be incompatible with the patients' interests; indeed the reverse may often be the case.

On the other hand, is it reasonable to recommend aggressive yet potentially toxic programs to patients who have a good chance of benefiting from them? We would all agree that it is, but the rationale has to be explained clearly so that it can be understood and remembered in those lonely times when the complications, and not the benefits, are confronting the patient. These are not new ideas but they bear repetition because they take far more time, effort, and thought than "plugging" a patient into a protocol of treatment which others have recommended. There are a lot of weak as well as good protocols that employ toxic doses of chemotherapy, and the thoughtful decision of how and when to use them may constitute the major contribution by the physician. Sometimes a second opinion is helpful at this point. Once the decision has been made by physician and patient to use a potentially toxic program, then the considerations described in the remainder of this chapter may be applicable to the circumstances.

With the advent of disease-related groups (DRG) there is great financial pressure to do as much of the treatment as possible outside of the hospital. Thus, patients will be treated in the clinic with toxic programs, some of which have very delayed side effects. This provides new challenges in anticipating and managing these potential problems, as reviewed in Chapter 3.

When considering the large subject of prevention of side effects of chemotherapeutic agents to the patient we must also protect the personnel during preparation, handling, and disposal of cytotoxic chemicals against possible hazards of these agents. Every health care worker who is exposed should remain informed about potential dangers and have guidelines for their use: this subject is discussed at the end of this chapter on chemotherapy.

II. NAUSEA, VOMITING, AND NUTRITIONAL DEPLETION: MAJOR COMPLICATIONS OF CANCER CHEMOTHERAPY

Nausea and vomiting have been associated with chemotherapy since the early use of alkylating agents such as intravenous nitrogen mustard. Nonetheless, there has been very little clinical antiemetic research until after the middle of the 1970s, perhaps because nausea and vomiting were not considered serious or life-threatening complications of chemotherapy, perhaps because the emetogenic chemotherapy programs were not as numerous or as potent, and perhaps because this field simply had less research appeal than did development of anticancer therapy. As an illustration of this point, Penta et al. (1981) found only 57 antiemetic studies in cancer patients reported between 1960 and 1981, and 47 of these were from between 1978 and 1981, indicating the recent interest in this subject (there have been innumerable reports since). There have been two books which review the mechanisms and treatments of this problem (Poster, Penta, and Bruno, 1981; Laszlo, 1983a) and a number of reviews (i.e., Stoudemire, Cotanch, and Laszlo, 1984).

There are three major consequences of inadequate antiemetic therapy, plus a myriad of miscellaneous ones. The most obvious concern is the problem of compliance with treatments such as the administration of high-dose cisplatin which causes serious nausea and vomiting in almost 100% of the patients, or by the more widely used cyclophosphamide-methotrexate-5-fluorouracil (CMF) program where there is roughly a 75% incidence of nausea and/or vomiting.

It is difficult to estimate the number of patients who drop out of lengthy
therapy programs, those who decline to participate in such programs as CMF
adjuvant chemotherapy, and those in whom therapy programs are postponed
beyond the desirable schedule. We had earlier estimated that less than
optimal compliance due to severe nausea and vomiting may be as high as
25-50% and on some occasions the patient actually declines potentially curative therapy (Laszlo and Lucas, 1981; Laszlo, 1983b). In such cases it is
literally a matter of life and death to prevent a patient with curable lymphoma or testicular cancer from opting out of proper therapy.

The second major concern is for the comfort of our patients, recognizing
the hardships that it causes to their mental and physical well-being, which
adversely affect their jobs and personal lives. How often have we seen
women receiving monthly adjuvant chemotherapy for breast cancer who are
debilitated by nausea and vomiting for 3 or 4 days, unable to work for at
least that long, and who want and need to maintain their jobs? *The issue
here is not one of compliance—they want to comply—but rather of attention
to the quality of life.* The third major concern of inadequate therapy is to
prevent the establishment of anticipatory nausea and vomiting, a particularly
refractory problem to manage (Morrow, 1982; Morrow and Morrell, 1982;
Morrow et al., 1982).

What is the reproducibility of nausea and vomiting when drugs are given
repeatedly, either on a daily basis or intermittently? With respect to the
former, a constant dose of highly emetogenic drug such as cisplatin, DTIC,
or nitrogen mustard can be given daily for 3 days and, almost invariably,
the most severe nausea and vomiting occurs on the first day, it tends to be
less on the second day, and by the third day the patient may have relatively
little nausea and vomiting. If, on the other hand, there is an interval of 3
or 4 weeks before this same 3-day course is repeated, then the identical
sequence of events is likely to transpire. Thus there is a kind of refractori-
ness in the nausea and vomiting mechanism when drug doses are given at
short intervals, whereas the system recovers completely when there is a lapse
of time between treatments (Laszlo, 1983a).

Another aspect is that with each repeated course of intermittent treatment
the patient will experience a comparable degree of nausea and vomiting; it
may even become worse, especially if complicated by anticipatory nausea and
vomiting on each occasion. Nausea and vomiting never go away spontaneously
upon repeated treatment unless successfully treated. This makes it possible
for some antiemetic studies to use the patient as his/her own control, and
crossover study designs are particularly powerful in comparing treatment A
versus treatment B in the same individual (Moertel and Reitemeier, 1973;
Sallan, Zinberg, and Frei, 1975; Sallan et al., 1980; Gralla et al., 1981; Laszlo
and Lucas, 1981). What can we predict about the efficacy of antiemetic drugs

when they are to be used repeatedly? It would seem that an antiemetic program which is effective in the first month will also be effective in subsequent months, although the dosage may at times have to be adjusted upward to maintain the desired degree of control (Laszlo, Lucas, and Huang, 1981; Laszlo, 1983a). Thus there is possibly a slight degree of tachyphylaxis but this is not absolute, and it may depend upon the antiemetic being used.

Indeed there are major medical consequences of severe nausea and vomiting; uncommonly violent retching may even result in esophageal tears (Mallory-Weiss syndrome) or in pathological bone fractures. Less dramatic but far more common is the prolonged anorexia and malnutrition which in turn compounds the problem of cachexia, which is frequently seen in patients with cancer and which makes it exceedingly difficult for the patient to tolerate normal dosages of chemotherapy.

The major metabolic derangements that result from vomiting include metabolic alkalosis, chloride and potassium depletion, and extracellular fluid contraction; the pathophysiology of this syndrome was reviewed by Dennis (1983). The overall magnitude of the disturbances depend upon the severity and duration of vomiting and the ability to take in fluid during that time, as well as in the compensatory renal mechanisms. It is the fluid and electrolyte losses in vomitus which induce metabolic alkalosis and chloride deficiency, but changes in renal function are responsible for maintaining the alkalosis and for developing the potassium deficiency. Thus extracellular volume contraction is the sum of gastric and renal losses as well as impaired fluid intake. The treatment of fluid and electrolyte derangements that accompany vomiting is aimed primarily at restoring extracellular volume and chloride, and this is most readily accomplished by providing intravenous saline. Saline also prevents further potassium wasting by the kidneys and, depending upon the severity of the previous potassium deficit, may or may not be necessary to correct the hypokalemia by means of oral or intravenous administration of potassium chloride.

What can we say about the *nutritional consequences* of nausea and vomiting in a patient with cancer? The general topic is discussed in Chapter 4 with particular reference to the surgical patient; here we will focus on nutritional problems related primarily to chemotherapy. We might arbitrarily divide the subject into three subheadings, depending upon whether the effects are acute, chronic, or psychologically but not physiologically significant. In general, different types of patients tend to get into these three classes of complications and it is well to think about them in advance. Frequent nausea and vomiting followed by prolonged anorexia can result in rapid nutritional depletion and weight loss. Furthermore, the patient who has endured major surgery, radiotherapy, or extensive prior chemotherapy may already be very debilitated even before receiving the next course of chemotherapy. *Failure to*

Table 1 Nutritional Problems of Patients with Cancer

Host factors	Nonspecific effects, anorexia, immobility, muscle depletion, hypercalcemia, nutritional deficiency
Tumor factors	Nitrogen, iron traps, glucose consumption, lactic acidosis, hyperuricemia
Host-tumor factors	Para-endocrine syndromes, cancer cachexia, excessive gluconeogenesis
Treatment effects	Surgery, radiation chemotherapy—decreased caloric and fluid intake, nausea and vomiting, taste aversion
Psychological effects	Dissatisfaction, loss of control

recognize the severity of inanition can mean that the patient may become so severely debilitated as to become dangerously intolerant to the effects of normal doses of chemotherapeutic drugs, or that further vomiting would exacerbate dehydration and the renal complications of hypokalemic alkalosis.

We know also that the patient with cancer is prone to have preexisting nutritional problems predicated on having a chronic illness which results in immobility and anorexia, the effects of the tumor itself as a nitrogen trap, consumer of glucose and producer of lactic acid, and of the peculiar host-tumor interactions which we refer to as para-endocrine syndromes. Among the latter is the cachexia which is sometimes associated with cancer, even when the size of the tumor is small. Some of these problems are outlined in Table 1. When these factors are compounded by gastrointestinal surgery, radiation therapy, or chemotherapy, then the patient may decompensate with respect to caloric or fluid balance. Failure to anticipate these problems can give rise to life-threatening complicaitons. The more chronic types of problems are seen in patients who are severely ill from a large burden of tumor and in those who lack the mechanism to compensate for the periods of nausea and vomiting which they undergo around the time of each course of chemotherapy. This results in progressive nitrogen depletion and muscle wasting. Clearly there is some overlap between the acute and chronic toxicities in this regard. Avoidance of unpalatable foods or unpleasant odors may be sufficient therapy, as may a change to frequent small meals rich in carbohydrates and adequate fluid intake.

The final classification of nutritional problem is that of the inconvenience and discomfort from the nausea and vomiting which is (incorrectly) perceived by the patient as inability to eat the proper nutrients. However, when the weight is checked repeatedly over time there may be no weight loss, or even weight gain. The explanation for this appears to be that although the patients endure 1-3 or more days of nausea, with or without vomiting, they overcompensate by eating frequent small meals and thereby actually gain weight. There may also be some analogy to the common experience by pregnant women that their nausea is relieved by eating, and patients with cancer may also experience some of this phenomenon. In any case, this perception of anorexia and malnutrition by the patient may not seem to be a problem for the physician but reassurance is necessary, for there is at least some lack of satisfaction when the patient believes his/her nutrition to be impaired. Patients frequently do not understand that it may be possible to fully compensate for the nutritional complications of nausea and vomiting in the days prior to the next treatment, and they may become alarmed if they equate a loss of taste for food that may be produced by chemotherapy with the effects of advancing cancer.

There are a number of general medical and pharmacological considerations that the doctor must be familiar with in developing an approach to the patient who either has suffered from these problems or is about to receive highly emetogenic chemotherapy. For example, there are many causes of nausea and vomiting that could be contributing in an individual patient who is being treated with chemotherapeutic drugs for cancer. It usually is not difficult to exclude some of the more common causes such as intestinal obstruction, peritonitis, and increased intracranial pressure. However, it *is important not to assume that nausea and vomiting are necessarily ascribable to the chemotherapy,* and a particularly prolonged duration of vomiting following a course of chemotherapy should suggest the possibility of alternative medical or psychological causes.

We should pay some attention to the difficult complications of anticipatory nausea and vomiting, problems for which there are no pharmacologic treatments at the present time. It may occur in as many as 25% of the patients who experience severe episodes of nausea and vomiting upon repeated (three or more) courses of chemotherapy (Morrow, 1982; Morrow et al., 1982). This experience can be sufficient to condition the patient to vomit from some "innocent" stimulus such as the view of the hospital parking lot, the smell of the treatment room or alcohol sponge, or the sight of the chemotherapy nurse. This problem is very reminiscent of the conditioned responses described in dogs by Pavlov. On rare occasions, after talking with other patients or friends, a new patient may be so apprehensive about starting chemotherapy that he/she begins vomiting even before the initial course of chemotherapy. Anticipatory problems may respond to behavioral desensitization as described by Morrow and Morrell (1982), but it is certainly refractory to antiemetic agents available today. The phenomenon of anticipatory nausea and vomiting makes it much more difficult to treat patients who have well-established patterns of nausea and vomiting as opposed to managing them effectively initially. *We suggest that the lesson to be learned is in not holding back on potent antiemetic agents in order to prevent the problem where it is likely to occur.* Some of the associated factors which are known about anticipatory nausea and vomiting make us confident that there must be higher centers of control which impinge upon the vomiting center.

A related concern in developing a program for a patient is whether the problem can adequately be managed in the outpatient clinic or whether the entire treatment episode should be dealt with during a brief period of hospitalization. The economic pressure for outpatient chemotherapy is also a strong factor in the process. It would seem that factors such as distance from the hospital and the extent of the delay of the nausea and vomiting following chemotherapy are factors which, if they permit the patient to go home to a supportive environment, make it preferable for the problem to be dealt with in that setting. At the same time we must be aware that some patients (fortunately this is no longer common), may be so incapacitated by retching every 5-10 minutes that someone needs to stay with them to minister to their needs and provide reassurance, and if that is not available at home, then it would be preferable to hospitalize such patients. For patients treated in the clinic, it is important to consider that most antiemetic agents produce sedation when given in the types of dosage needed to manage nausea and vomiting; thus, patients should refrain from driving vehicles or otherwise working with hazardous machinery while under the influence of some of our drugs. Simple and inexpensive treatments at home include the use of cold compresses, removing vomitus basins or smells after their use, food preparation in a separate room to minimize food odors, and the freedom to experiment with food and drink that may have some sudden interest to the patient.

When considering the chemotherapeutic drugs that induce nausea and vomiting, we have a general sense of which are more potent than others and a rough categorization of these is listed in Table 2. Clearly, drugs such as cisplatin and cylcophosphamide have a high potential for inducing nausea, vomiting, and retching, whereas vincristine and many antimetabolites are far less likely to do so. It is necessary to add that dosage considerations are extremely important because the nausea and vomiting produced by low doses of cisplatin may be counteracted by numerous antiemetics, whereas that from high doses of cisplatin responds poorly to most, though not all, antiemetics. No single classification scheme of emetogenic agents can consider all these variables nor that some antiemetics are more effective against one agent, whereas another may be preferable against a different agent (Neidhart et al., 1981a). The reasons for the latter discrepancies are undoubtedly related to the variable mechanisms of action which emetogenic chemotherapeutic drugs can exert on the specialized receptor organs in the brain and gut.

Table 2   Emetogenic Potency of Chemotherapeutic Drugs[a]

Worst	Moderate	Least
Cisplatin	Nitrosoureas	Vincristine
DTIC	Procarbazine	Vinblastine
Nitrogen mustard	Mitomycin-C	Bleomycin
Adriamycin		6-Mercaptopurine
Cyclophosphamide		Cytosine arabinoside

[a]Relationships based on usual doses.

Table 3   Antiemetic Drugs

Phenothiazines	Antihistamines
Chlorpromazine (Thorazine)	Hydroxyzine (Vistaril, Atarax)
Prochlorperazine (Compazine)	Cyclizine (Marizine)
Triethylperazine (Torecan)	Meclizine (Antivert)
Promethazine (Phenergan)	Dimenhydrate (Dramamine)
Triflupromazine (Vesprin)	Buclizine (Bucladin)
Perphenazine (Trilafon)	Diphenhydramine (Benadryl)
Miscellaneous	Investigational agents
Benzquinamide (Emete-Con)	Tetrahydrocannabinol (THC)
Haloperidol (Haldol)	Nabilone
Droperidol (Inapsine)	Levonantradol
Metoclopramide (Reglan)	Lorazepam
Trimethobenzamide (Tigan)	High-dose corticosteroids
Diphenidol (Vontrol)	Domperidone
Scopolamine hydrobromide	

There have been a number of reviews written about the pharmacological management of chemotherapy-induced nausea and vomiting (Penta et al., 1981; Penta, Poster, and Bruno, 1983; Laszlo, 1983a). Turning first to the standard antiemetic agents, we should begin any such listing with the classic antiemetics —the phenothiazines (Table 3). Most of these are very familiar and a good deal has been written about them since they were introduced in the early 1950s; their use has been critically reviewed by Lucas (1983) and Wampler (1983).

Moertel and colleagues at Mayo Clinic (Moertel, Reitemeier, and Gage, 1963; Moertel and Reitemeier, 1973) were among the early workers who studied emesis produced by anticancer agents, primarily by 5-fluorouracil, and they found that drugs such as prochlorperazine and thiopropazate were more effective than placebo in preventing 5-FU-induced nausea and vomiting. As a class the phenothiazines are the most widely used drugs in medical practice, being primarily employed in the management of patients with psychiatric disorders.

However, phenothiazines are also useful for their antiemetic, antinausea, and antihistaminic properties, as well as for their capacity to potentiate analgesics, sedatives, and other central nervous system depressant agents (Lucas, 1983). Phenothiazines seem to exert most of their antiemetic effects by means of blocking dopamine receptors, and drugs of this class have a marked protective action against the nausea- and emesis-inducing effect of apomorphine and certain ergot alkaloids, which can interact with central dopaminergic receptors in the chemoreceptor trigger zone (CTZ) of the medulla, with blockade of dopamine receptors in the CTZ in turn suppressing the vomiting center.

The most effective phenothiazine regimen at our institution is prochlorperazine (10 mg) or chlorpromazine (25 mg) given orally every 6 hours beginning at least 6-12 hours before starting chemotherapy and continuing for at least 24 hours. If the patient cannot tolerate oral medication or begins to vomit, then the oral dose is supplemented with rectal or parenteral doses. Mild emetogenic chemotherapeutic drugs such as 5-FU or radiation therapy generally respond nicely to these agents. However, more potent drugs rarely respond fully to phenothiazines. Furthermore, aggressive use of phenothiazines is associated with a considerable number of side effects, some of which are attributable to the actions of the drugs on the central and autonomic nervous systems while others are hypersensitivity reactions. More recent studies have compared various phenothiazines, mainly prochlorperazine, with several newer antiemetics such as tetrahydrocannabinol (THC) and nabilone, metoclopramide and high-dose steroids, and in most studies prochlorperazine was less effective (Sallan, Zinberg, and Frei, 1975; Sallan et al., 1980; Orr, McKernan, and Bloome, 1980; Steele et al., 1980; Gralla et al., 1981).

Antihistamines are often used as antinausea and antivomiting agents. Although they work extremely well in motion sickness (other than in space flights), they offer little protection against the nausea and vomiting produced by potent chemotherapeutic agents.

There are a variety of other agents which have been used in management of patients who are receiving cancer chemotherapy. Among these we might highlight the more potent drugs including butyrophenones such as haloperidol, benzquinamide derivatives, cannabinoids, and metoclopramide. Haloperidol is a major tranquilizer that appears to act as a membrane stabilizer blocking the action of dopamine at the postsynaptic membrane (Janssen, 1967). The drug decreases apomorphine-induced vomiting, suggesting its effectiveness at the CTZ as a major mechanism of action. In comparative studies against prochlorperazine or THC in patients receiving potent emetogenic chemotherapeutic agents, its overall efficacy was significantly better than benzquinamide and about the same as THC (Neidhart et al., 1981a; Neidhart et al., 1981b). A recent study showed that high-dose haloperidol given intravenously is almost as effective as metoclopramide against cisplatin given in large doses (Grunberg et al., 1984). We confirm that it is effective when given in high doses intravenously (circa 2-3 mg q4h) and we may use it in combination with phenothiazines and steroids.

Metoclopramide has been highlighted by the studies of Gralla and associates at Memorial Sloan-Kettering Institute in New York in which their randomized double-blind studies showed marked effectiveness of this agent in management of cisplatin-induced nausea and vomiting (Gralla et al., 1981) in followup to an earlier study by Kahn et al. (1978). This drug is now approved not only for cisplatin-induced nausea and vomiting, but also appears to be useful for other drugs. Metoclopramide is among the oldest of the antiemetics in use elsewhere in the world, having been introduced in 1964 by Justine-Besancon. However, the usual antiemetic doses were largely ineffective in preventing nausea and vomiting of potent emetogenic chemotherapeutic drugs. This procainamide derivative, a substituted benzamide, has attracted interest more recently when far higher doses were used than those used in other forms of emesis. It is not entirely clear whether the major effect of this agent is on the gastrointestinal tract or on the CTZ, it seems to have effects in both, but nonetheless it has been demonstrated that high doses of metoclopramide have efficacy against the most potent emetogenic agent, cisplatin. To date the toxicity has generally been manageable when it is given in the range of 1-2 mg/kg/dose by 15-minute I.V. infusion starting a half an hour before cisplatin and every 2 hours thereafter for 2-5 doses. Dyskineses do occur frequently as side effects in children, less frequently in adults and can be prevented or reversed by antihistamines such as diphenhydramine. Concomitant administration of 25 mg of diphenhydramine seems to be an effective preventative measure with the higher doses of metoclopramide. Another attractive way of giving metoclopramide is orally 50 mg q4h, and it can be used either alone or preferably with prednisone (Senn, Glaus, and Bachmann-Mettler, 1984). Since cisplatin may cause delayed emesis it is useful to have this available for patients after they leave the clinic.

There has been considerable research interest in the use of several cannabinoids, drugs that are still experimental in this country, and this field has been reviewed by Vincent et al. (1983). Delta-9-tetrahydrocannabinol (THC) is the best studied of these; it can be extracted from marijuana plants or synthesized. It is difficult to formulate even in capsule form and although its absorption is erratic, it is an effective antiemetic as originally reported by Sallan et al. and amply confirmed since (Sallan, Zinberg, and Frei, 1975; Sallan et al., 1980; Orr, McKernan, and Bloome, 1980; Neidhart et al., 1981a, Laszlo, Lucas, and Huang, 1981). Our studies using THC in 88 patients who had severe nausea and vomiting despite the use of other antiemetics found 18% complete responses and 48% partial responses and 34% who had less than a partial response; a response rate that could be enriched further with repeated courses of THC. A number of side effects have been reported, with the majority of patients experiencing somnolence, "high" and then to a lesser extent other side effects, among which we consider the dysphoric reactions, such as fear and anxiety, as the most serious ones. Interestingly, THC is not particularly helpful in counteracting cisplatin.

Nabilone was the first of the synthetic cannabinoid derivatives which Herman and colleagues described as a significant advance in the management of cisplatin-induced nausea and vomiting (Herman et al., 1979; Steel et al., 1980), studies now amply confirmed. Neither THC nor nabilone have been approved by the FDA at the time of this writing, although both are pending approval. One unresolved question about the cannabinoids is whether their dysphoric properties can be eliminated by chemical alterations of the parent molecule or whether doing so would also eliminate the antiemetic effect.

No review of any pharmacological program seems to be complete without mentioning the uses of high doses of corticosteroids, which seem to be good for just about everything. Indeed, there are a number of articles suggesting that high doses of steroids (methylprednisolone, dexamethasone), either alone or in combination with other antiemetics, may be very effective (Rich, Abdulhayoglu, and DiSaia, 1981; Winokur et al., 1981; Markman et al., 1984; Senn, Glaus, and Bachmann-Mettler, 1984). Steroids are quite attractive because, unlike all other agents, they do not cause sedation and can easily be combined with drugs such as metoclopramide, lorazepam, and phenothiazines. Lorazepam is technically still an experimental agent for nausea and vomiting, though it is on the market as a preanesthetic agent. We have found it to be of interest as a single drug because it not only possesses antiemetic effects but also is anxiolytic and blocks short-term memory. Thus a patient may vomit yet still be well-satisfied with the chemotherapy experience since the toxicity is not remembered and it may thereby block the imprinting of the conditioned reaction of anticipatory nausea (Laszlo et al., 1983, abstract; Laszlo et al., in press). There are an increasing number of recent reports that are favorably impressed with this agent as part of combination antiemetic therapy (Bishop et al., 1984; Gagen et al., 1984).

It is important to try to individualize the best antiemetic therapy for any given situation, though the means of achieving this are not firmly grounded scientifically because there are so many unknowns. We previously suggested a kind of algorithm depending on the intensity of the emetogenic stimulus and what is known about the effectiveness of certain therapeutic programs (Laszlo, 1983a). We might attempt to update and simplify the approach by outlining some guiding principles for the physician.

1. Become familiar with the usage of representative drugs from the major classes of antiemetics—doses, routes of administration, side effects.
2. Tailor the aggressiveness of antiemetic therapy to the intensity of the emetogenic stimulus and develop an initial strategy for mild, moderate, and maximal challenge.
3. Modify the dosage of the program as needed during the initial course of treatment. Escalate if not adequate; hold if there is excessive sedation, and reduce dosage thereafter.

4. Begin antiemetic therapy *before* starting chemotherapy, depending on route of administration (i.e., short lead time for I.V. metoclopramide; long for oral THC or phenothiazine).
5. If initial experience with the antiemetic program is satisfactory, then repeat it on subsequent courses. If not, change to a different program designed to maximize therapeutic ratio for this patient.
6. Consider the patients' preference—they may like a program which includes an amnestic and anxiolytic drug (i.e., lorazepam)—even if they did vomit.
7. Certain programs are better suited to in- or outpatient use depending on route, frequency of administration, and potential side effects. Aggressive therapy for outpatients requires initial parenteral administration followed by oral or rectal routes of suitable drugs; this requires that there be a responsible individual to take the patient home in a car.
8. Since the major consequences of vomiting are physical and psychological discomfort and dehydration, we need to pay attention to sedation, reassurance, and fluid replacement.
9. Cost can play a role in choice of agents.

We generally start with single antiemetics for mild challenges, larger doses of single doses or combinations for moderate challenges, and very large initial dose of drugs or antiemetic drug combinations for the most emetogenic programs, such as the high-dose cisplatin and doxorubicin combinations.

To assist the reader we will select some representative drugs and suggest initial doses, schedules and indications (Table 4). Clearly other mitigating medical circumstances such as liver, renal or brain disease, diabetes, and prior psychiatric disorders will enter into specific therapeutic selections.

The "bottom line" seems to be that newer chemotherapeutic programs are more emetogenic than they have been in the past, and fortunately, major studies in counteracting this problem have also taken place. Physicians do recognize that inadequate management of nausea and vomiting is deleterious to the health and well-being of the patient and that any delay in providing an aggressive approach merely aggravates the problem. Once the pattern of nausea and vomiting becomes established, or conditioned, during a period of ineffective antiemetic therapy, then the anticipatory nausea and vomiting become extremely difficult to manage. Judicious use of the available agents should make truly refractory nausea and vomiting a rare event in oncology practice.

The use of progressive muscle relaxation techniques and of hypnosis can be very helpful, particularly for children who are very responsive, for those who are refractory to antiemetics, or for those who are especially anxious. The methods are somewhat labor intensive and require special training, but they can

Table 4   Selected Antiemetic Programs

Drug	Dose (mg)-schedule (hr)-route	Indications
Prochlorperazine (Compazine)	10 q4-6, I.M. or p.o. 25 q4 p.r.	Mild challenge; when oral and parenteral Rx is appropriate, can be given at home
Metoclopramide (Reglan)	1 mg/kg q2 X 4 I.V. 2 mg/kg q2 X 4 I.V. 10-20 mg p.o. q4-6h p.r.n. X 24 hours: 50 mg p.o. at −4, 0, 4, 8, 12 hours	Moderate-dose chemotherapy; high-dose cisplatin: use with diphenhydramine (50 mg) or with dexamethasone; can use with oral prednisone
THC	5-7.5/M^2 q4 p.o. starting 8 hours before Rx	Moderate-high-dose chemotherapy (other than cisplatin)
Dexamethasone	20 mg I.V. 30 min. before Rx and 10 mg p.o. q6h X 4	Moderate-dose chemotherapy; useful in combination (i.e., metoclopramide, lorazepam) vs. aggressive emetogenic programs
Lorazepam (Ativan)	0.025-0.05 mg/kg I.V. q4 X 4	For anxiety, to prevent anticipatory symptoms
Haloperidol (Haldol)	1-2 mg q4-6 p.o. 1-3 mg I.V. q2h X 5 beginning before therapy	Moderate chemotherapy
Combination (metoclopramide, dexamethasone, lorazepam)	Full doses of each	Preferred for high-dose cisplatin

be very effective (Cotanch, 1983; Stoudemire, Cotanch, and Laszlo, 1984; Burish and Carey, 1984; Zeltzer et al., 1983). Burish and colleagues (personal communication) feel that not only will early relaxation training alleviate nausea and vomiting, but can significantly reduce associated anxiety; our group agrees with this conclusion.

III. BONE MARROW TOXICITY

A. General Principles of Drug Cytotoxicity to Bone Marrow

The adverse hematological effects that are associated with the use of cancer chemotherapy (and/or radiation therapy) can either be quite simple and straightforward or exceedingly complex. As a general rule patients who have hematological malignancies are likely to come in with the more complex problems, whereas previously healthy patients who have recently been detected to have a small tumor in the lung, breast, or elsewhere are likely to be hematologically normal prior to the use of myelosuppressive therapies and their response to therapy, unless that therapy is deliberately marrow ablative and requires autologous marrow transplantation, is fairly predictable. Between these two extremes are patients who do not have hematological malignancies but who have progressive metastatic cancer which has spread to other organs including bone marrow, which may give rise to myelophthisic anemia or to bone marrow fibrosis and myeloid metaplasia. Anemia itself is an exceedingly frequent finding in patients with neoplastic disease and physical replacement of marrow cells by tumor is neither essential nor even common in contributing to the pathogenesis of the anemia, even in patients with metastatic cancer. Study of the erythropoiesis of such patients has revealed multiple abnormalities in the various processes which are responsible for maintenance of an adequate hemoglobin concentration. The pathogenesis of anemia may include immune hemolytic varieties, aregenerative anemias, as well as those related to blood loss and vitamin deficiency, as have been reviewed previously (Laszlo, 1982). Anemia may occur alone or in association with mechanisms responsible for thrombocytopenia, thrombocytosis, thrombocytopathy, leukocytosis, and leukopenia.

If we restrict ourselves herein to discuss the complications of cancer chemotherapy in patients who are being treated for nonhematological malignancies, the problem is considerably simpler in scope. This arbitrary restriction is reasonable in that the chemotherapy of patients with leukemia is largely handled by oncology specialists who are very knowledgeable about these problems. Indeed, virtually every drug used in cancer chemotherapy has some adverse effect on the hematopoietic system and in fact it is these effects which often limit the dose of antimetabolite or alkylating agent that can be given.

We agree with Hoagland's review (1984) that myelosuppression by a course of cancer chemotherapy generally reverts spontaneously and without significant complications. It is often necessary to accept transient granulo- and thrombocytopenia as part of being sure that the patient is receiving maximal tolerated doses of chemotherapy. It is by knowing the propensities of the drugs and the clinical circumstances which modify their metabolic degradation that one is best able to avoid prolonged or life-threatening cytopenias. If these do occur then prompt antibacterial and specific blood product replacement will usually permit recovery in such cases. It is true that certain drugs characteristically elicit relatively more extreme granulocytopenia than thrombocytopenia, or vice versa, and that the type and severity of the marrow effect may depend not only on the drug, but on the dose, route, and schedule of administration. Indeed, it is the exploitation of some of these specific features which may be decisive in the rational selection of one or a combination of agents for a given clinical circumstance. The detailed effects of individual drugs has been previously reviewed (Laszlo and Kremer, 1973) and the concepts of myelosuppression and their effects on stem cell compartments have also been reviewed recently (Barr and Perry, 1982).

When the time comes to use a drug(s) it is necessary to know its primary hematological toxicity when used alone or in combination, the typical time for the nadir and recovery effects on the various blood elements, most notably granulocytes and platelets, and whether the drug tends to have cumulative suppressive effects when used on a repeated basis. For most drugs their characteristic effects are to produce pancytopenia, although the nadir of the counts varies considerably from class to class. Yet when the drug is readministered following a period of hematological recovery, the extent of myelosuppression tends to be quite comparable on each occasion. Certainly there is no evidence that bone marrow stem cells become "resistant" to the effects of chemotherapeutic drugs the way cancer cells may if they are not killed during the initial courses of treatment. Quite the contrary may be the case in that certain drugs, such as nitrosoureas and busulfan, may cause cumulative toxicity when used repeatedly over many months, an effect recognized by greater and lengthier myelosuppression following each course, and occasionally even permanent marrow aplasia. It is because of such vagaries that it is important to check the blood counts of patients on a repeated basis prior to each course of chemotherapy, particularly if one is using some of the more hazardous drug programs. When large numbers of cancer patients are being treated there is always the possibility of drug administration error, such as when a patient is or becomes confused about how much drug to take and for how long. One must always be on guard not to leave running orders for chemotherapy which can be followed blindly at home or when a patient is transferred to a nursing home.

If one looks closely at the blood films of patients being treated with anti-metabolites and/or alkylating agents, one commonly sees Dohle bodies, coarse and sparse (presumably primary) granules, and hypo- or hypersegmentation. Giant platelet forms may also be seen. Although the functional significance of these altered morphological blood cell forms is not known, they attest to the systemic nature of the metabolic effects and serve to remind one of the narrow window of drug selectivity, when one is fortunate enough to find and exploit it appropriately.

B. Myelosuppression

Over the course of repeated chemotherapy treatments with combination programs such as might be used for colon cancer, small cell lung cancer, or breast cancer, there tends to be a slow drop in hemoglobin and hematocrit which is a manifestation both of secondary marrow suppression due to the underlying disease and to the direct cytotoxic effects of drugs on erythroid precursors. Transient thrombocytopenias are rarely a problem unless very aggressive drug combinations are being used, and those are more likely to occur in the hematological malignancies such as acute leukemia where patients begin with an extremely low platelet count and limited marrow reserve. Far and away the most common complication of the use of our chemotherapeutic drugs is that of leukopenia and granulocytopenia with the associated increased risk for infection. An otherwise healthy patient who has a transient fall in granulocyte count to ca. 500 cells/mm^3 which lasts for 4-7 days is unlikely to be effected by an intercurrent infection, but the time at risk from more prolonged granulocytopenia and more severe granulocytopenia will be crucial in determining the occurrence of superinfection in the setting of the compromised host. The subject of infections occurring in patients undergoing chemotherapy is covered in Section IV, which describes the problems of neutropenia and associated infection and how these are usually dealt with by appropriate bacteriological techniques for making diagnosis, the use of antibiotics, and the period of waiting until the marrow recovers sufficiently to restore host immunity.

When radiation therapy or extensive prior chemotherapy has been given to a patient who is being considered for a course of aggressive combination chemotherapy, one can expect to produce an exaggeration of the normal cytopenic effects, and this is generally dealt with by an initial dose reduction (of the most cytopenic marrow suppressive agents) by a factor of perhaps one-third to one-half, gradually increasing the dosage on subsequent courses. For example, a patient who has had prior pelvic radiation for prostate cancer and who is now being considered for alkylating agent chemotherapy can be anticipated to have a lower than normal tolerance for the marrow suppressive agents on the basis of prior radiation, metastatic disease involving the bone marrow, plus the nonspecific secondary effects of cancer. Occasionally one does produce life-threatening granulocytopenia despite good treatment planning, and blood component therapy can be transiently used as an emergency measure to save the life of such a patient. The logistics of blood component therapy with white blood cells has been reviewed (McCredie and Freireich, 1982). We rarely utilize this modality now except in patients with leukemia or those undergoing bone marrow transplantation who have life-threatening infections at a time of prolonged neutropenia. Granulocyte transfusions are at times indicated in the febrile neutropenic patient who has not responded to vigorous antibiotic therapy in 2-3 days.

One conceptual point concerning the use of cytotoxic drugs is worth special emphasis. Although the hematological effects of drugs are commonly considered as untoward side effects, these very effects have been surprisingly useful in predicting specific diseases for which a given drug might be most effective. For example, the property of mustard agents to shrink normal lymph nodes was successfully exploited in the treatment of malignant lymphomas; the lymphopenic effects of chlorambucil were utilized for the treatment of chronic lymphocytic leukemia; and the granulocytopenic effects of busulfan were particularly desirable features in the treatment of chronic granulocytic leukemia. Suppression of the immune response is produced by most chemotherapeutic agents, and this property has been successfully applied in a variety of disorders, including autoimmune diseases and organ transplantation.

C. Cell Kinetics

A schematic outline of the sequence of hematopoietic depression is shown in Table 5. The type and duration of cytopenia produced by a drug should depend on its mechanism of action, the dose and schedule of administration, and the life-cycle kinetics of the affected cell. A drug that produces mitotic arrest by inhibiting the formation of spindle fibers, or one that produces a block in DNA synthesis, causes primarily a depletion of the most rapidly replicating cells. In this connection it is appropriate briefly to review hematopoietic cell division and maturation. In the case of erythropoiesis, there are probably four cycles of cellular division in the marrow, the last of which is the polychromatophilic normoblast which undergoes a cell cycle of about 30 hours in duration. Following that final step of cell division, the normoblasts require approximately 50 hours to lose their nuclei and turn into marrow reticulocytes. These are subsequently released into the blood, after a period of approximately 40 hours, to complete their maturation into erythrocytes during the course of an additional 40 hours. Thus, reticulocytopenia should begin some 4-6 days following the cessation of cell division;

Table 5 Examples of the Sequence of Hematopoietic Suppression and Recovery (in Days) Produced by Classes of Anticancer Agents

Treatment		Blood cell type			
		Polys	Lymphs	Platelets	Retics
Antimetabolite (cytosine arabinoside, methotrexate)	Maximum depression	10	0	12	5
X-ray ("mantle")	Recovery	15	0	20	14
	Maximum depression	14	7	14	10
Alkylating agent (HN$_2$)	Recovery	90	180	30	30
	Maximum depression	10	10	14	10
	Recovery	21	28	28	28

Note: Approximate times for maximal effect and recovery are listed. Time to maximum depression may vary by ±4 days.

a brief period of arrest of erythroid maturation would scarcely affect the red cell count, however, because of the length of survival of normal erythrocytes in the circulating blood (100-120 days). Prolonged or repeated arrest would ultimately result in anemia. Should there be a coexisting decrease in red cell survival (owing to hemolysis or hypersplenism, for example), the development of anemia may be quite rapid.

In *myelopoiesis* the final step of cell division is at the level of the myelocyte, and this apparently requires 60 hours. Earlier mitotic steps involve myeloblast and promyelocyte stages of approximately 1 day each. Thus it has been estimated by various authors that development of the myelocyte requires approximately 4-5 days, and subsequent maturation through the stages of metamyelocytes, stabs, and mature polymorphonuclear leukocytes, with release into the peripheral blood, may require an additional 3 days. Thus, if an agent were to affect cell division in a nonspecific fashion, granulocytopenia would result some 5 days later, representing the period for the final cell division plus subsequent maturation in the marrow and release into the peripheral blood. The brief survival of circulating granulocytes dictates that this will promptly be reflected as clinical neutropenia.

Less is known about the kinetics of lymphocyte production, although the cell is long lived, and may re-enter the circulation. Drugs that are phase and cycle specific, without general cytotoxic effects for lymphoid cells, cause less depression in lymphocyte than granulocyte counts. Such lymphopenia is most pronounced 10-20 days following drug administration. For drugs with direct effect on lymphoid cells, the nadir is more pronounced and occurs earlier.

Megakaryocyte endomitosis produces mature megakaryocytes that bud platelets more effectively than immature megakaryocytes. Multiplication from the megakaryoblast on 4n ploidy to the fully mature megakaryocyte with 8-32n takes at least 5 days and platelets appear in the circulation shortly after cytoplasmic budding is first seen in the marrow. Thrombocytopenia may appear from 3-30 days after drug administration, with the more delayed effect apparently related to injury of early megakaryocyte precursors.

These general considerations are intended to serve as guidelines for understanding drugs such as cytosine arabinoside, which primarily affect DNA synthesis within the cell cycle. For drugs that affect multiple targets, such as alkylating agents, hematological effects may be more rapid in onset and more generalized over all hematologic cell types. The hematological depression produced by certain drugs that appear to act predominantly on stem cells, such as nitrosoureas, may be substantially delayed.

It now seems clear that retreatment with the initial dose of chemotherapy may be lethal if given at a time prior to recovery of marrow stem cells, whereas the identical dose may be well-tolerated after the stem cells have recovered—possibly even prior to recovery of peripheral blood counts. Application of this principle of spaced dosages has been reported in the treatment of lung cancer in man (Bergsagel, Robertson, and Hasselback, 1968). These studies employing large doses of cyclophosphamide show beginning depression of leukocyte counts on the 6th day, with maximum depression on the 9th to 12th day and recovery toward normal by the 15th day. The primary effect of increasing the dose of cyclophosphamide would be to further lower the absolute leukocyte count rather than to change the time of fall or recovery. As the dose of cyclophosphamide is increased, the minimal leukocyte count falls in exponential fashion (Bergsagel, Robertson, and Hasselback, 1968). Retreatment with subsequent courses of cyclophosphamide following total recovery gave results similar to those of the initial treatment. Premature repetition of the dose, prior to the recovery of the marrow stem cell, however, may produce a much more profound leukocyte suppression than did the original dose.

D. Anemia

Slowly progressive anemia is infrequently a serious clinical problem, and when it occurs it can of course be handled with transfusion of red blood cells. In this regard the advantages of transfusing frozen red cells in the treatment of cancer patients has been pointed out (Sherwood and Yankee, 1982). If such patients were subsequently to require leukocyte or platelet transfusions, then they would be less likely to have become sensitized to these cells and therefore receive more benefit from those blood products. Likewise, the incidence of febrile, nonhemolytic reactions of patients given frozen cells are small, even when those same patients consistently react to fresh blood. The indications for red cell transfusions are not different in patients receiving myelosuppressive therapy than those who are not, except that the rate of fall and the degree of symptomatology may take a greater toll on patients who are simultaneously experiencing side effects of chemotherapy, and are therefore less tolerant to the cardiovascular adjustments which may pertain in an untreated patient.

Some drugs are particularly prone to produce anemia and this may be true for antimetabolites such as hydroxyurea and methotrexate given on a regular basis. Macrocytosis is commonly noted in patients treated with antimetabolites such as hydroxyurea, methotrexate, or cytosine arabinoside: mean corpuscular volumes can be astounding under such circumstances (>120) when such drugs are taken regularly. Then there are the more irregular and unusual types of hemolytic anemia produced by a drug such as mitomycin-C which can give rise to a picture similar to that of disseminated intravascular coagulation and which may be irreversible. The latter is worthy of separate mention since it is a life-threatening complication.

Microangiopathic hemolytic anemia combined with progressive renal failure (hemolytic-uremic syndrome) has occurred with the use of mitomycin-C. This drug has been used alone or in combination with drugs such as 5-fluorouracil in treatment of patients with gastrointestinal cancers. Most attempts to control this with steroids, salicylates, dipyridamole, and blood transfusions have been unsuccessful, but there have been occasional reports of recovery following prompt heparin, plasmapheresis, or hemodialysis for renal failure (Verwey et al., 1984; Hammer, Verani, and Winman, 1983).

E. Thrombocytopenia

Thrombocytopenia is also quite a common complication in patients with cancer and again, one needs to consider whether this is due to prior chemotherapy or radiation therapy, from the cancer itself as it involves the marrow, or from the current course of chemotherapy or radiation therapy. Judicious use of platelet therapy has made a tremendous impact on our ability to support patients with leukemia through lengthy induction courses and to minimize their risk of hemorrhage until their normal marrow cells have an opportunity to recover. However, platelet transfusion therapy is not often required in patients who do not have hematological malignancies and who are undergoing intermittent courses of chemotherapy, despite the fact that at their nadir the platelet count may fall to the range of 30,000-50,000. One does not need to treat an asymptomatic patient at that platelet level, although clearly the risk of hemorrhage is a function of the days at risk when the platelet count is <50,000, and there is a considerable risk of serious hemorrhage when the platelet count is <5,000.

Some of these practical aspects, particularly in regard to platelet component therapy, have been reviewed (Yankee and Sherwood, 1982).

F. Coagulation Defects

Coagulation deficits are rarely produced by drugs used for cancer chemotherapy. The most notable exceptions to this are from the use of L-asparaginase and mitomycin-C; to a lesser extent, mithramycin may produce transient bleeding diathisis as part of an acquired platelet disorder. Overt laboratory coagulation abnormalities result from L-asparaginase, which decreases the synthesis of fibrinogen and the factors produced by the liver. This process is usually self-limited, even upon continued drug use, and is not associated with clinical bleeding. The hemolytic-uremic syndrome that arises in a small fraction of patients treated with mitomycin-C has already been mentioned.

A brief discussion follows of the hematological effects of some of the important and interesting drugs used in clinical chemotherapy today. Table 5 summarizes the usual time at which specific cytopenia and recovery may be anticipated from the major classes of anticancer therapy.

G. Alkylating Agents

Nitrogen Mustard

Early pharmacological leads arising out of the experience of World War I on the effects of mustard gases on lymphoid tissues caused several clinical groups to study the use of mustard compounds in patients with malignant lymphomas during the 1940s. Dameshek and colleagues treated 50 patients with nitrogen mustard, and they reported hematological and other effects produced by therapy in addition to clinical responses (Dameshek, Weisfuse, and Stein, 1949). Reticulocytopenia following a single dose of nitrogen mustard occurred in 85% of the patients and reached its maximum effect by the 6th to the 10th day. Mild anemia began at 5-6 days following which there was a gradual return to normal levels at approximately 5 weeks. Leukocyte counts fell below baseline levels and instances of severe pancytopenia were observed in these patients. Thrombocytopenia was seen in a proportion of their patients, and this has been found to occur in a majority of patients in more recent studies. Clearly the incidence and relative severity of these reactions depend on the dose and schedule employed.

Serial bone marrow studies in patients treated with nitrogen mustard show decreased marrow cellularity and an increase in fat spaces, beginning within 24 hours after therapy. Erythropoiesis and myelopoiesis were also promptly suppressed. Bizarre, distorted myelocytes, metamyelocytes, polymorphonuclear neutrophils, and megakaryocytes were frequently noted. Marked hypoplasia occurred and bone marrow regeneration was observed following the cessation of treatment. Irreversible aplasia of the bone marrow was not encountered following therapy, although this fatal complication can occur with very intensive and frequent administration of nitrogen mustard. If such potentially lethal doses are contemplated in order to attempt curative therapy, then the marrow can be "rescued" by transfusion of preharvested autologous bone marrow which, 14-20 days after reinfusion, serves to repopulate bone marrow blood cell population.

Many studies have shown that intravenous nitrogen mustard produces prompt lymphopenia followed by reticulocytopenia, granulocytopenia, and thrombocytopenia; in most instances this is entirely reversible following the cessation of therapy. Generally the lymphocytopenia occurs within 24 hours and becomes more severe within 6-8 days. Granulocytopenia occurs within the first 3 days and lasts for 2-3 weeks following a single injection of nitrogen mustard. Variable degrees of depression in platelets and red cell counts occur during the 2nd and 3rd weeks after therapy, and hematological recovery is complete in 4-6 weeks; in fact, a rebound above baseline counts may occur in the 5th to 7th weeks. The rebounding of blood counts above baseline levels is quite common with other agents also.

Chlorambucil, Myleran, Alkeran, and Cyclophosphamide

A major advance in the use of alkylating agents occurred when compounds were synthesized which are well tolerated by oral administration. The question arose whether the hematological effects of different alkylating agents were basically identical and whether they were interchangeable in their usage when factors such as drug absorption were taken into account. Aromatic mustard agents, such as chlorambucil, had preferential effects on lymphocytes, causing only a brief granulocytopenia, which was followed by a granulocytosis with an "overshoot" in peripheral granulocyte counts reflecting the intense marrow regeneration following treatment. By contrast, busulfan (Myleran) had its predominant effect on granulopoiesis and a lesser effect on lymphocytes. In fact, a radiomimetic effect on marrow could be produced by the combined use of chlorambucil and busulfan, indicating that these agents are more selective in their hematopoietic effects than is radiation. In certain dosages, chlorambucil can cause lymphocytopenia without any significant effect on the other formed elements of the blood, whereas more intensive and prolonged therapy with daily or intermittent chlorambucil causes pancytopenia. Busulfan generally causes suppression of all marrow elements and variable degrees of pancytopenia; occasionally these effects may be extremely prolonged and rarely may lead to an irreversible state of aplastic anemia.

Cyclophosphamide (Cytoxan) is among the most widely used alkylating agents because of its broad spectrum of antitumor effectiveness. Its hematological effects are dose related but one of its attractions is that it is relatively platelet sparing when compared with other mustard agents. This feature of cyclophosphamide pharmacology is often useful, since thrombocytopenia is frequently a problem in patients having hematological neoplasms and in others who have received extensive prior radiation therapy or concurrent chemotherapy. Cyclophosphamide can also be effectively administered by intermittent intravenous injection.

An unusual effect that has been noted with cyclophosphamide, as well as with other mustards and chlorambucil, is the occasional occurrence of acute hemolysis. Such hemolytic episodes may appear abruptly and be associated with a positive direct Coombs' reaction.

H. Antimetabolites

Although the precise mechanism of action may not be known, most antimetabolites are generally considered to exert their inhibitory effects principally during the stage of DNA synthesis (S phase) of the cell cycle and to produce macrocytic or megaloblastic anemia. This would seem to be closely analogous to the unbalanced growth, or "thymineless-death," repeatedly described in cultured mammalian cells (or bacteria) that are grown in the absence of a thymine source or in the presence of inhibitors of DNA synthesis. Megaloblastosis is of no special concern except that attempts to treat it with vitamins such as B_{12} or leucovorin should be avoided unless that is part of a specific protocol design. The extent of cytopenia produced by antimetabolites varies by drug, dose, schedule of administration, and metabolic fate in plasma, liver, and other cells. The major details about each drug are found in pharmacology texts (Chabner, 1982) or package inserts and need not be repeated here except for some guidelines about avoiding excessive toxicity, as also discussed above in the case of alkylating agents.

Unlike alkylating agents or certain other types of drugs, very large single doses of antimetabolites (e.g., cytosine arabinoside, methotrexate, 5-fluorouracil, hydroxyurea) can be tolerated with little consequence of marrow injury. It is the repetitive use of much smaller doses [e.g., the recent popularity of continuous infusions (3-5 days at a time)] that causes progressive cytopenias. There are nuances in time to nadir and recovery, there may be biphasic drops with an early dip at 7 days and more morbid depression by 16-22 days in the case of *cytosine arabinoside,* and there may be specific ways to terminate the metabolite block by infusion of an endproduct of an inhibited pathway, as with leucovorin starting 48-72 hours after otherwise supralethal dose of *methotrexate,* the so-called leucovorin "rescue." This type of application is particularly noteworthy in that it depends upon frequent and *regular administration of leucovorin and, if the patient is at home and is experiencing nausea and vomiting as part of the G.I. toxicity, he/she may be unable or unwilling to take the rescue drug in oral form. This circumstance can be anticipated by some kind of planned checking of the patient by nurse, personal physician, or by phone report if necessary.* Lymphopenia is virtually never a problem with acute drug courses and severe or life-threatening hematological toxicity only occurs when truly massive doses of antimetabolites (alone or in combination) are given. High doses of *hydroxyurea* are occasionally used because of the rapid onset of action which may be desirable to lower leukemic cell counts or extraordinary platelet counts (>1 million) in chronic granulocytic leukemia or essential thrombocythemia. This drug requires closer supervision initially than do the others because of the rapid onset and rapid recovery by giving too much for too long or stopping abruptly, respectively. Nonetheless, once regulated by weekly blood counts, a relatively stable degree of myelosuppression can be induced over the course of a month or so of treatment and then bimonthly or monthly blood counts will suffice. Inexperienced physicians may give up on this drug prematurely by over- or underdosing, a result of not getting counts weekly during the initial month or two.

Nitrosourea compounds such as BCNU act partially as alkylating agents as discussed earlier and partially as antimetabolites. The major limitation to its use in man is the fear of developing severe and delayed and sometimes protracted marrow suppression. With doses of 200-300 mg/M^2 given intravenously over a 3-5 day period most patients experience granulocytopenia and thrombocytopenia with the nadir occurring 3-5 weeks after the start of therapy. The concern here is that the physician is assured that the patient has recovered from the last dose before giving the next course. That is sometimes not as easy to determine as it may seem because fluctuations in white count may occur during the recovery period and it is difficult to extrapolate until full recovery has occurred. Delayed secondary dips in the granulocyte count are particularly prone to occur with drugs such as nitrosoureas or in patients who have had extensive prior therapy, particularly radiotherapy, or myelophthisic tumors such as prostate or breast cancers. If the degree of cytopenia is not severe but is prolonged then most oncologists prefer to repeat the same dose but extend the intervals between treatment. Combination chemotherapy programs such as CMF for breast cancer and MOPP for Hodgkin's disease often present such dilemmas.

I. Radiation Therapy

Ionizing radiation has a depressant effect on both bone marrow function and lymphocyte production. A depression of hemoglobin concentration, neutrophils, lymphocytes, and platelets may be seen following radiation therapy. The degree of bone marrow impairment and the time required for recovery are dependent on the total effective dose administered and the fraction of total functional marrow included in the irradiated field. When a dose greater than 3000 rads is delivered to a particular anatomic site, regeneration of irradiated marrow may not occur (Sykes et al., 1964). Histological examination then reveals a fatty, fibrotic bone marrow containing a paucity of cells. With doses as low as 2500 rads, marrow regeneration can occur, but significant depression of bone marrow function in the irradiated marrow may persist.

Large doses of radiation to multiple areas, as are frequently administered in the treatment of patients with lymphomas, are associated with a significant degree of bone marrow depression. The "mantle field," which includes treatment to the cervical, axillary, and mediastinal nodes in contiguity, irradiates approximately 15% of the total bone marrow distribution. With doses ranging from 2000-4000 rads, a moderate drop in granulocytes and platelets is usually seen, with recovery to normal by 1 month for platelets and 3-5 months for granulocytes. The total bone marrow granulocyte reserve has been estimated by granulocyte response to endotoxin or etiocholanolone; is slightly decreased immediately following treatment; and returns to normal 4-5 months later. The transient nature of the marrow depression is illustrated by the fact that these patients are able to tolerate subsequent chemotherapy.

When total nodal irradiation is employed, the spleen, the para-aortic, pelvic, and inguinal nodes, and the "mantle" are included in the treatment field. This area covers approximately 65% of total bone marrow, and with doses greater than 2000 rads, considerable hematological toxicity can be expected. Neutrophil and lymphocyte counts are decreased during the 1st month after therapy has begun, and the fall in hemoglobin concentration and platelets is reached at approximately the 3rd month. By the 12th month the hemoglobin, lymphocytes, and platelets approach normal values, but granulocyte levels may still be slightly depressed. Bone marrow granulocyte reserve is markedly decreased immediately after therapy, with slow return to normal by the 5th month. To illustrate the degree of residual damage to the bone marrow, these patients have limited tolerance to subsequent chemotherapy for as long as one year or more after radiation therapy. If intensive chemotherapy and radiotherapy are both planned for a patient, the former may be given first because of the more transitory nature of the hematopoietic depression.

J. Bone Marrow Protection

The suppression of marrow growth by antineoplastic drugs is intrinsic to their anticancer effects as well, but attempts to achieve differential sensitivity of the tumor by use of folinic acid rescue, as with high-dose methotrexate infusions may be a case in point of some degree of selective marrow protection. There have been thoughts that splenectomy causes increased tolerance to chemotherapy, occurring generally as a byproduct of the staging procedure commonly used in Hodgkin's disease. However, although the white count does rise following splenectomy, the overall benefit of this in terms of greater tolerance to chemotherapy has not been well documented. Similar claims have been made that the lithium chloride to stimulate granulopoiesis may minimize the granulocytopenic effects of the chemotherapeutic drugs and thereby decrease the rates of infection, but this area remains controversial and furthermore the administration of lithium is not without its side effects.

Corticosteroid preparations such as prednisone are commonly used alone or in association with other drugs in the treatment of patients with lymphocytic leukemia, malignant lymphoma, and multiple myeloma, as well as occasional other types of cancer. Because prednisone does not have any depressive effect on the bone marrow, it is particularly useful in combination with myelosuppressive drugs. However, particularly when given in prolonged courses, prednisone generally causes granulocytosis, lymphopenia, impairment of the immune response, and sometimes erythrocytosis. The causes of these changes are not necessarily due to marrow effects of prednisone. Although not generally agreed upon, it is possible that concurrent administration of corticosteroids decreases the myelotoxicity of drugs such as alkylating agents, and thereby permits the utilization of larger doses than would otherwise be possible. The important subject of bone marrow protection has not been carefully investigated, and comparative studies of different steroid compounds are not available.

Androgenic hormones are sometimes helpful in the treatment of anemia in cancer patients. The most important attribute of the various androgenic preparations is their ability to stimulate erythropoiesis and to sustain a hemoglobin rise for the duration of therapy. Among several suitable methods, this may be accomplished by daily oral administration of fluoxymesterone (10-20 mg/day) or by biweekly injection of 400 mg of testosterone enanthate. Due to the virilizing effect of the prolonged use of androgens, which are required to produce a rise in hemoglobin, clinical application is usually limited to the severe anemia that may accompany multiple myeloma or chronic lymphocytic leukemia. In these circumstances a 1-3 gram rise in hemoglobin may be enough to convert a transfusion-dependent to an asymptomatic patient. This salutory effect on the bone marrow is limited to the erythroid series, since there is little stimulation of granulocytes or platelet production. It is interesting that this salutory increase in hemoglobin synthesis occurs in the absence of any effect on the underlying disease process.

IV. INFECTIONS

To the extent that there have been major advances in the management of patients with certain types of metastatic cancer and leukemia, the complications of chemotherapy, particularly infections, have emerged as a major impediment to survival. At least 50% of patients with cancer and leukemia ultimately succumb to infection, a point that is easily overlooked when confronted with many patients who appear healthy initially. Chemotherapy can produce transient defects in all aspects of host defense (phagocytosis and killing of bacteria by granulocytes, humoral immunity, and cell-mediated immunity) which individually and collectively increase the risk of infection caused by specific groups of microorganisms (Peterson, 1984). Although humoral and cell-mediated immunity are important defense mechanisms which are inhibited by chemotherapeutic drugs, quantitative deficiency of granulocytes (neutrophils) is the most common and serious problem in treated patients. Chemotherapy and steroids also impair phagocytic functions (granulocytes, monocytes) and lymphocyte-mediated immune functions.

The direct effects on host defense mechanisms are often compounded further. For example, the G.I. mucosa may become severely eroded, or infection may be introduced via catheters being used to deliver treatment. Further, patients with hematological malignancies such as chronic lymphocytic leukemia, Hodgkin's disease, and multiple myeloma compound their drug-induced propensity to infection by disease-related immunosuppression. Some of the specific and nonspecific potential infectious hazards that face the patient who has a progressive malignancy and is malnourished are being treated vigorously with chemotherapy, and are depicted in Figure 1; these problems are discussed in many excellent review articles (Bodey, 1982; Peterson, 1984; Brown, 1984; Armstrong, 1980; Bow et al., 1984).

Fever is usually the first sign of infection, although sometimes the temperature elevation is slight or even masked altogether by medications such as steroids. Of course fever can also be unassociated with infection, particularly with lymphoma and abdominal neoplasms (pancreas, kidney, G.I. tract). Neutropenia predisposes the patient to the infections caused by certain groups of extracellular bacteria and fungi (Table 6). Among neutropenic (absolute neutrophil count below $1000/mm^3$) patients with cancer, infection has been shown to be the major cause of death (Brown, 1984). Indeed the risk of infection generally rises as the count drops below 500, and the duration of suppression is also an important prognostic factor in that regard. An interesting point is that in one series 80% of febrile cancer patients had a granulocyte count $<500/mm^3$; infections accounted for fever in only 17% of patients whose count was >500 (Pizzo et al., 1984). Leukemia poses a special problem in that granulocyte counts are generally low prior to treatment of acute leukemia and will not improve unless a remission is achieved. The relationship between absolute granulocyte count and infection has been studied in acute leukemia (Bodey, 1982): the risk increases steadily at counts <1000. With cure rates for childhood leukemia approaching 60-70% it seems especially tragic to lose such patients to an infection. While effective antibacterial agents are available,

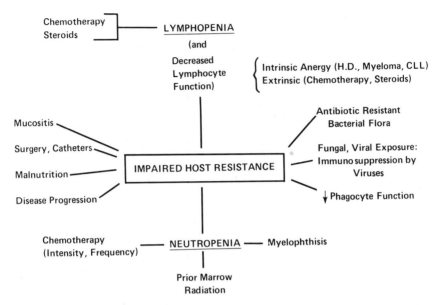

Figure 1 This schematic outline is intended to represent major factors which may be variably operative in a given patient who has both cancer and infection (or susceptibility to infections).

Table 6 Organisms in Patients with Neutropenia

Bacteria	Fungi
Streptococcus pyogenes	*Aspergillus* species
Streptococcus pneumoniae	*Mucorales*
Staphylococcus aureus	*Candida* species
Staphylococcus epidermidis	*Trichosporon* species
Viridans streptococci	*Pseudallescheria boydii*
Corynebacterium CDC-JK	*Fusarium* species
Enterococci	
Enterobacteriaceae	
Escherichia coli	
Klebsiella-Enterobacter-Serratia	
Proteus species	
Pseudomonas aeruginosa	

and antifungal and even antiviral agents are being developed, prevention seems to be the best approach for the infectious complications attendant to cancer chemotherapy. A look at the contributing factors (Figure 1) suggests some avenues for prevention.

The most common sites of infection in patients with cancer are lungs, G.I. tract, and skin (Bodey, 1982). Sometimes anatomic factors, such as bronchial obstruction, are important predisposing factors. Patients are at risk for infection from a variety of organisms: prior to being hospitalized the major pathogens are the so-called normal flora, of predominantly intestinal and respiratory origin, and those acquired organisms found in the external environment (air, food and water, etc.). Indeed, the majority of infections arise from the endogenous flora of the patient with cancer (Armstrong, 1980). While in the hospital the patient has the additional risk of hospital-acquired pathogens, and this varies with the ward, room, air circulation, etc. An effective hospital infectious disease committee will continually monitor these factors and may be able to recommend the safest hospital bed area. Careful hand washing by personnel is more important than so-called reverse isolation. Following one or more hospitalization events the normal flora may be unbalanced by both pathogenic and opportunistic organisms such as gram-negative bacilli (*Escherichia coli, Pseudomonas,* and *Klebsiella*) or by staphylococci (*aureus, epidermidis*). Important lessons are (1) if a patient is febrile at the time of presentation, then that problem should be evaluated and treated *before* starting chemotherapy, and (2) it may be advantageous to have the patient remain at home, monitoring temperature, during the period of transient granulocytopenia.

It has been emphasized repeatedly that the etiology of the febrile episode is likely to be very different for a patient being treated during the initial course of chemotherapy and granulocytopenia as opposed to repeated courses of chemotherapy and granulocytopenia, and even as a function of the duration of the granulocytopenia. With respect to the latter, Pizzo et al. (1984) indicate that the initial response to antibiotic therapy is usually successful because it is directed against bacterial pathogens, whereas with persistent granulocytopenia there is a continued risk for additional infectious complications which include not only resistant bacterial infections, but also fungal and viral infections. The emergence of these problems is schematized in Figure 2.

Several technological approaches have been developed to provide for total decontamination, which includes complete reverse isolation of the compromised patient to essentially sterile air (Schimpff et al., 1975; Bodey, Rodriguez, and Freireich, 1978) plus the addition of oral nonabsorbable antibiotics: granulocyte transfusion has been used both prophylactically and therapeutically. The initial expense and operating cost of laminar air flow units, however, have made them generally unavailable outside of research institutions, and some randomized studies have not confirmed their utility. On balance it would appear that laminar

ONSET OF
FEVER AND
GRANULOCYTOPENIA

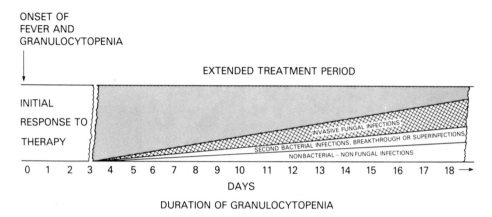

Figure 2   The efficacy of antibiotic regimens in cancer patients should be evaluated separately for initial empiric therapy (the first 72 hours after the initiation
of antibiotics) and during extended therapy (while the patient remains persistently
granulocytopenic and at continued risk for new infections). (From Pizzo et al.
(1984) by permission of the *American Journal of Medicine*.)

sterile air flow rooms have been shown to be of value for patients with acute
leukemia, or those with protracted neutropenia (i.e., bone marrow transplant)
but they are not suited for a clinical practice setting.

A number of alimentary tract sterilization programs have been derived to
protect the cancer patient from organisms in the internal environment. The
concept is to provide selective decontamination of aerobic gram-negative bacilli
without disturbing the normal anaerobes. While success has been seen in
prophylactic oral administration of gentamicin sulfate, vancomycin hydrochloride,
and nystatin, on a round-the-clock basis there are major problems associated with
these programs. These include the very unpleasant tastes of these medications,
their extreme expense, and the occasional acquisition of aminoglycoside-
resistant gram-negative rods. More recently it has been demonstrated that oral
sulfamethoxazole-trimethoprim may be as useful and much less costly than the
above agents in an infection prophylaxis program (Henry, 1984), and this has
been confirmed by 8-10 additional studies, although another review disputes
this approach (Schimpff et al., 1978; Schimpff, 1980).

Similarly, prevention of colonization of the upper respiratory tract by
bacterial pathogens should be a promising prophylactic approach. It does warrant study as suggested by Johanson (1984), but an effective remedy of this
problem is not yet at hand.

Table 7 shows a representative infection prevention program for profound
and prolonged granulocytopenia. The advocates propose that antibiotic therapy

Table 7 Infection Prevention Program for Profound and Prolonged Granulocytopenia

Isolation

1. Wash hands with hot water and disinfectant before examining patient.
2. Single patient room with reverse isolation.
3. Allow only cooked food in the diet.
4. Delay chemotherapy if patient is febrile.
5. Avoid instrumentation whenever possible (e.g., urinary catheter).
6. Avoid indwelling intravenous catheter and use butterfly-type needles instead.
   All intravenous tubing should be changed daily, and all intravenous catheters
   should be changed every 48 hours.

Monitoring

1. Take oral temperature every 6 hours before chemotherapy as well as during
   granulocytopenia.
2. Question patient about symptoms of infection every 6 hours.
3. Frequent examination of common sites of infection, i.e., pharynx, perirectal
   region, lungs.

Prophylactic Antibiotic Therapy

1. Trimethoprim, 160 mg, and sulfamethox-   Started at least 24 hours
   azole, 800 mg, orally every 12 hours.   before expected granulocyte
2. Nystatin tablets, 4 million units, and   count of $<1000/\mu L$.
   nystatin liquid, 1 million units, every
   4 hours; the latter should be swished
   around the mouth and then swallowed.

should be instituted for any patient who is expected to experience profound
granulocytopenia ($<1000/mm^3$) for a prolonged period (more than 7 days),
with treatment starting before the onset of granulocytopenia and continuing
until the count has risen above the danger level. Patients with transient
neutropenia need not be so treated. Thus, the patients who would benefit most
from this regimen are those with acute leukemia and those with more common
tumors who are receiving intensive combination chemotherapy. An early study
(Sickles, Green, and Wiernik, 1975) showed that this sulfamethoxazole-
trimethoprim combination decreased the incidence of *Pneumocystis carinii* and
bacterial infections in granulocytopenic patients with acute leukemia. Another
study using prophylaxis with oral sulfamethoxazole-trimethoprim showed decreased incidence of fever and antibiotic requirements for bacterial infection at
all levels of granulocytopenia (Hughes et al., 1977), and some other randomized

studies using this combination with other antibacterial or antifungal agents have shown similar benefits. However, not all studies have shown such benefit and the selection of drug-resistant gram-negative organisms during the course of prophylaxis is also possible. This controversy has been critically reviewed (Schimpff et al., 1978). Another study compared the two-drug combination against trimethoprim alone and suggested that the combination is more effective in preventing aerobic gram-negative bacillary infection; however, the authors also observed that myelosuppression may be prolonged by the use of this antibiotic combination (Gurwith et al., 1979). There is also the possibility of promoting overgrowth by *Aspergillus.*

Another recent randomized study of infection prophylaxis in acute leukemia patients receiving remission-induction therapy compared no prophylaxis, sulfamethoxazole and trimethoprim, ketoconazole, or the combination of all three drugs (Estey et al., 1984). No form of prophylaxis reduced infectious mortality or increased the complete remission rate but both antibiotic programs decreased the bacterial infection rate and lowered infectious mortality with also fewer fungal infections in the ketoconazole combination.

While this section is not appropriate for the discussion of specific treatment of proven infection, it must be mentioned that empiric therapy is important for patients who have temperature elevations in the setting of marked granulocytopenia. A patient in whom a temperature of 38.3°C develops in association with very severe granulocytopenia (<100 granulocytes/mm^3) has more than a 70% chance of being infected. An overall efficacy rate of 75-85% should be anticipated from an antibiotic or combination of antibiotics before considering its utility in the empiric treatment of febrile neutropenic patients. (That means, of course, that 15-25% of patients will not improve with the initial choice of antibiotics.) After efficacy, the choice of empiric therapy should be based on safety and the risk of superinfection in that particular hospital setting and/or emergence of resistance during therapy; also the cost versus benefit ratio must be considered with these expensive drugs. Patients who were possibly infected while granulocytopenic and who appear to respond to antibiotic usage are usually treated until they are afebrile for 4-5 days, then they are reevaluated.

Fungal infections constitute a second major risk of infection to the patient with cancer. These are being reported with increasing frequency in neutropenic patients, particularly those who are hospitalized and have been treated for prolonged periods both with chemotherapy and broad spectrum antibiotics (Bow et al., 1984). Because of this predictable setting, the physician should be especially alert to achieve an early diagnosis for the clinical manifestations of organisms like Candida, Aspergillus and Mucor species.

As advocated by de Jongh and Schimpff (1983), the basic approach to prevention of infection includes:

1. Improvement of host defenses
2. Minimizing use of invasive procedures
3. Reducing the acquisition of organisms
4. Suppressing colonizing organisms

There is not much that can be done to bolster host defense mechanisms once they are impaired. Prevention of life-threatening neutropenia can usually be accomplished by a knowledgeable approach to the hematological consequences of chemotherapeutic drugs as discussed earlier in this chapter and elsewhere (Laszlo and Kremer, 1973). Marrow suppressive drugs when used together will produce additive effects and the risk of overdosing can be minimized by combining drugs that do not cumulate this effect, by monitoring the granulocyte count (and platelet levels) during the nadir (usually 7-21 days depending on drugs), and remembering that subsequent courses will cause comparable degrees of cytopenia. Thus an initial course of chemotherapy which lowers the count excessively should be reduced in dosage for subsequent courses and titrated thereafter to produce the maximal "safe" response—defined as a granulocyte count not less than 500. Another potential modifying factor is that a patient who has had extensive prior radiation or one who has extensive bone marrow metastases will likely be unable to tolerate customary doses of myelosuppressive drugs; thus the initial course should be reduced by at least one-third. If this does not cause excessive marrow suppression, then the dose can be escalated on the second course.

Killed vaccines (influenza, pneumococcus) can be given to neutropenic patients during times of seasonal outbreaks but live viral vaccines should be avoided. Patients with Hodgkin's disease or those undergoing splenectomy should be immunized as early as possible in the course of their disease, preferably prior to receiving chemotherapy. Zoster immune plasma or globulin can be given to patients exposed to zoster or varicella. The use of corticosteroids should obviously be limited in neutropenic patients. It is of course difficult to avoid invasive procedures in very ill patients, but every catheter (I.V., urinary) introduces a hazard to the neutropenic patient. (Management of venous catheters is considered elsewhere in this chapter). Biopsies, surgical preparation, and dressing changes, should also receive special attention in these patients.

Since food is a common source of acquired infection, all uncooked items can simply be eliminated from the diet to prepare meals that are very low in microbial content. Thorough washing of hands is particularly important for personnel—so often hand washing seems to be done only after examination of the patient! Finally, careful dental care and oral and general hygiene should be part of the hospital routine for all immunosuppressed patients. This should include daily baths and skin antisepsis, particularly in axillary and perineal regions.

Surveillance cultures of the nose and stool (bacterial, fungal) may be predictive of subsequent infection and have been recommended in patients likely to experience prolonged neutropenia. There is a question of the cost effectiveness of such procedures. The use of prophylactic antibiotics has been discussed previously.

Infections of the central nervous system are a special threat to immunosuppressed patients with cancer and leukemia (Chernik, Armstrong, and Posner, 1973) and the limited means available for prophylaxis have recently been reviewed (Durack, 1984). Opportunistic organisms such as bacteria (i.e., *Listeria monocytogenes*), viruses (herpes, CMV), fungi (*Candida, Aspergillus, Cryptococcus neoformans*), and protozoa (toxoplasmosis, strongyloidiasis) are among the organisms that may infect the CNS. Unfortunately, no preventive measures are available for many of these infections, or are of unproved efficacy (Durack, 1984). Prophylactic antibiotics are usually given when shunts are implanted into the CNS for the purpose of delivering intrathecal antibiotics. This practice is intuitively attractive but limited trials, such as those of Odio et al. (1984), showed three shunt infections among 18 patients (17%) who received vancomycin prophylaxis versus 4 among 17 (23%) who received placebo.

There is little that can be done to prevent *Listeria monocytogenes* and herpes virus family (simplex, zoster, E-B) CNS infections. Screening of blood products and development of a vaccine are potential means of protecting against the more common virus infection, CMV; however, these are not in standard usage at this time. The most effective means of preventing CNS fungal infections is the prompt and aggressive treatment of pneumonia and septicemia produced by these organisms.

Periodontal disease is generally silent and effects almost all adults in the country. Clinically apparent periodontal and nonperiodontal oral infections increase in incidence with neutropenia, particularly when the absolute count is below 500/ml (Peterson, 1983). Bacteria, such as gram-negative bacilli, enter through the ulcerated lesions at times of myelosuppression or with leukemia. We recommend a clinical evaluation prior to chemotherapy and attention to oral hygiene measures beginning promptly. This generally involves brushing with a soft brush and flossing; intensive irrigation sprays are not recommended because they may induce bacteremia. Mouth washes are soothing to the gingiva and appear to limit mucositis in myelosuppressed patients. Some of these mouth wash mixtures contain antibiotics that may stimulate overgrowth by *Candida*. Overt dental pathology should be carefully evaluated and treated when likely to become exacerbated. Thus dental extractions are sometimes necessary before beginning an intensive program with myelosuppressive drugs.

Oral mucositis has a different etiology than periodontal disease but it represents a similar threat to afflicted patients. Fungi such as *Candida* and viruses such as herpes as well as bacteria of various types can be identified by wet smears, cultures, and cytological preparations. Prompt treatment uses antibiotics as well as supportive care with mouth washes and topical anesthetics. This recent availability of acyclovir makes it possible to treat cases of herpes simplex (or zoster) at very early stages.

V. DRUG EXTRAVASATION AND VEIN CARE

Most chemotherapeutic agents are given intravenously because of their pharmacological properties, such as variable gastrointestinal absorption, instability, etc. Preservation of veins is an extremely important issue for patients because of the multiple venipunctures which they must endure for laboratory tests, blood product administration, and antibiotic and anticancer drug therapy. When intensive and lengthy chemotherapy is indicated, as is predictable for a patient with acute leukemia, the early use of a central venous catheter is suggested, as this will alleviate most problems in venous access and venous care.

This section will discuss prevention and treatment of poor venous access and will give recommendations for prevention of drug extravasation. Many of the drugs used in cancer treatment may cause extensive debility if allowed to infiltrate local tissue and it is of great importance to minimize the risk of this happening. One must realize that while there are some guidelines for the treatment of extravasations, the treatment is controversial and, unfortunately, no single treatment has well-documented and consistent efficacy.

Given the seriousness of their other problems it may seem incongruous that patients often dread venipunctures more than almost any other aspect of their medical care. In turn they may judge the excellence of their medical care by the proficiency with which this is accomplished. The most important factor in the preservation of veins is to use experienced, well-trained professionals who deal with venipuncture techniques on a daily basis. The use of students or trainees for blood drawing (in our experience even medical house officers fall into this category) should be avoided for this patient population. It is also useful to discuss possible complications of intravenous chemotherapy with the patient in advance and/or provide a readable description.

With continued improvement in delivery systems for drugs and blood products, some devices that are frequently used include Hickman catheters, ventriculostomy reservoirs, totally implantable catheters, and pumps. One or more devices may be placed for the convenience of the therapy to be administered, thus reducing pain and discomfort; in so doing we should not fail to consider the importance of body image when these devices are recommended for use. Although these devices improve treatment, they are a constant reminder to patient, family, and friends that the cancer is present and that the treatment, with all the side effects, must continue. The devices should be recommended when absolutely necessary and a thorough discussion should take place with the patient to sufficiently reduce fears and concerns about his/her future with these mechanical devices.

Small gauge stainless steel needles for short-term I.V.s or blood drawing seem to decrease the irritation to the vein as well to reduce phlebitis and infection (Goldmann et al., 1973). The use of microfilters is now being evaluated as one promising means of diminishing this type of chemical irritation. Small gauge catheters should be used for long-term I.V. infusions. There are an increasing number of options for catheters; one recent large study has evaluated a dual-lumen catheter made of Silastic and finds it an excellent device when placed in the right atrium as a means of providing venous access for chemotherapy, as well as for parenteral nutrition and for blood sampling (Raaf, 1985). This article provides a good review of the practicalities of different methods and catheters. It goes without saying that thorough application of established skin cleansing methods will decrease the infection rate which can be serious in these patients.

Selection of the appropriate vein is most important not only for blood drawing, but also for drug and chemotherapy administration. Lower extremities should be avoided in all but life-threatening cases where venous access is critical. Upper extremities which are compromised by infection, lymphedema, or hemiparesis should be avoided; extremities where a drug extravasation has occurred should also be avoided.

Several (anecdotal) methods have been used by the authors with success in maintaining and improving venous integrity. These include hand exercising, e.g., squeeze small spongy ball or tubing several times daily and application of warm moist compresses to the extremity, such as a hot towel covered with plastic wrap, or moist heating pads for a minimum of 30 minutes four times a day. These techniques should be started at the beginning of intravenous therapy. When administering chemotherapy it is also useful to alternate the use of the arms or to use the limb opposite the one being used for venipuncture. When it is impossible to use the opposite limb, it is important not to select veins below a recent venipuncture site, as medication may leak through the perforated vein wall.

Extravasation is defined as infiltration of vesicant agent into the tissue outside of a vein. The vesicant agent can cause ulceration and/or tissue necrosis. A photo to document the damage can be useful when this occurs. It is often extremely painful and potentially disfiguring and may require surgical debridement and skin grafting, as shown in Figure 3a-c. This adds further discomfort, pain, and emotional trauma to the patient. The care of such an extravasation injury can be extremely expensive: for these reasons prevention is the best

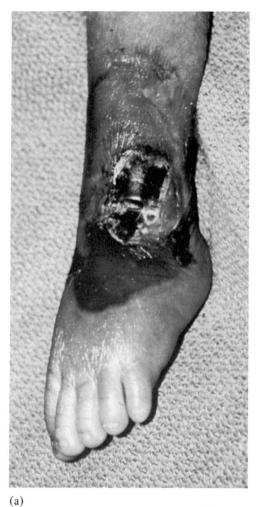

(a)

Figure 3 Necrosis induced by doxorubicin extravasation in a child. Before (a), during (b), and after (c) plastic surgery.

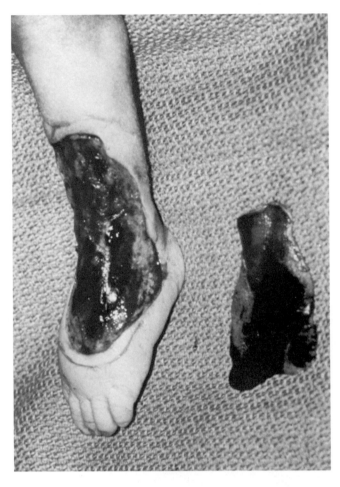

(b)

treatment, but unfortunately the incidence of reported extravasation injuries is on the order of 1-11% (Goldmann et al., 1973). The ulcers produced by extravasation can also be less severe and heal spontaneously, as one induced by vinblastine (Figure 4).

Another consideration in the choice of vein for drug administration is the particular antineoplastic being administered. Some agents, such as dacarbazine or carmustine, cause burning at the injection site and along the vein, even though the drug has not been extravasated. The use of a larger diameter vein or a decrease in drug concentration will serve to minimize this problem. There is some controversy concerning the choice of vein in an extremity: some feel that the

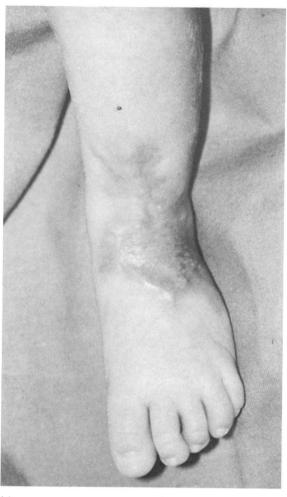

(c)

use of the veins in the dorsum of the hand and inside the wrist should be avoided, as there are major nerves and tendon sheaths just below these areas, and if an extravasation occurred, it could cause permanent damage to the areas. Others recommend using these areas as the choice site for short-term chemotherapy administration as the veins are easy to find and it is usually easy to spot any infiltration early. Another important aspect of extravasation prevention is the education of the patient as mentioned earlier. The patient should be advised that extravasation is a side effect of chemotherapy and that the prompt recognition of pain and discomfort can prevent serious problems. The patient should be instructed to report any pain or discomfort during the administration.

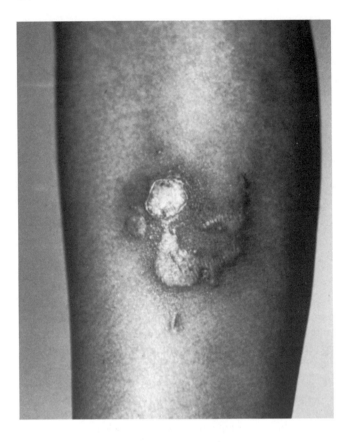

Figure 4   Skin ulcers produced by extravasation of vinblastine.

The technique of drug administration is very important in the prevention of extravasation. Data from this institution show that administration of all vesicant chemotherapeutic agents by "slow I.V. push" method reduces extravasation injuries to less than 1% (Stevenson et al., in press). This technique allows the constant monitoring by the chemotherapists for pain, swelling, and venous patency. When using this technique, the needle should first be checked for placement by flushing with normal saline/sterile water before administering chemotherapy and should be aspirated for blood return every 5-6 cc of medication. This type of one-on-one attention is beneficial not only for the prompt recognition of extravasation, but also is reassuring to the patient and builds a strong nurse-patient relationship from which the entire health care team can benefit.

Another aspect of extravasation prevention has to do with the order of drug administration. This is a controversial issue that has two diametrically opposing arguments. The first is that vesicant agents should be given first, since the initial assessment of vein patency is most accurate, the vein is less irritated at the beginning of therapy and it has been shown that vascular access decreases over time. The opposing argument is that these agents are irritating, may increase fragility, and cause the nonvesicant agents to infiltrate. We cannot resolve this controversy. However, chemotherapy should be administered in a quiet room without interruptions so that the chemotherapists' full attention will be on the patient. It is important to rinse the tubing and vein between drugs, especially at the end of the infusion. This will decrease potential physical drug interaction and reduce venous irritation. If a vesicant drug is to be given by continuous infusion, it should be administered via a central venous line if there is no one to observe the patient during the entire administration. New devices are currently available to aid in this technique (Gyvers et al., 1984; Raaf, 1985).

The use of totally implanted arterial and central venous access devices (e.g., Infusaport, Port-a-cath, etc.) for blood sampling, intermittent or continuous chemotherapy administration can cause some unique problems. Access to these totally implanted devices is performed under sterile conditions using a Huber needle inserted into the skin through a rubber-like septum. There is a possibility that the needle may slip out and the drug would then infiltrate into the tissue. In this instance, the needle can be secured with appropriate sterile adhesive strips and covered with transparent sterile dressing, which allows visibility of the needle site. The site should be monitored closely, particularly if a vesicant agent is being infused. A separate issue is that when inexperienced surgeons are implanting these devices for the first time it is relatively common for them to fit too tightly into the skin "pocket" and cause inflammation and skin erosion, quite independently of the use of drugs. At the time of insertion of these devices, radiographic confirmation of proper placement of the catheter is performed, but it must be remembered that inadvertent withdrawal of the catheter can occur at a later date. This has been referred to as Twidder's syndrome. Instruct the patient to report any discomfort during drug administration; preinjection radiography may be considered (Gebarski and Gebarski, 1984). The totally implanted catheters, unlike the external central venous catheters (e.g., Hickman, Quinim, etc.), do not require site care or frequent heparinization. Observing for site infection and "flushing" after usage is the only care required. With the increasing use of long-term central venous catheters for the oncology patient, a new entity, iatrogenic superior vena cava syndrome, has been reported (Bertland et al., 1984) and occurs without evidence of mediastinal tumor involvement.

Table 8 Vesicant, Irritant, and Non-Vesicant Chemotherapeutic Drugs

Drugs commonly associated with severe local necrosis (vesicants)[a]	Drugs uncommonly associated with severe local necrosis (non-vesicants or irritants)[b]	
Actinomycin-D	L-asparaginase	Imidazole carbox-
Chromomycin-A[3]	Azacytidine	amide (DTIC)**
Daunomycin	Bleomycin	Iphosphamide
Doxorubicin	Carmustine (BCNU)**	6-Mercaptopurine
Mechlorethamine	Cyclocytidine	Methotrexate
Mithramycin	Cyclophosphamide	Cisplatin
Mitomycin-C	Cytarabine (ARA-C)	Thiotepa**
Streptozotocin	5-Fluorouracil	VM-26
Vinblastine	Ftorafur	Etoposide (VP-16)
Vincristine		

[a]Vesicant—an agent that when extravasated produces local necrosis.
[b]Irritant—an agent that when extravasated produces burning or inconsequential inflammation without necrosis. Non-vesicant—an agent devoid of significant vesicant or irritant effects.

Another group of chemotherapeutic agents are those classified as irritants. While these do not cause frank extravasation injuries, they can cause pain and phlebitis and irritate the vein. These agents should be administered by slow intravenous push, as above, but can be administered as continuous infusions if certain precautions are taken. The drug should be administered through a large, high blood volume (flow) vein in a large volume of fluid. This will cause rapid dilution of the drug and thus decrease burning or chemical phlebitis. The patient should be instructed for the signs of infiltration and should be able to call the nurse quickly. The therapy must also be closely monitored. Table 8 classifies the currently used agents into vesicants, irritants, or neither. Table 9 lists the vesicant and irritant agents and provides a suggested treatment for their extravasation. The reader will note that in few instances are these remedies well documented in the clinic.

A procedure for treating a local extravasation of a vesicant agent is as follows: (1) stop infusion; (2) while cannula is in place, aspirate drug from site, if possible; (3) remove cannula; (4) using a 25-27 gauge needle, inject the recommended antidote intradermally around the infiltrated site; (5) apply ice (warm compresses with vinca alkaloids).

Table 9 Antineoplastic Drug Associated with Local Reactions

Drugs	Type of Reaction	Onset of Inflammation	Symptoms	Duration of Reaction	Treatment (Dorr & Fritz, 1980)
Mechlorethamine (nitrogen mustard), HN_2	Vesicant	12-24 hours	Pain	4-6 weeks	Instill vein and tissue area with 10-20 ml of 1/6 M Sodium thiosulfate* followed by cold (hydro-cortisone)
	Vein Discoloration	2 weeks	-	3-4 weeks	None
Doxorubicin (Adriamycin)	Vesicant, recall	1-2 weeks	Pain	Several weeks	Cold packs (hydrocortisone) Followed by early surgical consultation (debridement)
Daunomycin (Cerubidine)	Vesicant	1-2 weeks	Pain	Several weeks	Cold packs (hydrocortisone) Followed by early surgical consultation (debridement)
Dactinomycin (Cosmegen)	Vesicant, recall	1-2 weeks	Pain	Several weeks	Cold packs (hydrocortisone) Followed by early surgical consultation (debridement)
Mitramycin (Mithracin)	Vesicant	1 week	Pain	Several weeks	Cold packs (hydrocortisone) Followed by early surgical consultation (debridement)
Mitomycin-C (Mutamycin)	Vesicant, ?recall	1 week	Pain	Several weeks	Cold packs (hydrocortisone) Followed by early surgical consultation (debridement)

Drug					
Vinblastine (Velban)	Vesicant	12-24 hours	Pain	Several weeks	Cold packs (hydrocortisone) Followed by early surgical consultation (debridement)
Vincristine (Oncovin)	Vesicant	12-24 hours	Pain	Several weeks	Cold packs (hydrocortisone) Followed by early surgical consultation (debridement)
Carmustine (BiCNU)	Burning, even if in vein	Minutes	Pain	During infusion	Cold packs, slow infusion use large vein
Bleomycin (Bleoxane)	Discoloration at SC injection site	-	-	Several weeks	None
Dacarbazine (DTIC)	Pain during infusion	Minutes	Pain	During infusion	Cold packs, slow infusion use large vein
Fluoruracil	Vein Discoloration	-	-	Several weeks	None
Thiotepa	Pain during infusion	Minutes	Pain	During infusion	Cold packs, slow infusion use large vein

*1/6 M solution is made by aseptically combining 4 ml 10% Sodium thiosulfate USP with 6 ml sterile water for injection.

VI. ALOPECIA

Chemotherapy-induced alopecia can be a devastating event to a patient, depending on the importance of one's body image. It constitutes a definite change in physical appearance which is a constant reminder to the patient, family, and friends that cancer has invaded his/her body. Many patients cannot deal with this emotionally and they may withdraw socially, or may even refuse chemotherapy. Emotional support and physical interventions are required to aid the patient in adjusting to this adverse effect.

Hair loss is a result of the effect of antineoplastic drugs on the rapidly dividing cells of the hair follicle that weakens the shaft and causes the hair to break (Munro, 1971). Hair loss usually begins 2-3 weeks after the initial dose of chemotherapy, and usually regrowth begins 4-8 weeks after discontinuing therapy. Scalp hair is primarily affected, but pubic, facial, and axillary hair loss may also occur.

The amount of hair loss from chemotherapy is related to the drug, dosage, and combination of agents received. Doxorubicin and intravenous cyclophosphamide, two agents which are commonly used to treat a variety of malignancies, are notorious for causing alopecia. Other antineoplastic agents that can cause hair loss are vincristine, methotrexate, VP-16, mitomycin-C, daunomycin, cytosine arabinoside, dacarbazine, 5-fluorouracil, and vinblastine. Current studies on methods to decrease alopecia usually include doxorubicin, with reports of 33-75% hair protection, although the best results occur when <50 mg of doxorubicin is used.

Techniques which will totally prevent alopecia are, unfortunately, not available at this time. Scalp tourniquets and/of scalp hypothermia are two methods that have been reported to decrease or prevent alopecia. The rationale is that blood circulation to the scalp vessels will be temporarily constricted, thus decreasing the peak (and total) load of chemotherapy to the hair follicles. The scalp tourniquet can be applied by a variety of methods: by using a Penrose tourniquet in place for 5 minutes prior and 5 minutes after the drug is administered; and by using a pressure cuff in place at 10 mmHg above systolic blood pressure to 300 mm Hg pressure, from just before to 5-30 minutes after the drug is administered (Cline, 1984).

Scalp hypothermia also has been achieved by a variety of cooling methods ranging from crushed ice to gel packs. The devices are applied 5-15 minutes prior to chemotherapy and kept in place for 10-40 minutes after drug administration (Cline, 1984; Dean et al., 1983; Satterwhite and Zimm, 1984). Patients who have impaired liver function and who are receiving doxorubicin have had a decreased effect from scalp hypothermia (Anderson, Hunt, and Smith, 1981). This is probably related to the inability of the liver to clear doxorubicin normally.

Certain factors concerning the neoplastic process must be kept in mind when considering the prevention of alopecia by the above methods. By decreasing the circulation to the scalp it provides a sanctuary site for any malignant cells which happen to be in the field. In general, caution is recommended in using these techniques for patients with hematological malignancies such as leukemia and lymphomas, and in solid tumors such as melanoma which carry a high incidence of scalp metastases (Whitman, Cadman, and Chen, 1981).

Since prevention of chemotherapy-induced alopecia is not always possible, it is of utmost importance to prepare the patient for possible hair loss. Suggesting the use of wigs, scarves, or hats and possible places for their purchase can often be helpful. The hair color and style can be more closely matched by selecting a wig prior to the advent of hair loss.

The health care team must be sensitive to the importance that society places on hair. We must provide the emotional support required to help the patient adapt to this alteration in physical appearance.

VII. CARDIOTOXICITY

Cardiotoxicity is not a common side effect of chemotherapy but when it occurs it can be devastating, particularly in a patient who was cured by the drug. Table 10 summarizes the agents that can cause cardiotoxicity. Although these cardiotoxic effects should be considered whenever a treated patient with cancer presents with a cardiac disorder, there are a multitude of more common etiologies for cardiac disease which should be considered first, such as a preexisting disease (i.e., atherosclerotic cardiovascular disease), involvement of the heart of pericardium by tumor, infection, and others (Rozencweig, Piccart, and Von Hoff, 1981).

The anthracyclines (doxorubicin, Adriamycin, daunorubicin, Cerubidine) are both active against a wide range of tumors, but it is cardiotoxicity which limits their long-term clinical use. The cardiotoxic effects of both drugs can be divided into two categories: (1) acute effects on the heart manifested by electrocardiographic abnormalities, and (2) a cumulative dose-dependent cardiomyopathy.

The incidence of EKG changes associated with the administration of doxorubicin and daunorubicin ranges from 0-41 and 0-1% respectively (Von Hoff, Rozencweig, and Piccart, 1982). Because most of the investigators who report abnormalities have not performed continuous cardiac monitoring the incidence (especially for daunorubicin) may be underestimated. Also, many patients with cancer are febrile, anemic, and malnourished, all of which can contribute to cardiographic changes. Electrocardiographic changes have been noted during and after drug administration and these include virtually every possible arrhythmia. They are reversible and of little consequence except under unusual

Table 10   Cardiotoxicity of Antineoplastic Agents

Drug	Toxicity
Known cardiotoxic drugs	
Doxorubicin	EKG changes, cardiomyopathy
Daunorubicin	EKG changes, cardiomyopathy
Cyclophosphamide (high dose)	Cardiac necrosis
Diethylstilbesterol	Increased cardiovascular deaths
Possibly cardiotoxic drugs	
Mitoxantrone	EKG changes, cardiomyopathy
5-Fluorouracil	Angina, myocardial infarction
Busulfan	Endocardial fibrosis
Mitomycin-C	Myocardial damage (rare)
Cisplatin	EKG changes (rare)
Methotrexate (high dose)	EKG changes
Vincristine	Myocardial infarction
Vinblastine	Precordial pain
Etoposide	Myocardial infarction
Alpha interferon	EKG changes

circumstances. Continuous monitoring of the patient is not warranted. These changes appear to be unrelated to total dose and apparently are not associated with the development of cardiomyopathy (Von Hoff, Rozencweig, and Piccart, 1982). The one exception may be the diminished QRS voltage which some investigators believe is related to total dose of drug.

The development of transient, benign electrocardiographic changes is usually not an indication to discontinue therapy with these agents. On the other hand, one cannot feel secure even with a normal recent EKG since life-threatening ventricular arrhythmias and sudden death have been reported during or just after doxorubicin administration (Wortman et al., 1979).

The most serious cardiotoxicity that is associated with anthracycline therapy is drug-induced cardiomyopathy. This toxicity has a mortality of up to 61%. The incidence ranges from 0.4-9% of all patients receiving doxorubicin and is less well-defined for daunorubicin. Anthracycline cardiomyopathy is discussed extensively in the literature and details of pathology, clinical presentation and treatment are beyond the scope of this chapter. For purposes of this book however, it will be useful to review the predisposing factors, means of early detection, and experimental methods of prophylaxis.

There is no doubt that the total dose of the anthracyclines is the most significant known risk factor for development of drug-induced cardiomyopathy; this recognition has led to the recommendation that the administration of doxorubicin be stopped when the cumulative dose of 550 mg/M^2 has been reached (600 mg for daunomycin). This absolute cutoff has caused worry among investigators because there are certainly a sizable number of patients who reach these doses when their tumor is still responding, and the clinician is faced with the dilemma of stopping an effective drug. In a study of more than 4000 patients there was no absolute point where drug should be stopped under any circumstances (Von Hoff et al., 1979). This information has lent support to the concept that the clinician caring for the patient must balance the benefit of discontinuing the drug at a predetermined point against the risk of progressive tumor when the drug is discontinued.

Dose schedule is also a risk factor with studies showing that lower weekly doses may be less cardiotoxic yet as efficacious as higher doses given every 3 weeks (Von Hoff et al., 1979). Continuous infusion therapy is another good alternative to high-dose bolus therapy. Other important predisposing risk factors are the patient's age, prior cardiac disease, prior mediastinal radiation, and the use of other cardiotoxic drugs such as cyclophosphamide. Depending on the circumstances some change in strategy such as dose reduction (e.g., by 100 mg/M^2) or the substitution of alternative drugs are usually indicated.

A variety of monitoring techniques has been employed in an attempt at early detection of cardiomyopathy and before irreversible changes have taken place. Noninvasive methods to detect heart failure have included physical examination, serial chest x-rays, electrocardiograms, cardiac enzyme measurements, echocardiography and systolic time intervals, QRS-Korotkoff interval measurements, and radionuclide cineangiography. Although none are uniformly successful in early detection, QRS-Korotkoff interval measurements may reflect subclinical cardiomyopathy (Greco et al., 1975; Greco, 1978). Radionuclide cineangiography studies are ongoing but this technique seems to be the most accepted noninvasive method of predicting CHF. Further work is needed to establish workable guidelines for obtaining the scans and accurate criteria for the discontinuation of the anthracycline. Percutaneous endomyocardial biopsy to monitor the myocardium for damage, although not widely available, has demonstrated a direct relationship between the total dose administered and the severity of the pathological changes in the myocardium. The value of this technique and its optimal use has not yet been established on a routine basis.

A variety of agents have been used preclinically and clinically in attempts to prevent the occurrence of anthracycline-induced CHF. These agents include prednisone, digitalis, coenzyme Q10, alpha tocopherol (Vit. E) adenosine, ICRF-187, and liposome encapsulation of the anthracycline. Whereas this continues to be an active area of research, no truly convincing data have proved that any of these agents do in fact prevent anthracycline-induced CHF.

Although cardiotoxicity is not uncommon with the anthracyclines, it is rare for most other antineoplastic agents. Table 10 summarizes the cardiotoxic potential of the other agents.

VIII. PULMONARY TOXICITY

Although pulmonary toxicity has been associated with a variety of antineoplastic agents, its occurrence is generally infrequent and sporadic except with
the cumulative dose-related toxicity that is recognized with bleomycin and the
nitrosoureas (Comis, 1978; Ginsberg and Comis, 1982; Aronin et al., 1980).
Table 11 summarizes the toxicity of antineoplastic agents and their known or
associated risk factors. It is beyond the scope of this chapter to detail all of
the clinical signs, symptoms and treatment of chemotherapy-induced pulmonary
toxicity; there are several excellent reviews covering the total scope of this
problem, an example of which is by Ginsberg and Comis (1984). The purpose
of this section is to suggest preventive measures.

A. Bleomycin

Bleomycin pulmonary toxicity is often heralded by the development of a dry
hacking cough, followed by exertional dyspnea. Progressive pulmonary involvement may be associated with dyspnea at rest, tachypnea, fever, and cyanosis.
Emergence of the problem can be insidious in that symptoms may develop as
late as 1-3 months *after* discontinuing bleomycin. The earliest physical finding
associated with bleomycin toxicity is the presence of fine crackling bibasilar
rales that progress to coarse rales involving the lower third of the lung fields.
Rhonchi, and occasionally a pleural friction rub, may be heard. On standard
chest radiogrpahy the earliest sign of bleomycin toxicity is that of fine reticu-
lar bibasilar infiltrates which may progress to bibasilar alveolar and interstitial
infiltrates.

Numerous studies have shown that abnormalities in pulmonary function
tests may precede the onset of clinically detectable bleomycin pulmonary
toxicity and because of this it is recommended that patients receiving bleomycin
be tested periodically. Although guidelines for discontinuing therapy based upon
test information have not been absolutely defined, further bleomycin therapy
should be withheld if the diffusing capacity (DLCO) falls to <40% of the initial
value, if the forced vital capacity (FVC) falls to <25% of the initial value, or if
any of the signs, symptoms, or radiographic features associated with bleomycin
pulmonary toxicity occur. Patients with the following increased risk factors of
bleomycin pulmonary toxicity should be observed for toxicity particularly
closely: (1) age >70; (2) prior or concomitant radiotherapy to the lungs; (3)
hypoxia; (4) use of high oxygen concentrations (i.e., anesthesia) subsequent to
bleomycin; (5) previous exposure to bleomycin (within 6 months); (6) past
history of smoking or pulmonary disease; (7) Hodgkin's lymphoma and/or concurrent use of cyclophosphamide. Although there is not a clear dose-response
curve for the incidence of pulmonary toxicity, the incidence increases significantly as cumulative doses rise to doses above 500 units. Figure 5a,b illustrate

Table 11 Pulmonary Toxicity

Agent	Nature of toxicity	Incidence	Risk factors
		Known Pulmonary Toxins	
Bleomycin	Fibrosis	Fatal: 1-2%	Age >70; pulmonary radiation therapy
		Non-fatal: 2-3%	High oxygen concentration; prior bleomycin or concurrent cyclophosphamide; non-Hodgkin's lymphoma
Mitomycin-C	Fibrosis	3-12%	Prior mitomycin-C Rx; high oxygen concentration
Nitrosoureas	Fibrosis	20-30% with doses >1000 mg/M^2	Preexisting lung disease, smoking; ?concurrent chemo- and radiotherapy
Busulfan	Fibrosis; occasional calcification and pulmonary ossification	3%	Radiotherapy to lung
		Possibly Pulmonary Toxins	
Cyclophosphamide	Fibrosis	Unknown at present	Most often reported in Hodgkin's disease and non-Hodgkin's lymphoma
Chlorambucil	Fibrosis	Unknown at present	None identified
Melphalan	Fibrosis	Only 7 cases to date	None identified
Methotrexate	Allergic Delayed pneumonitis	Probably uncommon	None identified
	Immediate pulmonary edema	3 cases reported	None identified
	Severe pleuritic chest pain	4-8%	None identified
Cytosine arabinoside	Pulmonary edema	Unknown at present	None identified
Procarbazine	Hypersensitivity	Rare	None identified

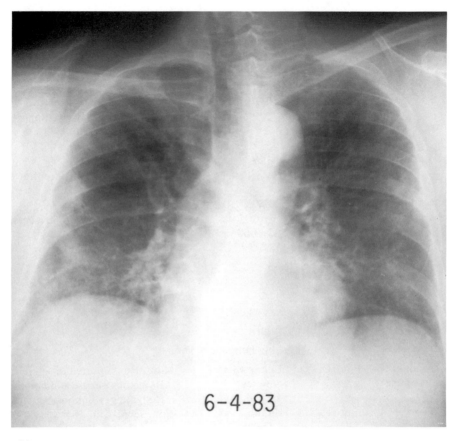

(a)

Figure 5 Bleomycin-induced pulmonary toxicity (a) followed by total resolution (b).

the chest x-ray of a patient who was being treated for head and neck cancer with bleomycin when he rapidly became dyspneic and severely hypoxic. He was treated with high-dose corticosteroids and after a few weeks had returned back to baseline and his x-ray findings disappeared permanently. There was no attempt to further use the drug.

B. Mitomycin-C

Although not frequently reported, pulmonary toxicity from mitomycin-C is definitely a risk in use of this agent. The pathology is similar to that of bleomycin.

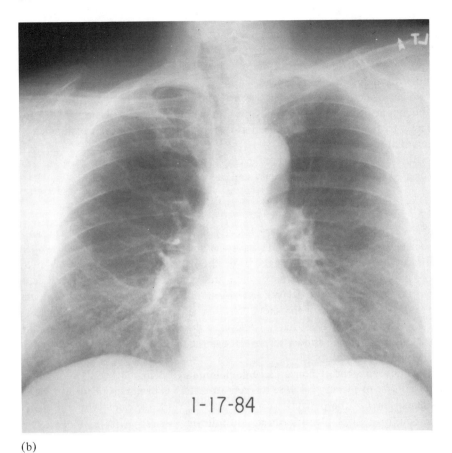

1-17-84

(b)

Serial pulmonary function studies have not been studied prospectively but a decrease in DLCO has been reported in a few patients. Risk factors similar to those associated with bleomycin, particularly the use of supportive oxygen therapy, can predict for toxicity risk with cumulative doses ranging between 40 and 350 mg: symptoms have even been reported following the initial course of therapy.

C. Alkylating Agents

Busulfan (Myleran) was the first chemotherapeutic agent to be associated with pulmonary toxicity. The symptoms of busulfan pulmonary toxicity include the insidious onset of dyspnea, dry cough, and fever that may progress over a period of weeks to months. Weakness and weight loss are also frequently described.

Tachypnea and bilateral crepitant basilar rales are characteristically described, and cyanosis has occasionally been noted. Most commonly the chest radiograph shows a diffuse linear infiltrate. The DLCO is decreased and a restrictive ventilatory defect has sometimes been seen.

No clear relationship exists between the total busulfan dose and the incidence of pulmonary toxicity. There may be a threshold of 500 mg however. Radiotherapy to the chest prior to busulfan therapy may enhance the development of interstitial pneumonitis.

Other alkylating agents such as cyclophosphamide and carmustine have been associated with pulmonary toxicity and are described in Table 11.

D. Methotrexate

Three distinct types of pulmonary toxicity have now been described that can be associated with methotrexate. There is the delayed parenchymal disease which curiously has headache and malaise as prodromal symptoms and there are two more immediate types of toxicity: noncardiogenic pulmonary edema and acute pleuritic chest pain. The delayed toxicity is not associated with total dose, but there does appear to be a threshold effect since patients receiving weekly doses of less than 20 mg are not likely to develop the syndrome. Leucovorin administration has not been shown to protect against this (or any) pulmonary toxicity of methotrexate.

The development of noncardiogenic pulmonary edema occurring 6-12 hours after an oral or intrathecal dose of methotrexate has been described in three patients: two of the patients have died and the third recovered within 3 days. The development of pleuritic chest pain following therapy with methotrexate occurred in 4-8% of patients from two series. The pain lasted for 3-5 days and did recur following some but not all subsequent doses. Interestingly, none of the patients experienced any late pulmonary toxicity.

Pulmonary toxicity associated with the administration of antineoplastic agents is increasing in frequency as more effective combination regimens lead to increased survival and remissions, thus allowing the administration of higher total doses of drugs and sufficient time to observe late manifestations. Another factor that may contribute to the increase is better supportive therapy (platelets, antibiotics, antiemetics), thus allowing higher doses to be given acutely. Table 11 summarizes the drugs associated with this toxicity.

IX. ALLERGIC REACTIONS

Antineoplastic agents can cause a hypersensitivity response and some of these agents are more notorious for anaphylactic reactions and local hypersensitivities than others. They are as follows: L-asparaginase, bleomycin, doxorubicin, cisplatin, cyclophosphamide, VP-16, and VM-26.

When discussing allergic reactions it is necessary to describe the reaction that each drug may produce. L-asparaginase can cause anaphylaxis during the first course of treatment and the likelihood of that happening increases with subsequent courses. Performance of an intradermal skin test is recommended prior to giving the initial dose and when there has been a lapse of a week or more between doses, although the skin test is not totally predictable (Elspar Merck, Sharp and Dohme, 1983). Because of the high risk of anaphylaxis the drug should be administered via a "running" intravenous line, with antihistamines and/or steroids being readily available.

Bleomycin reactions are characterized by fever and chills that are usually self-limiting. These may be prevented by using diphenhydramine (Benadryl) and acetaminophen (Tylenol) as premedication. Anaphylactic reactions occur primarily in lymphoma patients and these may be delayed up to 24 hours (Dorr and Fritz, 1980; Bristol Laboratories, 1982). A pretreatment test dose of 1-5 units subcutaneously is recommended.

Doxorubicin may produce urticaria along the course of the vein during drug administration. If this occurs, hydrocortisone and/or diphenhydramine is recommended. If anaphylaxis has occurred, though infrequently, this agent should be administered with caution and then only if there is no suitable alternative (Dorr and Fritz, 1980; Adria Laboratories, 1982).

Intravenous cyclophosphamide can produce posterior pharyngeal sensations, dyspnea and facial flushing (Arena, 1972). These problems are self-limited and no treatment is required. This drug also has been reported to produce anaphylactic reactions (Karchmer and Hansen, 1977), although infrequently. There is a possible correlation between an allergic reaction to cyclophosphamide and that seen in mechlorethamine-sensitive patients (Ross and Bruce, 1977).

Cisplatin is an interesting agent since anaphylaxis usually does not occur until several doses have been administered (Bristol Laboratories, 1983a). Therefore, it is necessary to keep up-to-date records and be alert for an allergic response.

VM-26 has also been associated with hypersensitivity reactions in up to 10% of patients. Such allergic reactions usually occur after several doses, but may require only one (Weiss, 1982): the treatment consists of the use of hydrocortisone and diphenhydramine.

VP-16 anaphylactoid reactions have been reported in 0.7-2% of the patients receiving this agent (Bristol Laboratories, 1983b). Anaphylactic reactions are characterized by tachycardia, wheezing, shortness of breath, urticaria, and hypotension. Routine treatments for anaphylaxis using epinephrine (1 mg 1:1000), corticosteroids and diphenhydramine (25-50 mg I.V.), and hydrocortisone (100 mg I.V.) are generally effective. Since the above antineoplastic agents can potentiate anaphylactoid reactions, they should be given in a setting with emergency equipment nearby and be administered by personnel who have knowledge of the side effects and their treatments.

X. SKIN TOXICITY

Skin eruptions that occur in patients who are receiving cancer chemotherapeutic
agents may have a variety of causes. Direct toxic effects of the agent on skin
and cutaneous appendages cause the most frequent and distinctive reactions
and these are discussed elsewhere in this chapter. Hypersensitivity reactions do
occur to many of these agents, although much less commonly than drugs such
as penicillin, and these are also discussed separately. Chemotherapeutic
agents may indirectly cause unpredictable rashes by destroying tumor cells, affecting circulating immune complexes, affecting suppressor mechanisms of immune reactions, and releasing mediators of inflammation from necrotic tumor
masses (Dunagin, 1982). Such reactions are highly variable, are difficult to
study, and may account for many of the "one of a kind" rashes that do not
fit regularly reported patterns. Table 12 summarizes reported reactions for the
commonly used agents.

Changes in finger- and toenails during the course of chemotherapy may include pigmentation, Beau's lines (transverse lines usually seen after wasting
diseases), Muehrcke's lines (paired white transverse bands), brittleness, and
slowed growth. Pigmentation is the most frequent change. Dark coloration
of the nail during chemotherapy is much more common and more intense in
black patients than in whites. The pigment is deposited at the base of the
nail and advances outward as the nail grows. With regular or continuous
therapy a diffuse and even darkening occurs whereas with intermittent therapy,
transverse dark bands alternating with bands of normal color appear to correlate
with the time of administration of the offending agents. The agents most likely
to effect nails are cyclophosphamide, doxorubicin and mitomycin-C (Lockich
and Moore, 1984). Others include melphalan, 5-fluorouracil, daunomycin, and
bleomycin. Combinations of drugs increase the likelihood of producing band-
ing of nails even when each of the individual agents may rarely do so alone.
Often the increased pigmentation of nails is associated with hyperpigmentation
of the skin. There is nothing much that can or need be done about these
cosmetic changes save to reassure the patient that they are not harmful and that
they could reverse slowly if these drugs were discontinued.

Many of the cancer chemotherapeutic agents can cause hyper- or hypopig-
mentation of the skin and mucous membranes, but the patterns and mechanisms
vary widely (Dunagin, 1982). Sometimes the pigmentation is temporary, and
often resolves after stopping therapy. After prolonged use, however, the pigmentation may be more persistent (Figure 6). Photosensitivity reactions to
methotrexate and 5-fluorouracil leave residual tanning in the distribution of
sunlight exposure. Hyperpigmentation may follow enhanced reactions to
ionizing radiation. 5-Fluorouracil and BCNU also are capable of causing a
peculiar pigmentation of the veins into which the drug is administered. The
veins underlying the pigment remain patent, nontender, and nonsclerosed.

Table 12 Reported Skin Reactions for Commonly Used Agents

Agent name	Pigmentation	Radiation recall	Nail problems	Erythema	Allergic	Miscellaneous
Mechlorethamine					Occasional	
Cyclophosphamide	Occasional	Occasional	Frequent		Occasional	Occ. sq. cell Ca. of skin
Chlorambucil					Occasional	
Melphalan			Occasional		Occasional	
Busulfan	Frequent				Occasional	
Thiotepa	Occasional				Occasional	
Methotrexate	Occasional	Frequent		Occasional	Occasional	
5-Fluorouracil	Frequent	Frequent	Occasional		Occasional	
6-Mercaptopurine		Occasional			Occasional	
Vinblastine		Occasional			Occasional	
Doxorubicin	Occasional	Frequent	Frequent	Occasional	Occasional	
Daunorubicin			Occasional		Occasional	
Bleomycin	Frequent	Occasional	Occasional		Occasional	Fibrosis and skin edema
Dactinomycin	Occasional	Frequent			Occasional	Folliculitis
Mithramycin				Frequent	Occasional	
Carmustine	Occasional			Frequent		
Cisplatin	Occasional			Occasional	Occasional	
Hydroxyurea		Frequent	Occasional	Occasional	Occasional	
Dacarbazine				Frequent		
Procarbazine	Occasional			Occasional	Occasional	
L-asparaginase					Frequent	

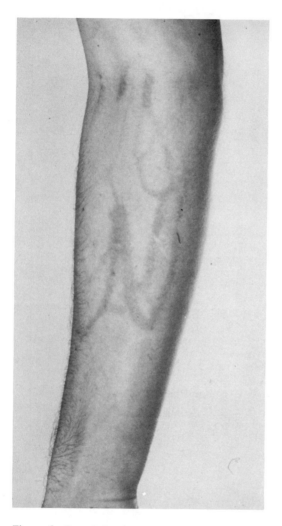

Figure 6 Serpentine hyperpigmentation produced by continuous infusion of 5-fluorouracil.

Several chemotherapeutic drugs are capable of severely damaging tissues that have received radiation exposure. These reactions which differ from a drug's usual toxicity on nonirradiated tissues are often termed "radiation recall" reactions; however, the radiation may be before, concurrent with, or even after administration of the drug in some cases. Sometimes these reactions can be exploited therapeutically to enhance tumor destruction, but more often, they are a complication of therapy. Certain drugs are much more likely to produce these effects than others because they interfere with cellular processes of radiation repair. These reactions occur most commonly in the skin and secondly in the mucous membranes. Drugs that are most associated with radiation enhancement are doxorubicin and actinomycin-D, and less commonly with 5-fluorouracil, bleomycin, and hydroxyurea.

The usual result of radiation-drug interaction is erythema followed by a dry desquamation of the skin. However, more severe cases develop vesicles and oozing. Necrosis with persistent, painful ulceration occurs in the most severe cases. Milder cases can be treated with steroid creams, but radiation ulcers are extremely slow to heal and difficult to treat.

A more recent side effect, palmar-plantar erythrodysesthesia syndrome, has been reported when administering systemic continuous chemotherapy (particularly 5-FU) over an extended period of time (Lokich and Moore, 1984). This is characterized by tingling of hands and feet, followed by pain with the palms and soles being swollen and erythematous. When chemotherapy is interrupted there is gradual resolution over 5-7 days with desquamation of the skin on the hands and soles. We have observed this syndrome in a patient receiving Floxuridine for 14 days each month by hepatic artery infusion via an implanted infusion pump (Figure 7). Reducing the dosage or using an analog drug has not always been successful in continuing to use the treatment.

Most of the reactions above cannot be predicted or prevented. Careful explanation of possible reactions will help decrease the patient's anxiety if a minor reaction occurs and may help the patient recognize more serious reactions and hasten treatment. Patients receiving drugs that may cause photosensitivity reactions should be warned to reduce their sun exposure by staying out of the sun, wearing clothes that cover all exposed areas, or covering the areas with sun screens containing high concentrations of PABA. Careful radiation port planning can reduce the severity of radiation recall effects. Prompt treatment of these reactions can reduce morbidity.

XI. GASTROINTESTINAL AND LIVER TOXICITY

A. Gastrointestinal Toxicity

The gastrointestinal and oral epithelium is a normal physiological model of rapid cell turnover. Thus it is commonly a target for the action of many anticancer

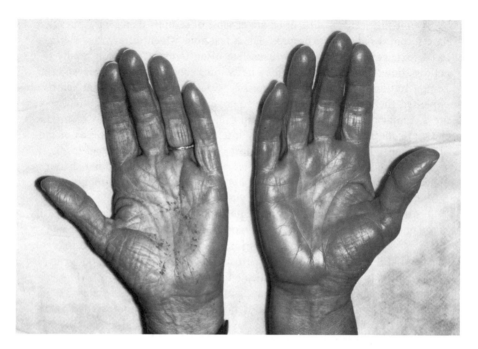

Figure 7 Foot-hand syndrome is associated with repeated infusions of chemotherapy.

agents (Dorr and Fritz, 1980; Lucarelli, 1984). Proctitis or small intestinal ulcerations with bleeding may be observed on occasion. The possibility of unmasking
a latent or indolent peptic ulcer is present when corticosteroids are used chronically or in high doses. Stress ulcers may occur in severely ill cancer patients
and these may be aggravated by chemotherapy. However, in general, a history
of peptic ulcer disease does not represent a contraindication to the use of anticancer drugs.

Stomatitis produced by cancer drugs is a painful irritation to the oral mucosal
tissues. There is relatively little that can be done to prevent this side effect,
however, the following suggestion may reduce morbidity. For several drugs (i.e.,
bleomycin, fluorouracil, and methotrexate), the early onset of severe oral lesions
may herald impending serious systemic toxicity and the need for prompt dose

reduction or discontinuance. The occurrence of moderate or severe stomatitis requires some reduction of drug dosage on subsequent courses. The cytotoxic effects of the agent on rapidly dividing mucosal cells are dose related and usually appear a few days to a week or more following treatment. The frequency of drug administration can also be crucial and is with the high incidence of oral ulcers following frequent administration of even small doses of methotrexate. Thus, an actual loss of cells occurs with minute ulcerations and denuded mucosa. The cell cycle-specific agents, such as methotrexate, are more likely to cause this toxicity than other drugs (Table 13) (Dorr and Fritz, 1980; Lucarelli, 1984). The long-term complications of stomatitis can contribute to malnutrition if severe and may be the dose-limiting toxicity. Curiously, the mucositis of high doses of 5-FU, particularly by the 5-consecutive-day regimen, is also likely to produce bloody diarrhea.

A good oral hygiene regimen is of vital importance in the prevention and treatment of stomatitis and oral infections in chemotherapy patients. A regimen for patients at risk is to remove dentures or keep them meticulously clean to prevent irritation. Routine, gentle brushing with a soft toothbrush or toothette (disposable foam stick) after meals and every 4 hours removes dental plaque. Normal saline is used as a mouthwash after brushing. Mouthwashes containing alcohol are not used because they may promote oral ulceration. Hydrogen peroxide should not be used because it can cause an overgrowth of white papillae on the tongue (an excellent substrate for *Candida*) and may be damaging to tissues. When mucositis occurs then we add a mouthwash containing an antibiotic such as Nystatin or tetracycline, depending on the situation. The regimen outlined above may be increased to every 2 hours for patients who have moderate to severe stomatitis.

Dry mouth or xerostomia is a common complication of chemotherapy. Lubricants can keep the membranes moist and pliable for up to two hours. Commercially available artificial saliva preparations contain electrolytes in a carboxymethylcellulose base. They loosen mucus and prevent mucous membranes from stocking together. Mineral oil and petroleum jelly, which were used in the past, should not be used if the patient is receiving oxygen because they can be aspirated. They should be used only on the lips. Water-soluble jellies that form a film on the skin make excellent lip lubricants and can be used by patients receiving oxygen.

Pain in the oral cavity from stomatitis can hamper the maintenance of oral hygiene and nutrition. This pain can be managed by local anesthetics, such as dyclonine HC1, lidocaine, diphenhydramine, and cocaine solution. Patients should be cautioned not to eat or drink for 1 hour after using a local anesthetic because of the danger of aspiration and to allow it to remain in longer contact with the mucosal surface.

Table 13   Chemotherapeutic Agents Commonly Associated with Mucositis

Drug	Notes
Methotrexate	May be quite severe with prolonged infusions or compromised renal function Severity is enhanced by irradiation May be prevented with adequate and timely leucovorin rescue
5-Fluorouracil	More severe with higher doses, frequent schedule, arterial infusions
Dactinomycin	Very common and may prevent oral alimentation Severity is enhanced by irradiation
Doxorubicin	May be severe and ulcerative Increased with liver disease Severity is enhanced by irradiation
Bleomycin	May be severe and ulcerative
Vinblastine	Frequently ulcerative

We have mentioned the mucositis and diarrhea that may result from administration of antimetabolites such as methotrexate and 5-fluorouracil and this may also be observed with hydroxyurea, nitrosourea, and alkylating agents. The contrary problem of constipation and even adynamic ileus can be noted in patients receiving vinca alkaloids such as vincristine in particular. This can be particularly insidious in the older age group and it should therefore be anticipated and treated prophylactically with mild laxatives and the use of stool softeners.

Gastrointestinal infections secondary to neutropenia following chemotherapy have been discussed earlier, but are particularly common in patients with leukemia and lymphoma. When the combination of potent cytotoxic agents, radiation to the gastrointestinal tract, antimicrobial therapy, and corticosteroids are used, then one must be particularly vigilant against infections throughout the G.I. tract.

B. Hepatotoxicity

The liver plays a central role in drug metabolism because of the differentiated role of hepatocytes and also partly because of its unique dual blood supply from the portal vein and the hepatic artery. Intravenously administered drugs reach the liver via the hepatic artery, and drugs given orally arrive via the portal vein from the gastrointestinal tract. The potential susceptibility of the liver to toxic drug reactions is thus not surprising.

Determining whether or not a chemotherapeutic agent is hepatotoxic is often difficult because of the multiplicity of potentially toxic events that can affect the liver of a patient with cancer. Patients are usually exposed to a variety of medications in treating the direct and indirect effects of the tumor. This makes it difficult to pinpoint any one drug as the cause of a particular side effect. For example, the immunosuppressive effects of chemotherapy may predispose to complicating infections involving the liver, transfusion of blood products adds the risk of viral hepatitis, the liver is a common site of metastases that can alter its function (Zimmerman, 1978), and so on. A further complicating factor is that the metabolism of many chemotherapeutic agents in man is unclear, as is the potential for metabolites to cause hepatotoxicity. It is important that those drugs known to regularly cause hepatic toxicity be identified so that they can be replaced (if possible) or used at a lower dose, if necessary. Table 14 shows chemotherapeutic agents and the type of hepatic toxicity which they produce.

A separate but also important issue is to recognize that drugs which are not toxic to the liver but which are metabolized there may require dose adjustment in the face of hepatic dysfunction, regardless of the cause. This is generally attributable to the sustained blood levels resulting from impaired hepatic clearance. Impaired liver function due to alcoholic liver disease or other forms of liver disease make it particularly difficult to use chemotherapy on a chronic basis, and not particularly against non-neoplastic conditions such as with the use of methotrexate in severe psoriasis. There are no absolute guidelines except to tailor the therapy to the individual and monitor quite closely if chemotherapy is used in such cases. Table 15 summarizes dose reduction suggestions in the presence of hepatic toxicity (Perry, 1984).

Among the more controversial issues, particularly in patients who have non-neoplastic diseases such as psoriasis, is that of chronic hepatotoxicity from long-term use of methotrexate. Clearly, fibrosis and cirrhosis of the liver can result from use of this drug, more so when it is used on a daily oral basis than the more commonly used intermittent intramuscular administration (Weinstein, 1977). This type of problem is rarely associated with liver failure, but whether or not the risk of hepatotoxicity should dictate the long-term use of a drug in an older patient with very severe psoriasis is the subject of some debate. Very often these very same patients also have a history of chronic alcoholism and may have baseline liver disease: this is best documented by an initial liver biopsy and probably by periodic biopsies, since liver function tests are not sufficient predictors of the degree of hepatic toxicity. High doses of 6-mercaptopurine may also induce hepatotoxicity, either due to hepatocellular disease or to obstructive liver disease: this is also true of azathioprine, which is often used in the prevention of organ transplantation rejection. For more extensive information concerning hepatotoxicity, the reader is referred to the chapter by Perry (1984).

Table 14 Chemotherapeutic Agents Producing Hepatic Toxicity

Drug	Effects
Nitrosoureas	
Carmustine	Elevated liver enzymes
Lomustine	Elevated liver enzymes
Streptozotocin	Elevated liver enzymes
Antimetabolites	
Methotrexate	Fibrosis, cirrhosis
6-Mercaptopurine	Cholestasis, necrosis
Azathioprine	Cholestasis, necrosis
Cytosine arabinoside	Elevated liver enzymes
Antibiotics	
Mithramycin	Acute necrosis
Enzymes	
L-asparaginase	Fatty metamorphosis

Table 15 Dose Modification with Hepatic Dysfunction

	Percent of usual dose to administer:			
Drug	Bilirubin $<$1.5 mg% and SGOT $<$60 IU	Bilirubin = 1.5-3.0 or SGOT = 60-180	Bilirubin = 3.1-5.0 or SGOT $>$180	Bilirubin $>$5.0
5-Fluorouracil	100	100	100	Omit
Cyclophosphamide	100	100	75	Omit
Methotrexate	100	100	75	Omit
Daunorubicin	100	75	50	Omit
Doxorubicin	100	50	25	Omit
Vinblastine	100	50	Omit	Omit
Vincristine	100	50	Omit	Omit
Etoposide	100	50	Omit	Omit

Source: Modified from Perry and Yarbro (1984).

XII. TOXICITY TO THE URINARY TRACT

Patients treated with many antineoplastic and immunosuppressive agents are at increased risk of developing renal and metabolic derangements. These may be secondary to the disease process or to therapy. Pathophysiologic mechanisms of disease-induced nephrotoxicity include hyperuricemia, hypercalcemia, immune complex deposition, renal vascular obstruction, amyloidosis, direct tumor invasion, and paraproteinemic nephropathy. The rapid tumor lysis syndrome with its attendant hyperuricemia and hyperphosphatemia is a cause of renal dysfunction which relates to the treatment of neoplasms, but not specifically to any particular agent. Fortunately the prophylactic use of allopurinol (300-900 mg/day) has largely eliminated the problem of hyperuricemic nephropathy in patients who have bulky tumors which are expected to lyse rapidly with chemotherapy (i.e., lymphoma). As distinct from such general processes, a number of immunosuppressive and antineoplastic agents may be directly associated with severe nephrotoxicity and these are listed in Table 16, along with suggested protective measures (Shilsky, 1984; Raymond, 1984).

Renal dysfunction induced by these agents may be evidenced by a reduction in glomerular filtration rate (GFR) or by defects in the tubular reabsorption of single or multiple solutes. In addition, chemotherapy may have indirect effects on renal function via changes in antidiuretic hormone (ADH) or volume and electrolyte status caused by vomiting or other gastrointestinal effects. Chemotherapy-induced renal defects generally effect the tubular cells but some agents (anthracyclines, mitomycin-C) induce glomerular damage (Harden et al., 1982), some cause vascular changes (cyclosporin-A, mitomycin-C), and some induce metabolic derangements (vincristine, cyclophosphamide).

Very significant risks are associated with certain agents such as the short-term use of cisplatin, streptozotocin, high-dose methotrexate, and high-dose mithramycin. Indeed, the formidable problems of nephrotoxicity stalled the development of cisplatin for some years until safe and relatively simple ways of infusing it were found, a decisive point in the ability to use this drug to cure testicular cancer.

In particular, the cumulative renal toxicity associated with cisplatin can be very severe and the tendency for this to happen is increased by lack of ample hydration and diuresis in advance of drug administration, a patient having pre-existing elevation in serum creatinine or creatinine clearance, and also as the drug is used in higher doses and more frequent intervals with repeated courses. It is important for renal function tests to return to normal before repeat courses of cisplatin are given. Since nausea and vomiting are also common complications of the use of this drug and may persist long after the patient leaves the clinic, it is important to insure adequate hydration, such as by the use of pretreatment hydration with 1-2 L of fluid during the hours preceding

Table 16 Nephrotoxic Antitumor Agents

Drug	Azotemia	Tubular dysfunction	Site of pathology	Reversible	Protection
Streptozotocin	Yes	No	Tubular	Yes	None
Nitrosoureas	Yes	No	Glomerular and tubular	No	Limit dose to 1500 mg/M²
Methotrexate	Yes	No	Tubular	Yes	Hydration and urinary alkalinization
Cisplatin	Yes	Yes	Tubular	Yes	Saline hydration, mannitol diuresis
Mitomycin-C	Yes	No	Glomerular and tubular	No	None
Azacytidine	No	Yes	?	?	?
Mithramycin	Yes	No	Tubular	No	None
Cyclophosphamide (cystitis)	No	Yes	–	Yes	Limit free water intake
	–	–	Bladder	Yes	Increase fluid intake, void frequency, especially before sleep

chemotherapy, diluting the drug in 2 L of 5% dextrose in half-normal saline containing 37.5 g of mannitol and infused over a period of 4-6 hours, and providing
for adequate hydration and urinary output during the subsequent 24 hours.

Agents such as the nitrosoureas and cyclophosphamide can induce nephrotoxic effects after long-term use, and there is even a risk of developing bladder
cancer. Cyclophosphamide-induced chemical cystitis is a particularly troublesome problem with estimates of some degree of hemorrhagic cystitis occurring
in approximately 10% of patients who receive an average dose therapy and going
up several fold in patients who receive very high-dose cyclophosphamide as part
of an ablative bone marrow transplantation program. The cornerstone of prevention again is vigorous hydration, maintaining a consistent urinary flow. Once
hemorrhagic cystitis occurs, it is necessary to stop the therapy; a variety of
agents have been used to sclerose the bladder, including even the use of formalde-
hyde. More recently, bladder irrigation with N-acetyl cysteine has been encouraging as has the substitution of ifosphomide in place of cyclophosphamide. When
the complication is very severe, it can last for months and even require cystectomy
in extreme cases.

Analogous to the situation with liver disease, a number of drugs which themselves may not induce nephrotoxicity need to have dosage adjustments made
when renal function is reduced, and these are indicated in Table 17. Depending on the drug and the extent of renal impairment the dose adjustment can
vary from 0-100%, and fatal reactions have occurred from lack of attention to
this fact.

Table 17   Dose Modification with Renal Dysfunction

| Drug | Percent of usual dose to administer if, on day of treatment, GFR is: | | |
	>50 ml/min	10-50 ml/min	<10 ml/min
Doxorubicin	100	100	100
Bleomycin	100	75	50
Cytarabine	100	50	0
Cyclophosphamide	100	100	50
Cytarabine	100	100	100
5-Fluorouracil	100	100	100
Melphalan	100	100	100
Methotrexate	100	50	0
Mithramycin	100	75	50
Nitrosoureas	100	0	0
Vincristine	100	100	100
Vinblastine	100	100	100

XIII. ENDOCRINE

Many antineoplastic drugs produce gonadal dysfunction, including azoospermia and amenorrhea. We recommend that such potential consequences be discussed prior to initiating the treatment program and as often as indicated thereafter since it is a long-term side effect of chemotherapy that can cause sexual dysfunction, possible sterility, and decrease the quality of life. The severity of the effect is usually related to age of the patient and the total dose of drug received in both males and females (Chapman, 1982). If this highly emotional subject can be discussed early, and this is admittedly difficult at times, the patient can begin to consider alternatives and have a better understanding of emotional and physical problems that may arise during treatment. Recommending support resources and counseling can be helpful to many patients. Men should be informed of the likelihood of decreased libido and the possibility of impotence during therapy and that these usually resolve after treatment has stopped. The extent of discussion is best documented in the chart in the event that a dispute arises years later when memories have faded and witnesses have moved or lost interest.

The effect on spermatogenesis varies with the drugs that are given and their cumulative dosage; we also are aware that after puberty males are at a higher risk of impaired endocrine function (Chapman, 1983). Reversible azoospermia has occurred in some instances, but infertility may be an end result. Therefore sperm banking prior to initiating therapy may be an option if the semen is not affected by the malignancy. In this regard it is interesting that azoospermia may be present in the patient even before starting the chemotherapy. If infertility has resulted in the male, then artificial insemination by donor may be an option if both partners agree.

The reproductive capacity of females after chemotherapy is somewhat brighter than males, since amenorrhea may be reversible (Kumar, Biggart, and McEvoy, 1972; Chapman, Sutcliffe, and Malpas, 1979). Protection of ovarian function with the use of oral contraceptives has been reported (Chapman and Sutcliffe, 1981) and may be a possibility if the use of hormones are not contraindicated due to the malignancy. Once irreversible ovarian failure and sterility are documented, then the possibility of adoption can be raised, and the symptoms of menopause, if they occur, should be treated by hormone replacement.

Open communication regarding sexual activity is important to patient and partners to alleviate fears and concerns. It is surprising how often a problem in this realm does exist which has not been discussed with the physician. Sexual counseling should be made readily accessible.

For those patients who remain fertile after being treated there is apparently no higher risk for spontaneous abortion or mutation to the offspring (Li and Jaffe, 1974; McKeen, Rosner, and Zarrob, 1979).

In discussing gonadal function, it is useful to consider the issue of treatment to the pregnant female who has a malignancy. Since antineoplastic agents effect rapidly dividing cells the developing fetus is at risk to untoward effects. The fetus is most vulnerable during the first trimester when principal development is taking place. If damage to the fetus is great, it obviously can result in spontaneous abortion or fetal malformation.

Treatment with chemotherapy should be withheld during the first trimester unless immediate therapy is required to the mother: even so fetal malformation is not inevitable. When therapy is necessary during the first trimester treatment with combination drugs should be avoided to decrease the risk of malformation. During the second and third trimester the drug regimen does not appear to increase the risk of congenital anomalies. There may be a slightly higher incidence of spontaneous delivery during the second trimester (Barber, 1981).

There is an instructive recent report of a 21-year-old woman with lymphoma who received combination chemotherapy for 16 months before conception and throughout the first and second trimesters with procarbazine and BCNU, and with streptozotocin in the third trimester (Schapira and Chudley, 1984). The literature regarding the administration of chemotherapeutic drugs was reviewed by Sweet and Kinzie (1976) and with other case reports it would appear that the use of single agents, such as alkylating agents, in the first trimester causes fetal malformations in about 10% of cases, that with drug combinations in the first trimester this rises slightly to 12.7% (9 of 71) but that chemotherapy used in the second and third trimester did not yield any abnormality among 76 treated patients. We agree with the suggestion of Schapira and Chudley to offer to terminate a pregnancy for patients exposed to chemotherapy around the time of conception or during the first trimester. Clearly there is an increased hazard in teratogenicity, approximately fivefold, though not as high as might have been anticipated. Though teratogenicity may not be a significant risk thereafter, one cannot exclude a potential hazard to an infant for development of a childhood malignancy.

Breast feeding is discouraged for mothers who are currently undergoing or have recently received chemotherapy, due to the possibility of transmitting toxic chemical through the milk.

XIV. LATE COMPLICATIONS, INCLUDING SECONDARY MALIGNANCIES

It has been pointed out that the mere occurrence of late complications of chemotherapy points to the great success in achieving long-term survival of patients treated with cytotoxic drugs (Kardinal, 1985). The risks are well illustrated in children who are cured of acute lymphocytic leukemia or

Table 18 Unusual Delayed Complications of Chemotherapy

Side effect(s)	Drug(s)
Cardiomyopathy, arrhythmia	Anthracyclines, high-dose cyclophosphamide
Inappropriate ADH syndrome	Vincristine, cyclophosphamide
Peripheral neuropathy	Vincristine
Hepatic fibrosis	Methotrexate
Cholestatic jaundice	6-Mercaptopurine
Cushing's syndrome, osteoporosis	Corticosteroids
Cataracts	Corticosteroids, busulfan
Bladder cancer	Cyclophosphamide
Raynaud's phenomenon	Bleomycin, vinblastine
Hemolytic-uremic syndrome	Mitomycin-C
Hypoadrenalism	Busulfan
Encephalopathy	Methotrexate, high-dose ARA C
Aplastic anemia	Busulfan, nitrosourea

Source: Modified from Perry and Yarbro (1984).

Hodgkin's disease but who face potentially serious complications of impaired growth and development (D'Angio, 1978), infertility, learning and psychological disabilities, cardiopulmonary impairment, and increased risk of a second malignancy, particularly acute nonlymphocytic leukemia. These various problems are discussed further in Chapter 9.

There are a great many unwanted effects of chemotherapy which may not be expressed for months or years. These have been carefully summarized by Perry and Yarbro (1984). Many agents are capable of producing hypogonadism in males and females, liver damage, pulmonary fibrosis, prolonged marrow aplasia, and secondary malignancies (discussed below). The effects on gonads have been discussed earlier in this chapter. Then there is a large assortment of unusual effects generally produced by only a small number of drugs, as listed in Table 18.

Being aware of potential late effects can be helpful in several ways. First, one can inform the patient that there is a significant risk, though it may be rare, and the physician can discharge some of the obligation and share the responsibility, which can prevent surprise and anger. Second, one can be stimulated to search for preexisting conditions which might make a particular patient more vulnerable to late untoward effects. Examples of this are to try to avoid the use of long-term methotrexate in patients with preexisting liver disease, anthracyclines in patients with severe myocardial disease and bleomycin in those with compromised pulmonary function. The timely use of sperm banking is another measure, as discussed earlier in this chapter, which can

circumvent a serious problem of infertility in young men who may be cured
of testicular cancer or Hodgkin's disease. Obviously this is not the first
thought to arise in an 18-year-old student with stage IV Hodgkin's disease,
but it should be part of orderly treatment planning and discussion.

As a general rule the hormonal or metabolic changes associated with long-
term drug use are usually fully reversible, the neurological changes may be
reversible (not leukoencephalopathy), but fibrosis, collagenosis, cardiopulmonary damage, secondary cancer, and hemolytic-uremic syndrome are not.

The causation of leukemia by ionizing radiation has long been documented
but the possible relationship to chemotherapy, particularly alkylating agents,
has been known only since 1970 when the use of melphalan in treatment of
multiple myeloma was later associated with development of acute leukemia
(Kyle, Pierre, and Bayrd, 1970). Since the mid-1970s there have been numerous series of reports of leukemia developing following the use of chemotherapy
for Hodgkin's disease, cancer of the ovary, breast, lung, sarcoma, and even for
nonmalignant conditions such as rheumatoid arthritis and renal transplantation.
The true incidence of developing leukemia following chemotherapy, with or
without radiation therapy, is still not known but estimates place it at 1-5%.
Discussions of the various reports pertaining to patients with Hodgkin's disease place it at slightly less than 1%, but this is still some 50-fold higher than
the expected (Kardinal, 1985). Increase in the incidence of other cancers are
also being reported (Berk et al., 1981). An extensive review of the types of
treatment associated with leukemia was recently presented (Dorr and Coltman,
1985).

Some of the hallmarks of the late development of leukemia are the prolonged use of cytotoxic agents (median 3.5 years), the latency of 3-7 years
after onset of treatment, and usually a preleukemic phase characterized by
pancytopenia with a myelodysplastic bone marrow picture. Unfortunately, we
know of no way to reverse the preleukemic phase once it occurs and the treatment of frank leukemia rarely results in remissions, unlike acute leukemia which
arises de novo.

Now that the potential for causing a second malignancy is well recognized,
the question again is whether it is possible to reduce or eliminate the risk.
Clearly the use of chemotherapy cannot now be eliminated since as a result of
its use many patients are living longer and only a small fraction of them will
then succumb to this complication. Although all cytotoxic agents have some
potential for causing mutagenesis and carcinogenesis, clearly the long-term use
of alkylating agents such as melphalan, chlorambucil, and cyclophosphamide
in addition to procarbazine are among the more commonly implicated drugs
(Dorr and Coltman, 1985). Whenever there are adequate substitutes for their
use then that should enter into the decision-making process.

An example of the evolving thought being given to this problem comes from the recognition that polycythemia vera is a chronic disease which may spontaneously terminate as leukemia but which is much more likely to do so when treated with chlorambucil (Berk et al., 1981). Now it has been found that the disease can usually be well controlled with hydroxyurea, a drug that is probably far less carcinogenic. Another area of concern stems from the use of adjuvant chemotherapy in patients who are at high risk for recurrence after surgical removal of breast cancer. Here the problem is highlighted by the possibility that some of the women exposed to increased risk of second malignancy are already cured of their primary cancer and, if one could identify them with certainty, would not need to be exposed to any chemotherapy. The approach that is most appealing is to find chemotherapy programs which are potent enough to rid the body of residual breast cancer, where that exists, yet have less danger of leukemogenesis. Such clinical trials involve long-term study of efficacy and safety and it is premature to recommend changing the standard CMF programs at this time. Surprisingly, the larger CMF trials have not yet reported a major problem with second malignancies.

XV. NEUROTOXICITY OF CHEMOTHERAPY

There is a large range of neurological complications that may be associated with cancer and, unfortunately, chemotherapy can add to the list of complications. The potential for nervous system toxicity produced by drugs adds a degree of complexity to differential diagnosis of central and peripheral nervous system changes in the patient with cancer. The cancer-induced complications are described in Chapter 7 and the reader is referred to that discussion.

XVI. OCULAR SIDE EFFECTS

Although ophthalmological side effects from chemotherapy are uncommon, they are important to the practitioner and patient because of the disability produced by the loss of vision. Busulfan is one of the few agents with a definite incidence of ocular toxicity, usually manifest by posterior subcapsular cataracts. These are apparently dose related but seldom produce enough visual impairment to require surgical extraction. Corticosteroids also produce cataracts and this can be a problem to patients who require prolonged use of such drugs.

Excessive lacrimation may result from 5-fluorouracil and the drug may cause cicatrical ectropion and arborization of tear ducts. Methotrexate may add to the excessive tearing produced by 5-FU and may potentiate optic nerve atrophy from cranial irradiation. Methotrexate also causes conjunctivitis, and toxic levels of drug have been reported in tears from patients who are receiving high-dose therapy. High doses of cytosine arabinoside such as may be used in acute leukemia may produce conjunctivitis (Ritch, Hansen, and Heuer, 1983). Both vincristine and vinblastine may cause diplopia and other cranial nerve palsies that affect vision (Dorr and Fritz, 1980).

Tamoxifen has been reported to cause a retinopathy, primarily affecting the region about the macula, which can result in significant decrease in visual acuity (Kupfer-Kaiser and Lippman, 1978).

XVII. REDUCTION OF RISK TO PERSONNEL HANDLING ANTINEOPLASTIC AGENTS

We need to be concerned about the physical and mental well-being of doctors, nurses, and technicians who work with patients who have cancer. The first article pertaining to any potential danger to personnel who are mixing chemotherapeutic drugs appeared in 1979 when Falck et al. (1979) reported finding mutagenic activity in the urine of oncology nurses who had mixed and administered chemotherapy. Since that time there has been increasing concern regarding the risks of mutagenesis or carcinogenesis, particularly among nurses and pharmacists. Waksvik, Klepp, and Brogger (1981), from Norway, did chromosome studies on nurses who had worked daily with such drugs. Chromosome damage was assessed by three methods: the number of breaks per 100 cells, the number of gaps per 100 cells, and the number of sister chromatid exchanges per 30 cells from each subject. Results showed that compared to nonexposed controls, there was an increase in the frequency of chromosome gaps and a slight increase in sister chromatid exchange frequency among the nurses who had experienced long-term exposure. The authors concluded that the handling of cytostatic drugs constitutes a *possible* health hazard, and therefore protective measures should be used.

Data from M.D. Anderson Hospital and Tumor Institute (Anderson et al., 1982) showed that there was uptake of mutagenic substances by persons who were handling antineoplastic agents while using horizontal laminar flow hoods, either when using no protection or while wearing gloves or masks. On the other hand, when using vertical flow biological safety cabinets and wearing gloves, no mutagenic substances were detected. Although there are controversial points in this study it does indicate that exposure risks can be reduced.

A number of review articles have made practical recommendations about the ways in which cytotoxic drugs should be prepared and handled in order to minimize the risk to personnel (Davis, 1980; Hoffman, 1980; Knowles and Virden, 1980; Harrison, 1981; Zimmerman et al., 1981; Stolar, Power, and Viele, 1983). From various sources we have prepared an example of a set of guidelines.

A. Recommended Practices for Personnel Preparing Injectable Antineoplastic Drug Products

1. All procedures involved in the preparation of injectable antineoplastic drugs should be performed in a class II laminar flow biological safety cabinet. A class II, type A cabinet will provide product protection and prevent exposure of the operator to aerosols. The filtered exhaust from this type of cabinet is normally discharged into the room environment. Where possible, however, it is desirable to discharge the filtered exhaust air to the outdoors. This can be accomplished by installing an exhaust canopy over the class II, type A cabinet or by the use of a class II, type B biological safety cabinet, which discharges exhaust air to the outdoors.

2. Personnel should be familiar with the capabilities, limitations, and proper use of the biological safety cabinet selected. Careful consideration should be given to selecting a cabinet size with space that will accommodate the work load.

3. The safety cabinet work surface should be covered with plastic back absorbent paper. This will reduce the potential for dispersion of droplets and spills and facilitate cleanup. The paper should be changed after any overt spills and after each workshift.

4. Professionally acceptable standards concerning the aseptic preparation of injectable products should be followed.

5. Personnel preparing the drugs should wear surgical gloves and a closed front surgical type gown with knit cuffs. Gowns may be washable or disposable. Overtly contaminated gloves or outer garments should be removed and replaced. In case of skin contact with the drug product, the affected area should be washed thoroughly with soap and water. Flush affected eyes with copious amounts of water.

6. A sterile alcohol-dampened cotton pledget should be carefully wrapped around the needle and vial top during withdrawal from the vial septum. Similarly, a sterile alcohol-dampened cotton pledget should be placed at the needle or syringe tip when ejecting air bubbles from a filled syringe. This method will control the drippage and aerosol production that may occur during these procedures.

7. Luer lock syringes and tubing should be used to prevent separation of tubing and needles, thereby causing leakage of drug solution.

8. Vials containing reconstituted drugs should be vented to reduce internal pressure. This will help to reduce the possibility of spraying and spillage when a needle is withdrawn from the septum.

9. The external surfaces of syringes and I.V. bottles should be wiped clean of any drug contamination.

10. Avoid self-inoculation. Take care when conducting any procedure that involves the use of needles.

11. When breaking the top off of a glass ampule, wrap the ampule neck at the anticipated break point with a sterile alcohol-dampened cotton pledget to contain the aerosol produced and also to protect fingers from being lacerated by the broken glass.

12. Syringes and I.V. bottles containing antineoplastic drugs should be properly identified and dated. When these items are delivered to a nursing unit, an additional label such as, "Caution—Cancer Chemotherapy, Dispose Properly," is recommended.

13. Wipe down the interior of the safety cabinet with 70% alcohol using a disposable towel after completing all drug preparation operations.

14. Needles, syringes, vials, bottles, gloves, absorbent paper, pledgets, gauze, etc., used during the drug preparation and cleanup operations should be placed in a box lined with a plastic bag, appropriately labeled, sealed, and incinerated. Needles should be carefully recapped before disposal rather than clipped because of the aerosol generated by clipping. Washable gowns may be laundered in a normal fashion.

15. Hands should be washed after removing gloves: gloves are not a substitute for hand washing.

16. Unused chemotherapy drug products should be considered toxic chemical waste and should be disposed of in accordance with applicable federal, state, and local codes and ordinances.

17. Only properly trained personnel should handle drug products. Training sessions about safe handling should be offered to new professionals as well as technical and maintenance personnel who may come in contact with the agents.

B. Recommended Practices for Personnel Administering Injectable Antineoplastic Drug Products

1. A protective outer garment, such as a closed front surgical-type gown with knit cuffs, should be worn. Gowns may be washable or disposable.

2. Disposable surgical gloves should be worn during those procedures where leakage of the drugs may result (i.e., removing air bubbles from syringes and I.V. tubing, injecting drugs, disconnecting I.V. tubing, and fixing leaking tubing or syringe connections). Gloves should be discarded after each use.

3. When bubbles are removed from syringes or I.V. tubing, a sterile alcohol-dampened cotton pledget should be placed carefully over the tips of needles, syringes or I.V. tubing in order to collect any of the antineoplastic drug product that may be inadvertently discharged.

4. Drug-contaminated gloves, needles, syringes, pledgets, I.V. bottles, etc.,
    should be placed in a box lined with a plastic bag, appropriately
    labeled, sealed, and incinerated. Needles should be carefully recapped
    before disposal rather than clipped because of the aerosol generated by
    clipping. Washable gowns may be laundered in a normal fashion.
5. In case of skin contact with an antineoplastic drug product, the
    affected area should be washed thoroughly with soap and water. Flush
    affected eyes with copious amounts of water. Hands should be washed
    after administering any antineoplastic drug product.

Such guidelines are to a great extent a matter of common sense and are
based on the simple principle of using and designing equipment and work techniques to ensure that personnel have minimal contact with antineoplastic drugs
(D'Arcy, 1983). Guidelines should include measures to protect the personnel
who handle waste generated from the preparation and administration of antineoplastic agents. Separate waste containers, labeled for careful handling and
disposal, are critical. There is some controversy regarding the method of disposal of cytotoxic waste, and as yet no guidelines have been forthcoming from
the Environmental Protection Agency. Most sources recommend incineration
whenever feasible.

Although we have given detailed safety recommendations it should be said
that there is a tendency to overreact to concerns involving carcinogenesis
(Ballentine, 1982). While reduction of risk to health care personnel is
important, care must be taken not to alarm patients and families. For example,
how would one expect a patient to feel if a nurse dressed in mask, gloves, etc.
approached bearing their chemotherapy? Another example is the case where,
due to space constraints, drugs must be prepared in the same room where they
are given and patients question the protective equipment and clothing the
personnel use to prepare their medication. Careful explanation and open communication are essential in order to allay fears.

REFERENCES

Adria Laboratories. (1982). Adriamycin, Package Insert.

Anderson, J. E., Hunt, J. M., and Smith, I. E. (1981). Prevention of doxorub-
    icin-induced alopecia by scalp cooling in patients with advanced breast
    cancer, *Brit. Med. J., 282*:423-424.

Anderson, R. W., Puckett, W. H., Dana, W. J., Nguyen, T. V., Theiss, J. C., and
    Matney, T. S. (1982). Risk of handling injectable antineoplastic agents,
    Am. J. Hosp. Pharm., 39:1881-1887.

Arena, P. J. (1972). Oropharyngeal sensation associated with rapid intravenous
    administration of cyclophosphamide (NSC-26271), *Cancer Chemother. Rep.,
    56*:779-780.

Armstrong, D. (1980). Infections in patients with neoplastic disease, in *Infections in the Immunocompromised Host—Pathogenesis, Prevention and Therapy* (J. Verhoef, P. K. Peterson, and P. G. Quie, eds.), Elsevier/North-Holland, Amsterdam, pp. 129-158.

Aronin, P. A., Mahaley, M. S., Rudnick, S. A., Dudka, L., Donohue, J. F., Selker, R. G., and Moore, P. (1980). Prediction of BCNU pulmonary toxicity in patients with malignant gliomas. An assessment of risk factor, *New Engl. J. Med., 303*:183-191.

Ballentine, R. (1982). Cancer phobia—or whatever happened to red M and Ms? (editorial), *Drug Intell. Clin. Pharm., 16*:60-61.

Barber, H. R. (1981). Fetal and neonatal effects of cytotoxic agents, *Obstet. Gyn., 58*:41-46.

Barr, R. D., and Perry, C. (1982). Hematologic effects of antineoplastic therapy, in *Cancer Medicine,* 2nd Edition, Lea & Febiger, Philadelphia, pp. 1288-1302.

Bergsagel, D. E., Robertson, G. L., and Hasselback, R. (1968). Effect of cyclophosphamide on advanced lung cancer and the hematological toxicity of large intermittent intravenous doses, *Canad. Med. Assoc. J., 98*:532-538.

Berk, P. D., Goldberg, J. D., Silverstein, M. N., Weinfeld, A., Donovan, P. B., Ellis, J. T., Landaw, S. A., Laszlo, J., Najean, Y., Pisciotta, A. V., and Wasserman, L. R. (1981). Increased incidence of acute leukemia in polycythemia vera associated with chlorambucil therapy, *New Engl. J. Med., 304*: 441-447.

Bertland, M., Present, C. A., Klein, L., and Scott, E. (1984). Iatrogenic superior vena cava syndrome, *Cancer, 54*:376-378.

Bishop, J. F., Oliver, I. N., Wolf, M. M., Matthews, J. P., Long, M., Bingham, J., Hillcoat, B. L., and Cooper, I. A. (1984). Lorazepam: A randomized, double-blind, crossover study of a new antiemetic in patients receiving cytotoxic chemotherapy and prochlorperazine, *J. Clin. Oncol., 2*:691-695.

Bodey, G. P. (1982). Infections in patients with cancer, in *Cancer Medicine* (J. F. Holland and E. Frei, III, eds.), Lea & Febiger, Philadelphia, pp. 1329-1372.

Bodey, G. P., Rodriguez, V., and Freireich, E. J. (1978). The prevention of infection in patients with acute leukemia, *The Infection-Prone Hospital Patient* (J. Burke and G. Y. Hildrick-Smith, eds.), Little, Brown, Boston, pp. 143-156.

Bow, E. J., Louie, T. J., Riben, P. D., McNaughton, R. D., Harding, G. K. M., and Ronald, A. R. (1984). Randomized controlled trial comparing trimethoprim/sulfamethoxazole and trimethoprim for infection prophylaxis in hospitalized granulocytopenic patients, *Am. J. Med., 76*:223-233.

Bristol Laboratoreis. (1982). Bleomycin Package Insert.

Bristol Laboratories. (1983a). Platinol Package Insert.

Bristol Laboratories. (1983b). Vepesid Package Insert.

Brown, A. E. (1984). Neutropenia, fever and infection, *Am. J. Med., 76*: 421-428.

Burish, T. G., and Carey, M. P. (1984). Conditioned responses to cancer chemotherapy: Etiology and treatment, in *Impact of Psychoendocrine*

Systems in Cancer and Immunity (B. H. Fox and B. H. Newberry, eds.), C. J. Hogrefe, Toronto, pp. 147-178.

Chabner, B. (1982). *Pharmacologic Principles of Cancer Treatment,* W. B. Saunders, Philadelphia.

Chapman, R. M. (1982). Effect of cytotoxic therapy on sexuality and gonadal function, *Semin. Oncol., 9*:84-90.

Chapman, R. M. (1983). Gonadal injury resulting from chemotherapy, *Am. J. Indust. Med., 4*:149-161.

Chapman, R. M., and Sutcliffe, S. M. (1981). Protection of ovarian function, contraception in women receiving chemotherapy for Hodgkin's disease, *Blood, 58*:849-851.

Chapman, R. M., Sutcliffe, S. B., and Malpas, J. S. (1979). Cytotoxic induced ovarian failure in women with Hodgkin's disease. I. Hormone function, *JAMA, 242*:1877-1881.

Chernik, N. L., Armstrong, D., and Posner, J. B. (1973). Central nervous system infections in patients with cancer, *Medicine, 52*:563-581.

Cline, B. W. (1984). Prevention of chemotherapy-induced alopecia: A review of the literature, *Cancer Nursing, June*:221-228.

Comis, R. L. (1978). Bleomycin pulmonary toxicity, in *Bleomycin: Current Status and New Development* (S. K. Carter, S. T. Crooke, and H. Umezawa, eds.), Academic Press, New York, pp. 279-291.

Cotanch, P. H. (1983). Relaxation techniques as antiemetic therapy, in *Antiemetics and Cancer Chemotherapy* (J. Laszlo, ed.), Williams & Wilkins, Baltimore, pp. 164-176.

Dameshek, W., Weisfuse, L., and Stein, T. (1949). Nitrogen mustard therapy in Hodgkin's disease, *Blood, 4*:338-379.

D'Angio, G. J. (1978). Complications of treatment encountered in leukemia-lymphoma longterm survivors, *Cancer, 42*:1015-1022.

D'Arcy, P. F. (1983). Reactions and interactions in handling anticancer drugs, *Drug Intell. Clin. Pharm., 17*:532-538.

Davis, M. R. (1980). Handling and preparation of cytotoxic drugs—minimising the risk, *Aust. J. Hosp. Pharm., 10*:127-130.

Dean, J., Griffith, K. S., Cetas, T. C., Mackel, C. L., Jones, S. E. and Salmon, S. E. (1983). Scalp hypothermia: A comparison of ice packs and the Kold Kap in the prevention of doxorubicin-induced alopecia, *J. Clin. Oncol., 1*: 33-37.

deJongh, C. A., and Schimpff, S. C. (1983). Prevention and management of infectious complications of cancer, in *Supportive Care of the Cancer Patient* (P. H. Wiernik, ed.), Futura Publishing Company, Mt. Kisco, N.Y., pp. 75-108.

Dennis, V. W. (1983). Fluid and electrolyte changes after vomiting, in *Antiemetics and Cancer Chemotherapy* (J. Laszlo, ed.), Williams & Wilkins, Baltimore, pp. 34-42.

Dorr, F. A., and Coltman, C. A., Jr. (1985). Second cancers following antineoplastic therapy, in *Current Problems in Cancer* (F. A. Dorr and C. A. Coltman, Jr., eds.), Year Book Medical Publishers, Chicago, pp. 1-43.

Dorr, R. T., and Fritz, W. L. (1980). *Cancer Chemotherapy Handbook,* Elsevier, New York, pp. 112, 134-135.

Dunagin, W. G. (1982). Clinical toxicity of chemotherapeutic agents: Dermatologic toxicity, *Semin. Oncol., 9*:14-22.

Durack, D. T. (1984). Prevention of central nervous system infections in patients at risk, *Am. J. Med., 76(5A)*:231-237.

Elspar Merck, Sharp and Dohme (1983). Package Insert.

Estey, E., Maksymiuk, A., Smith, T., Painstein, V., Keating, M., McCredie, K. B., Freireich, E. J., and Bodey, G. P. (1984). Infectious prophylaxis in acute leukemia, *Arch. Intern. Med., 144*:1562-1568.

Falck, K., Grohn, P., Sorsa, M., Vainio, H., Heinonen, E., and Hulsti, L. R. (1979). Mutagenicity in urine of nurses handling cytostatic drugs, *Lancet, 1*:1250-1251.

Gagen, M., Gochnour, D., Young, D., Gaginella, T., and Neidhart, J. (1984). A randomized trial of metoclopramide and a combination of dexamethasone and lorazepam for prevention of chemotherapy-induced vomiting, *J. Clin. Oncol., 2*:696-701.

Gebarski, S. S., and Gebarski, K. S. (1984). Chemotherapy port "Twiddler's syndrome," *Cancer, 54*:38-39.

Ginsberg, S. J., and Comis, R. L. (1982). The pulmonary toxicity of antineoplastic agents, *Semin. Oncol., 9*:34-51.

Ginsberg,. S. J., and Comis, R. L. (1984). The pulmonary toxicity of antineoplastic agents, in *Toxicity of Chemotherapy* (M. C. Perry and J. W. Yarbro, eds.), Grune & Stratton, Orlando, Fla., pp. 227-268.

Goldmann, D. A., Maki, D. G., Rhame, F. S., Kaiser, A. B., Tenney, J. H., and Bennett, J. V. (1973). Guidelines for infection control in intravenous therapy, *Ann. Intern. Med., 79*:848-850.

Gralla, R. J., Itri, L. M. Pisko, S. E., Squillante, A. E., Kelsen, D. P., Braun, D. W., Jr., Bordin, L. A., Braun, T. J., and Young, C. W. (1981). Antiemetic efficacy of high-dose metoclopramide: Randomized trials with placebo and prochlorperazine in patients with chemotherapy-induced nausea and vomiting, *New Engl. J. Med., 305*:905-909.

Greco, F. A. (1978). Subclinical Adriamycin cardiotoxicity: Detection by timing the arterial sounds, *Cancer Treat. Rep., 62*:901-905.

Greco, F. A., Merrill, R. M., Brereton, H. D., and Robard, D. (1975). Noninvasive monitoring of subclinical Adriamycin cardiotoxicity by "sphygmo-recording" of the QRS-Korotkoff interval, *Clin. Res., 23*(Abstr.):595.

Grunberg, S. M., Gala, K. V., Lampenfeld, M., Jamin, D., Johnson, K., Cariffe, P., Strych, D., and Krailo, M. (1984). Comparison of the antiemetic effect of high-dose intravenous metoclopramide and high-dose intravenous haloperidol in a randomized double-blind crossover study, *J. Clin. Oncol., 2*:782-787.

Gurwith, M. J., Brunton, J. L., Lank, B. A., Harding, G. K. M., and Ronald, A. R. (1979). A prospective controlled investigation of prophylactic trimethoprim/sulfamethoxazole in hospitalized granulocytopenic patients, *Am. J. Med., 66*:248-256.

Gyvers, J. W., Ensminger, W. D., Niederhuber, M. D., Dent, T., Walker, S., Gilbertson, S., Cozzi, E., and Saran, P. (1984). A totally implanted injection port system for blood sampling and chemotherapy administration, *JAMA, 251*:2538-2541.

Hammer, R. W., Verani, R., and Weinman, E. J. (1983). Mitomycin-associated renal failure, *Arch. Intern. Med., 143*:803-807.

Harden, E., Lucas, V. S., Proia, A., and Silberman, H. R. (1982). Hemolytic uremic syndrome during therapy with mitomycin-C (MMC) plus 5-fluorouracil (5-FU), *Proc. ASCO, 1*:93 (C-360).

Harrison, B. R. (1981). Developing guidelines for working with antineoplastic drugs, *Am. J. Hosp. Pharm., 38*:1686-1693.

Henry, S. A. (1984). Chemoprophylaxis of bacterial infections in granulocytopenic patients, *Am. J. Med., 76*:645-651.

Herman, T. S., Einhorn, L. H., Jones, S. E., Nagy, C., Chester, A. B., Dean, J. C., Furnas, B., Williams, S. D., Leigh, S. A., Dorr, R. J., and Moon, T. E. (1979). Superiority of nabilone over prochlorperazine as an antiemetic in patients receiving cancer chemotherapy, *New Engl. J. Med., 300*:1295-1309.

Hoagland, H. C. (1984). Hematologic complications of cancer chemotherapy, in *Toxicity of Chemotherapy* (M. C. Perry and J. W. Yarbro, eds.), Grune & Stratton, Orlando, Fla., pp. 433-448.

Hoffman, D. M. (1980). The handling of antineoplastic drugs in a major cancer center, *Hosp. Pharm., 15*:302-304.

Hughes, W. T., Kuhn, S., Chaudhary, S., Feldman, S., Verzosa, M., Aur, R. J., Pratt, C., and George, S. L. (1977). Successful chemoprophylaxis for *Pneumocystis carinii* pneumonitis, *New Engl. J. Med., 297*:1419-1426.

Janssen, P. A. J. (1967). The pharmacology of haloperidol, *Int. J. Neuropsych., 3*:S10-S18.

Johanson, W. G., Jr. (1984). Prevention of respiratory tract infection, *Am. J. Med., 76(2)*:69-77.

Justin-Besancon, L., and Laville, C. (1964). Action antiemetic du metoclopramide vis-a-vis de l'apomorphine et de l'hydergine, *C. R. Soc. Biol. (Paris), 158*:723.

Kahn, T., Elias, E. G., Mason, G. R., and Herbel, J. R. (1978). The study of a single dose of metoclopramide in the control of nausea and vomiting from cis-platinum (II) therapy in man, *Cancer Treat. Rep., 62*:1106-1107.

Karchmer, R. K., and Hansen, V. L. (1977). Possible anaphylactic reaction to intravenous cyclophosphamide, *JAMA, 237*:475.

Kardinal, C. G. (1985). Complications of treatment for advanced colorectal cancer, in *Complications of Colon and Rectal Surgery: Prevention and Management* (B. T. Ferrari, J. E. Ray, and J. B. Gathright, eds.), W. B. Saunders, Philadelphia, pp. 283-290.

Knowles, R. S., and Virden, J. E. (1980). Handling of injectable antineoplastic agents, *Brit. Med. J., 281*:589-591.

Kumar, R., Biggart, J. D., and McEvoy, J. (1972). Cyclophosphamide and reproductive function, *Lancet, 1*:1212-1214.

Kupfer-Kaiser, M. I., and Lippman, M. E. (1978). Tamoxifen retinopathy, *Cancer Treat. Rep., 62*:315-320.

Kyle, R. A., Pierre, R. V., and Bayrd, E. D. (1970). Multiple myeloma and acute myelomonocytic leukemia: Report of four cases possibly related to melphalan, *New Engl. J. Med., 283*:1121-1125.

Laszlo, J. (1982). Hematologic effects of cancer, in *Cancer Medicine,* 2nd Edition, Lea & Febiger, Philadelphia, pp. 1275-1288.

Laszlo, J. (1983a). *Antiemetics and Cancer Chemotherapy,* Williams & Wilkins, Baltimore.

Laszlo, J. (1983a). Methods for measuring clinical effectiveness of antiemetics, in *Antiemetics and Cancer Chemotherapy* (J. Laszlo, ed.), Williams & Wilkins, Baltimore, pp. 43-52.

Laszlo, J. (1983b). Closing remarks: Selecting an antiemetic for the individual patient, *Drugs, 25(1)*:81-83.

Laszlo, J., and Kremer, W. B. (1973). Hematologic effects of chemotherapeutic drugs and radiation, in *Cancer Medicine,* (J. F. Holland and E. Frei, III, eds.), Lea & Febiger, Philadelphia, pp. 1099-1115.

Laszlo, J., and Lucas, V. S. (1981). Editorial: Emesis as a critical problem in chemotherapy, *New Engl. J. Med., 305(16)*:948-949.

Laszlo, J., Lucas, V. S., and Huang, A. T. (1981). Iatrogenic emesis model in cancer: Results of 120 patients treated with delta-9-tetrahydrocannabinol, in *Treatment of Cancer Chemotherapy-Induced Nausea and Vomiting* (D. S. Poster, J. S. Penta, and S. Bruno, eds.), Masson Publishing, New York, pp. 61-74.

Laszlo, J., Clark, R. A., Hanson, D. C., Tyson, L., Crumpler, L., and Gralla, R. (1985). Lorazepam in cancer patients treated with cisplatin: A drug having antiemetic, amnesic and anxiolytic effects, *J. Clin. Oncol., 3*:864-869.

Laszlo, J., Hanson, D. C., Lucas, V. S., Clark, R., Tyson, L., Gralla, R., and Derivan, A. (1983). Lorazepam as an antiemetic against cisplatin, *Proc. ASCO, 2*:95.

Li, F. P., and Jaffe, N. (1974). Progeny of childhood-cancer survivors, *Lancet, 2*:707-709.

Lockich, J. J., and Moore, C. (1984). Chemotherapy-associated palmar-plantar erythrodysesthesia syndrome, *Ann. Intern. Med., 101*:798-799.

Lucarelli, C. D. (1984). Chemotherapy-induced oral mucositis: Causes and treatment, *Cancer Chemother. Update, 2*:1-4.

Lucas, V. S., Jr. (1983). Phenothiazines as antiemetics, in *Antiemetics and Cancer Chemotherapy* (J. Laszlo, ed.), Williams & Wilkins, Baltimore, pp. 93-107.

Markman, M., Sheidler, V., Ettinger, D. S., Quosky, B. S., and Mellits, E. D. (1984). Antiemetic efficacy of dexamethasone, *New Engl. J. Med., 311*: 549-552.

McCredie, K. B., and Freireich, E. J. (1982). Blood component therapy: White blood cell transfusion, *Cancer Medicine,* 2nd Edition, Lea & Febiger, Philadelphia, pp. 1309-1319.

McKeen, E. A., Rosner, F., and Zarrob, M. H. (1979). Pregnancy outcome in Hodgkin's disease, *Lancet, 2*:590-593.

Moertel, C. G., and Reitemeier, R. J. (1973). Controlled studies of meto-
primazine for the treatment of nausea and vomiting, *J. Clin. Pharmacol.*,
13:283-287.
Moertel, C. G., Reitemeier, R. J., and Gage, R. P. (1963). A controlled
clinical evaluation of antiemetic drugs, *JAMA, 186*:116-118.
Morrow, G. R. (1982). Prevalence and correlates of anticipatory nausea and
vomiting in chemotherapy patients, *JNCI, 68*:585-588.
Morrow, G. R., and Morrell, C. (1982). Behavioral treatment for anticipatory
nausea and vomiting induced by cancer chemotherapy, *New Engl. J. Med.*
307:1476-1480.
Morrow, G. R., Arseneau, J. C., Asbury, R. F., Bennett, J. M., and Boros, L.
(1982). Anticipatory nausea and vomiting in chemotherapy patients, *New
Engl. J. Med., 306*:431-432.
Munro, D. (1971). *Dermatology in General Medicine,* McGraw-Hill, New York,
pp. 297-331.
Neidhart, J. A., Gagen, M. M., Wilson, H. E., and Young, D. C. (1981a).
Comparative trial of the antiemetic effects of delta-9-THC and haloperidol,
J. Clin. Pharmacol., 21:38S-42S.
Neidhart, J. A., Gagen, M., Young, D., and Wilson, H. E. (1981b). Specific
antiemetics for specific cancer chemotherapeutic agents: Haloperidol versus
benzquinamide, *Cancer, 47*:1439-1443.
Odio, C., Mohs, E., Sklar, F. H., Nelson, J. D., and McCracken, G. H. (1984).
Adverse reactions to vancomycin used as prophylaxis for CSF shunt pro-
cedures, *Am. J. Dis. Child., 138*:17-19.
Orr, L. E., McKernan, J. F., and Bloome, B. (1980). Antiemetic effect of
tetrahydrocannabinol, *Arch. Intern. Med., 140*:1431-1433.
Penta, J. S., Poster, D., and Bruno, S. (1983). The pharmacologic treatment
of nausea and vomiting—a review, in *Antiemetics and Cancer Chemotherapy*
(J. Laszlo, ed.), Williams & Wilkins, Baltimore, pp. 53-92.
Penta, J. S., Poster, D. S., Bruno, S., Abraham, D., Perinna, K., and MacDonald,
J. S. (1981). Cancer chemotherapy-induced nausea and vomiting: A review,
in *Treatment of Cancer Chemotherapy-Induced Nausea and Vomiting* (D.
S. Poster, J. S. Penta, and S. Bruno, eds.), Masson Publishing, New York,
pp. 1-31.
Perry, M. C. (1984). Hepatotoxicity of chemotherapeutic agents, in *Toxicity
of Chemotherapy* (M. C. Perry and J. W. Yarbro, eds.), Grune & Stratton,
Orlando, Fla., pp. 297-315.
Perry, M. C., and Yarbro, J. W. (1984). Complications of chemotherapy: An
overview, in *Toxicity of Chemotherapy* (M. C. Perry and J. W. Yarbro, eds.),
Grune & Stratton, Orlando, Fla., pp. 1-19.
Peterson, D. E. (1983). Dental care, in *Supportive Care of the Cancer Patient*
(P. H. Wiernik, ed.), Futura Publishing Company, Mt. Kisco, N.Y., pp.
145-171.
Peterson, P. K. (1984). Host defense abnormalities predisposing the patient to
infection, *Am. J. Med., 76*:2-10.

Pizzo, P. A., Commers, J., Cotton, D., Gress, J., Hathorn, J., Hiemenz, J., Longo, D., Marshall, D., and Robichaud, K. J. (1984). Approaching the controversies in antibacterial management of cancer patients, *Am. J. Med., 76*:436-449.

Poster, D. S., Penta, J. S., and Bruno, S. (1981). *Treatment of Cancer Chemotherapy-Induced Nausea and Vomiting* (D. S. Poster, J. S. Penta, and S. Bruno, eds.), Masson Publishing, New York.

Raaf, J. H. (1985). Results from use of 826 vascular access devices in cancer patients, *Cancer, 55*:1312-1321.

Raymond, J. R. (1984). Nephrotoxicities of antineoplastic and immuno-suppressive agents, *Current Problems in Cancer, 8(16)*:3-32.

Rich, W. M., Abdulhayoglu, G., and DiSaia, P. J. (1981). Methylprednisolone as an antiemetic during cancer chemotherapy, in *Treatment of Cancer Chemotherapy-Induced Nausea and Vomiting* (D. S. Poster, J. S. Penta, and S. Bruno, eds.), Masson Publishing, New York, pp. 221-224.

Ritch, P. S., Hansen, R. M., and Heuer, D. K. (1983). Ocular toxicity from high-dose cytosine arabinoside, *Cancer, 51*:430-432.

Ross, W. E., and Bruce, A. C. (1977). Allergic reaction to cyclophosphamide in a mechlorethamine-sensitive patient, *Cancer Treat. Rep., 61*:495-496.

Rozencweig, M., Piccart, M., and Von Hoff, D. D. (1981). Cardiac disorders in cancer patients, in *Medical Complications in Cancer Patients* (J. Kastersky and J. J. Staquet, eds.), Raven Press, New York, pp. 211-229.

Sallan, S. E., Zinberg, N. E., and Frei, E., III. (1975). Antiemetic effect of delta-9-tetrahydrocannabinol in patients receiving cancer chemotherapy, *New Engl. J. Med., 293*:795-797.

Sallan, S. E., Cronin, C., Zelen, M., and Zinberg, N. E. (1980). Antiemetics in patients receiving chemotherapy for cancer. A randomized comparison of delta-9-tetrahydrocannabinol and prochlorperazine, *New Engl. J. Med., 302*: 135-138.

Satterwhite, B., and Zimm, S. (1984). The use of scalp hypothermia in the prevention of doxorubicin-induced hair loss, *Cancer, 54*:34-37.

Schapira, D. V., and Chudley, A. E. (1984). Successful pregnancy following continuous treatment with combination chemotherapy before conception and throughout pregnancy, *Cancer, 54*:800-803.

Schimpff, S. C. (1980). Infection prevention during granulocytopenia, in *Current Clinical Topics in Infectious Diseases* (J. S. Remington and M. N. Swartz, eds.), Vol. 1, McGraw-Hill, New York, pp. 85-106.

Schimpff, S. C., Green, W. H., Young, V. M., Fortner, C. L., Jepsen, L., Cusack, N., Block, J. B., and Wiernik, T. H. (1975). Infection prevention in acute nonlymphocytic leukemia: Laminar air flow room reverse isolation with oral nonabsorbable antibiotic prophylaxis, *Ann. Intern. Med., 82*: 351-358.

Schimpff, S. C., Hahn, D. M., Brouillet, M. D., Young, V. M., Fortner, C. L., and Wiernik, T. H. (1978). Comparison of basic infection prevention techniques, with standard room reverse isolation plus added air filtration, *Leukemia Res., 2*:231-240.

Senn, H. J., Glaus, A., and Bachmann-Mettler, I. (1984). Effective control of chemotherapy-induced nausea and vomiting with oral prednisone and metoclopramide, *J. Clin. Oncol., 2*:320-322.

Sherwood, G. K., and Yankee, R. A. (1982). Red cell therapy and transfusion reactions, in *Cancer Medicine*, 2nd Edition, Lea & Febiger, Philadelphia, pp. 1302-1308.

Shilsky, R. L. (1984). Renal and metabolic toxicities of cancer treatment, in *Toxicity of Chemotherapy* (M. C. Perry and J. W. Yarbro, eds.), Grune & Stratton, Orlando, Fla., pp. 317-342.

Sickles, E. A., Green, W. H., and Wiernik, P. H. (1975). Clinical presentation of infection in granulocytopenic patients, *Arch. Intern. Med., 135*:715-719.

Steele, N., Gralla, R. J., Braun, D. W., and Young, C. W. (1980). Double-blind comparison of the antiemetic effects of nabilone and prochlorperazine on chemotherapy-induced emesis, *Cancer Treat. Rep., 64*:219-224.

Stevenson, D. F., Emmerich, B. F., and Lucas, V. S. (1985). Preventing extravasation during administration of antineoplastic drugs, *Oncol. Nursing Forum, 12*:83.

Stolar, M. H., Power, L. A., and Viele, C. S. (1983). Recommendations for handling cytotoxic drugs in hospitals, *Am. J. Hosp. Pharm., 40*:1163-1171.

Stoudemire, A., Cotanch, P., and Laszlo, J. (1984). Recent advances in the pharmacologic and behavioral management of chemotherapy-induced emesis, *Arch. Intern. Med., 144*:1029-1033.

Sweet, D. L., and Kinzie, J. (1976). Consequences of radiotherapy and anti-neoplastic therapy for the fetus, *J. Reprod. Med., 17*:241-246.

Sykes, M. P., Chu, F. C. H., Savel, H., Bonadonna, G., and Mathis, H. (1964). The effects of varying dosages of irradiation upon sternal marrow regeneration, *Radiology, 83*:1084-1088.

Verwey, J., Boven, E., van der Meulen, J., and Pinedo, H. M. (1984). Recovery from mitomycin C-induced hemolytic uremic syndrome, *Cancer, 54*:2878-2881.

Vincent, B. J., McQuiston, D. J., Einhorn, L. H., Nagy, C. M., and Brames, M. J. (1983). Review of cannabinoids and their antiemetic effectiveness, *Drugs 25(1)*:52-62.

Von Hoff, D. D., Rozencweig, M., and Piccart, M. (1982). The cardiotoxicity of anticancer agents, *Semin. Oncol., 9*:23-33.

Von Hoff, D. D., Layard, M. W., Basa, P., Davis, H. L., Jr., Von Hoff, A. L. Rozencweig, M., and Muggia, F. M. (1979). Risk factors for doxorubicin-induced congestive heart failure, *Ann. Intern. Med., 91*:710-717.

Waksvik, H., Klepp, O., and Brogger, A. (1981). Chromosome analyses of nurses handling cytostatic agents, *Cancer Treat. Rep., 65*:607-610.

Wampler, G. (1983). The pharmacology and clinical effectiveness of pheno-thiazines and related drugs for managing chemotherapy-induced emesis, *Drugs, 25(1)*:35-51.

Weinstein, G. D. (1977). Methotrexate, *Ann. Intern. Med., 86*:199-204.

Weiss, R. B. (1982). Hypersensitivity reactions to cancer chemotherapy, *Semin. Oncol., 9*:5-13.

Whitman, G., Cadman, E., and Chen, M. (1981). Misuse of scalp hypothermia, *Cancer Treat. Rep., 65*:507-508.

Winokur, S. H., Baker, J. J., Lokey, J. L., Price, N. A., and Bowen, J. (1981). Dexamethasone as an antiemetic during cancer chemotherapy, in *Treatment of Cancer Chemotherapy-Induced Nausea and Vomiting* (D. S. Poster, J. S. Penta, and S. Bruno, eds.), Masson Publishing, New York, pp. 225-228.

Wortman, J. R., Lucas, V. S., Schuster, E., Thiele, D., and Logue, G. L. (1979). Sudden death during doxorubicin administration, *Cancer, 44*:1588-1591.

Yankee, R. A., and Sherwood, G. K. (1982). Platelet transfusions, *Cancer Medicine*, 2nd Edition, Lea & Febiger, Philadelphia, pp. 1319-1325.

Zeltzer, L., Kellerman, J., Ellenberg, L., and Dash, J. (1983). Hypnosis for reduction of vomiting associated with chemotherapy and disease in adolescents with cancer, *J. Adolescent Health Care, 4*:77-84.

Zimmerman, H. J. (1978). *Hepatotoxicity: The Adverse Effects of Drugs and Other Chemicals on the Liver*, Appleton-Century-Croft, New York.

Zimmerman, P. F., Larsen, R. K., Barkley, E. N., and Gallell, J. F. (1981). Recommendations for the safe handling of injectable antineoplastic drug products, *Am. J. Hosp. Pharm., 38*:1693-1695.

6

Radiation Therapy: Acute and Late Morbidity

Gustavo S. Montana
Duke University Medical Center, Durham, North Carolina

I. INTRODUCTION

Approximately half of the patients afflicted with cancer will receive radiation therapy during the course of their illness. In some instances the therapy is given with curative intent, but at other times it is given for palliation of symptoms or in anticipation of symptoms that are likely to occur. Finally, there are some patients who are given radiation therapy, despite the fact that the likelihood of benefit is low, when all other measures have failed or cannot be used. These patients are treated sometimes at the request of referring physicians, relatives, or sometimes are "self-referred" since denial of any kind of cancer treatment may be viewed as hopeless and unacceptable by the patient, relatives, and the health care team. The complex circumstances surrounding all the types of decisions regarding therapy inhibit objective analysis of the possible cost-benefit ratio of the treatment. Nevertheless, whenever a patient is considered for radiation therapy an attempt should be made, inasmuch as possible, to inform the patients, their relatives, as well as the referring physicians of the potential gain and side effects of the therapy.

Whenever treatment is intended to achieve a cure, then a higher risk of morbidity may be acceptable. It seems obvious that treatment given for symptom relief or purely psychological reasons should not cause more symptoms and distress than the untreated condition. Although radiation does cause morbidity and complications, when carefully prescribed and administered it can certainly cure some patients for whom no comparable curative treatment may be available or preferable (i.e., carcinoma of the cervix stage II or III, medulloblastoma, Hodgkin's disease, carcinoma of the larynx). With radiation some patients can be cured who could also be cured by surgery, but the surgery may have more functional or esthetic sequalae to which the patient may have serious objections. Lastly, although achieving a cure of a patient with cancer cannot be overemphasized, it should be kept in mind that palliation of symptoms is an equally important objective, and most rewarding to all concerned.

In the last few decades there has been a definite change in the practice of oncological subspecialties. The radiation oncologist, like his/her counterpart in surgical and medical oncology, participates in the evaluation of patients before definitive therapeutic measures are undertaken and helps to formulate a multidisciplinary therapeutic approach. In this way the relative merits, advantages and disadvantages, and sequence of use of the different therapeutic modalities are brought forth and the most rational and appropriate plan is then chosen for the individual patient.

In this chapter we will describe the acute and late effects of radiation according to anatomical sections. The effect on the central nervous system and the effects in children will be discussed within the context of separate chapters.

II. HEAD AND NECK

Head and neck cancers represent approximately 5% of the new cancer cases per year in the United States. They are, however, quite important because of their anatomical location and the specific function that the different organs of the head and neck area perform. The therapeutic approach to the tumors in the head and neck area can differ significantly depending upon the location, histologic type, and extent of the tumor. In some instances, either surgery or radiation therapy would be utilized. In other instances, the combination of these two modalities, with or without chemotherapy, may be necessary for optimal results. The morbidity of the therapy would obviously depend upon the type and extent to which these modalities are utilized.

A. Orbit

Radiation to the orbit is given most often for the treatment of retinoblastomas in children, sarcomas originating from the orbital contents, and, less frequently, for metastatic disease to the choroid or for other primary tumors. In some instances, depending upon the nature of the tumor and the purpose of the treatment, the entire orbit and orbital contents are radiated whereas in other cases the treatment is confined to a more limited area. If the entire orbit is radiated not only the eye but the surrounding structures are also affected. In the latter, the early manifestations of radiation are epilation of the lashes and of the eyebrows. Normally this can be handled by cosmetic applications and it does not have any serious consequences except when the eyelashes regrow inwardly and produce corneal and conjunctival irritation. Epiphora can be seen following relatively low doses of radiation due to edema causing obstruction of the lacrimal duct.

Radiation of the lacrimal gland induces a decrease in the quantity and quality of the tears which can lead to eye irritation (Lederman, 1980; Nakissa et al., 1983; Parsons et al., 1983). This condition can be ameliorated with (nonprescription) tear substitutes.

Radiation of the globe is relatively well tolerated. The cornea is an avascular structure and does not manifest the acute, inflammatory changes seen in vascular structures. However, pericorneal injection may occur at the limbus as well as corneal edema. These findings are not obvious and the only early manifestation is that of a decreased corneal reflex. The edema may on rare occasions be followed by keratitis. More commonly there is conjunctivitis that can be painful and may be aggravated by secondary infection. This conjunctivitis can be treated with topical analgesic, anti-inflammatory preparations, and specific antibacterial medications.

Radiation of the other intraocular structures has minimal, if any, acute manifestations. The iris and ciliary body are not radiosensitive. The most sensitive structure is the lens, which does not display the acute effects of radiation but rather the late effect of cataract formation. The lens is quite radiosensitive and cataract formation may occur after a single dose of 200 rads (Merriam and Focht, 1957). The retina and choroid membranes of the eye are resistant to radiation and very little, if any, acute effects are observed.

High doses of radiation can cause permanent changes on the orbital soft tissue structures and the eye. Permanent epilation of the eyelashes and eyebrows occurs but this is generally of no clinical consequence. Epiphora due to fibrosis of the lacrimal duct is bothersome though not of major significance; it does not improve by duct dilatations (Parsons et al., 1983). High doses of radiation may cause lid deformity secondary to fibrosis and atrophy of the tarsal plate resulting in ectropion.

The cornea is avascular and therefore relatively radioresistant. Depending upon the amount of radiation received by the cornea, necrosis and ulceration may develop though this is not usually seen unless the doses used are in the range of 7000 rads (Parsons et al., 1983). Corneal ulceration may also be related to trauma associated with the loss of the lubricating and cleansing effect of the tears secondary to radiation of the lacrimal glands. Furthermore, this corneal irritation may be solely caused or aggravated by ectropion of the lower eyelid.

The internal structures of the eye tolerate therapeutic doses of radiation quite well. The iris and ciliary body seem to be resistant to radiation and the late effects of radiation are rarely manifested. Glaucoma secondary to radiation is a rare occurrence.

Of the intraocular structures the lens is the most sensitive structure and cataract formation will, inevitably, develop even with doses well below the therapeutic range. Doses as low as 200 rads (Merriam and Focht, 1957) are considered potentially cataractogenic. Thus cataracts are inevitable unless the lens is protected. Cataracts are correctable surgically. Perhaps more significant are the irreversible, late effects of radiation on the retina. The retina does not appear to be very sensitive to radiation and does not manifest any acute effects. The late effects of radiation are seen with doses in the therapeutic range (in excess of 4500-5000 rads) (Nakissa et al., 1983; Thompson, Midgal, and Whittle, 1983) and are manifest as perimacular exudates and petechial hemorrhages. This can lead to gradual loss of vision and eventual blindness. Vitreous hemorrhages may occur due to damage of the retinal vasculature but this is a rare occurrence. In some instances when the entire eye has been irradiated with high doses, the eye can become painful and nonfunctional and may have to be removed.

B. Ear

The acute and late effects of irradiation on the ear have not been well documented. Generally the ear is not intentionally exposed to radiation since primary tumors of the ear are rare. On the other hand, the ear is frequently exposed to radiation when patients are treated for primary or metastatic tumors of the central nervous system or when patients are treated for head and neck tumors. Radiation of the ear lobe for skin tumors should have no effect on the auditory canal and middle ear structures.

When the external auditory canal and the middle ear are exposed to radiation in the therapeutic dose range, the patient may experience discomfort due to the acute epithelial reaction of the ear canal. This is manifested by erythema, dry desquamation, and itching. Patients may also have partial hearing loss but this frequently subsides spontaneously. If there is a superimposed infection of the external ear canal topical antibiotics are indicated.

The only significant, long-term effect of irradiation to the ear pertains to the middle ear structures. Progressive loss of hearing occurs with therapeutic doses of radiation but the reason for this is not clear. Undoubtedly, the loss of mobility of the middle ear fine structures due to fibrosis could account for this, but it is also possible that hearing loss may be due to damage to the receptor cells in the middle ear. The threshold dose level for this to occur is not known. Once the hearing loss has occurred there is no treatment available. However, loss of hearing may be avoided by protecting the middle ear structures, if

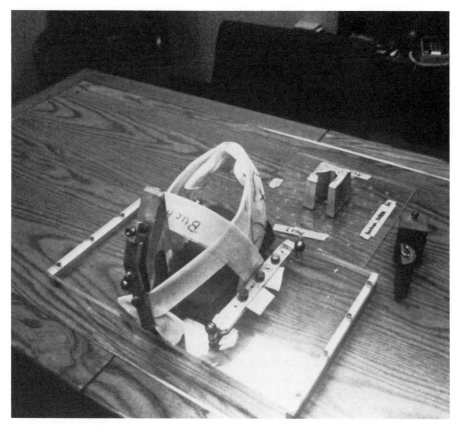

Figure 1 Head immobilization is essential for accurate, reproducible x-ray therapy. This device is used to immobilize the head. Shown are also custom-made cerrobend blocks designed to "shape the fields" thus sparing unaffected normal structures.

possible, from high doses of radiation with appropriate treatment planning and field shaping (Figure 1).

The majority of skin tumors in the ear lobe are treated surgically. The delayed effects of radiation on the skin and supportive tissues of the ear lobe are, therefore, rarely seen. When tumors in this location are treated with radiation now, the time-dose-fractionation schemes are better understood (Von Essen, 1980) and are used with high probability of success and negligible potential for complications.

C. Nasal Cavity and Paranasal Sinuses

The nasal cavity and paranasal sinuses may be radiated for primary tumors in these structures or they may be included in the field of radiation because they are adjacent to other structures harboring tumors. Primary tumors of the nasal cavity itself are rare but tumors of the paranasal sinuses are more common.

Mucositis of the nasal cavity usually occurs with doses of around 3000 rads delivered in 3 weeks. The mucositis is manifested by nasal stuffiness, increased mucous production, and bloody nasal discharge. The patient experiences discomfort and difficulty with nasal breathing and the degree of reaction may be such that a treatment interruption may be required. Radiation of the paranasal sinuses, on the other hand, rarely has acute, clinical manifestations per se. The symptoms that the patients may experience are often, if not always, overshadowed by the reaction of the adjacent structures. In instances when there is tumor or necrotic debris blocking the outlet of sinus secretions, drainage of the cavity contents may have to be achieved surgically with a Caldwell-Luc procedure. This condition may mimic acute sinusitis and may require antibiotics if a superimposed infection is also present.

The delayed effects of radiation are primarily seen in the nasal cavity. Irradiation of the nasal cavity to doses in the therapeutic range will cause atrophy of the mucosa which may lead to chronic irritation. Whether this interferes with olfactory function or not is not determined. Delayed sequelae of irradiation may be manifested by ulceration of the mucosa, leading to necrosis of the nasal septum or ala nasi. When it does happen it is likely to be in patients who have received treatment with a combination of external beam and interstitial radiation therapy. Primary tumors of the nasal cavity are rare and the effects of radiation in the nasal cavity are thus encountered infrequently. Post-therapy, the atrophic mucosa of the nasal cavity may have to lubricated and protected from extreme temperatures and irritants. Cauterization may be necessary for chronic, repeated bleeding. Caution must be exercised because this can conceivably cause further necrosis.

D. Oral Cavity

Radiation therapy of the oral cavity affects not only the mucosa and soft tissues of the oral cavity, but the teeth and osseous structures as well. The oral cavity is obviously of great importance in the maintenance of adequate nutrition and sense of well-being of the patient. The acute and chronic effects of treatment on the oral cavity can have a significant impact on the patient's ability to complete therapy as well as to recover thereafter. Physicians, dentists, nurses, and nutritionists who treat cancer patients must be aware of these effects and provide the patients with preventive and supportive care to

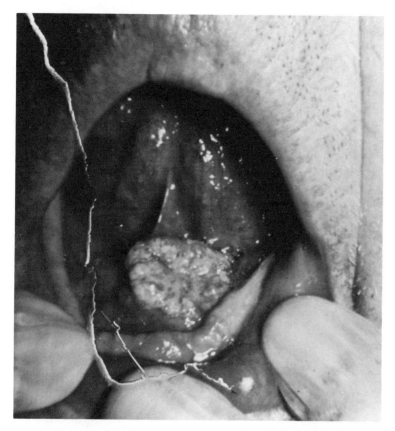

Figure 2a Patient with epidermoid carcinoma lesion in the floor of the mouth.

minimize the impact of therapy. Furthermore, it is extremely important to give utmost attention to the use of appropriate radiotherapy equipment, techniques, and the judicious utilization of interstitial therapy (Figure 2). Since the advent of high energy beams for external beam therapy (supervoltage units), cancercidal doses can be delivered with a low incidence of bone necrosis. The reason for this is that with supervoltage units there is no difference in the absorption of energy between bone and soft tissues. With low energy units (orthovoltage), the bone absorbs more energy relative to the soft tissues.

Radiation of the oral cavity produces a mucosal reaction which is dose-dependent and begins as erythema of the mucosa after a dose as low as approximately 2000 rads given in 2 weeks. As the dose is carried to higher levels, the mucosa exhibits punctuate, yellowish areas that gradually become larger and ultimately form a confluent pseudomembrane. This yellowish pseudomembrane sloughs leaving a hemorrhagic surface.

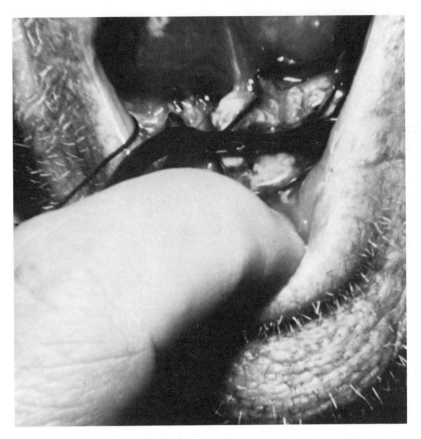

Figure 2b Lesion in floor of the mouth was treated with interstitial therapy (radium needles). With interstitial therapy a high dose of radiation can be given to a limited volume.

Salivary glands are very sensitive to radiation. The acute effects of radiation follow a similar dose response to that of the oral mucosa (Mosseman, 1983). The serous, acinar cells of the salivary glands are quite sensitive to irradiation As the cumulative dose increases they are affected and the saliva diminishes in quantity and becomes more viscous and adherent (William, 1983). As the mucositis and the changes in the salivary glands progress in increasing doses, the patient may become dehydrated, compounding the problem. Xerostomia begins to appear at a dose of about 1500 rads and is generally more pronounced at night. After higher doses are reached, xerostomia is also experienced during the day. The extent to which production of saliva is impaired depends upon the radiation dose as well as the volume of the salivary glands being radiated.

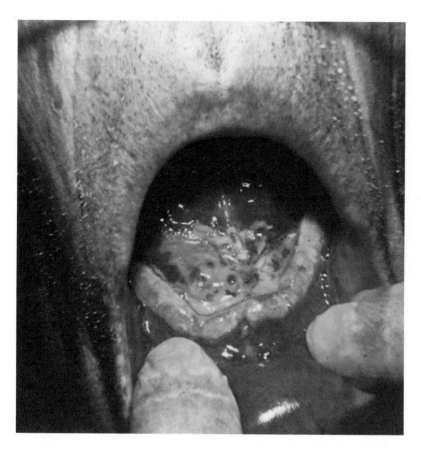

Figure 2c Marked, homogeneous reaction seen in the floor of the mouth and tumor corresponding to the volume of the implant.

In addition to the quantitative change of the saliva, there is also a qualitative change. The pH of the saliva decreases from a normal of 6.8 to approximately 5.5 and perhaps even lower. These salivary changes are very significant as the saliva which is normally a buffering, lubricating, and bactericidal agent no longer performs these functions and this in turn plays a direct role in the changes that occur in the teeth and gums. In addition to the effects of radiation on the salivary glands the taste buds of the tongue, and along with the oral mucosal changes, there is also a loss of taste sensation. The mucosal reaction, salivary gland dysfunction, and loss of taste make it very difficult for patients to maintain adequate nutrition.

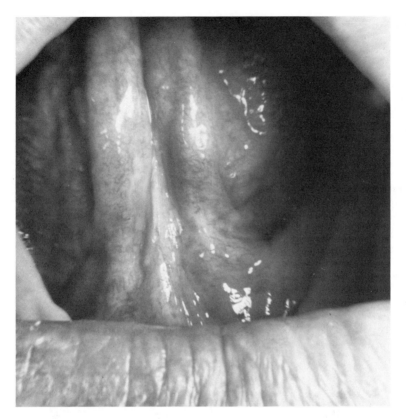

Figure 2d Follow-up 2 years later. The tumor has been controlled with excellent cosmetic and functional results.

The acute effects of radiation on the teeth and bones are not obvious except that the mucosal and salivary changes make it difficult for patients to maintain good oral hygiene and this can lead to or accelerate tooth decay. Ulcerated tumors which overlie or are in proximity to the bone can be the portal of entry of infection, leading to osteomyelitis and potentially to bone necrosis.

The late effects of radiation on the oral cavity are dose-volume related. They are also related to the use of interstitial therapy (iridium seed or radium needle implants). With interstitial therapy smaller volumes of tissue are exposed to a higher dose, whereas with external beam larger volumes of tissue are exposed to a lower dose. With doses above 5000 rads there is some atrophy of the mucosa manifested by paleness, telangiectasia, and dryness. With doses of 6500-7000 rads, these changes are more pronounced and superficial ulceration may occur. Frequently it is not possible to spare the salivary glands which compounds the problem. Since salivary glands do not recover from radiation, the xerostomia produced by exposure to radiation of the glands is significant and permanent with doses above 4000 rads. The degree of xerostomia depends upon the volume of the glands carried to a high dose. As a result of the mucosal and salivary gland changes taking place in the mouth, the teeth are indirectly affected. Dental caries develop frequently, particularly in the crown of the teeth and eventually the teeth may break off. Prior to radiation treatment the patients need to be evaluated carefully and should be handled according to the I-IV prognostic categories recommended by Daly (1980). Edentulous patients (category I) should still have x-rays of the oral cavity as there may be tooth fragments or cysts which should be cared for before treatment begins. Patients with teeth in poor condition (category II) should have full mouth extraction. Patients with carious but restorable teeth (category III) should have restorations and, if necessary, removal of nonrestorable teeth. Patients with teeth in good condition (category IV) and patients with the restored teeth (category III) need a program of careful hygiene and prophylaxis including the construction of custom-made fluoride carriers for fluoride treatment. Such a program needs to be adhered to rigorously during treatment and for an indefinite period afterwards. Soft tissue and bone necrosis occurs with significant frequency among long-term survivors of treatment for oropharyngeal malignancies (Larson et al., 1983). Such necrosis is painful and slow to heal. Conservative management consisting of topical application of 1% neomycin solution, analgesics, and maintaining the ulcer bed clean are very important measures, but surgery may ultimately be required. Hyperbaric oxygen has been used for bone necrosis with some success. The surgery needs to be quite radical to remove devitalized tissue. This may have a substantial functional and aesthetic impact. Trismus due to fibrosis of the muscles of mastication and ankylosis of the temporomandibular joints may also be observed. Trismus is usually more pronounced in patients treated with a combination of surgery and preoperative or postoperative radiotherapy and it may be advisable to put these patients on an intensified exercise program post-treatment. It is helpful to obtain an interarch measurement before trismus develops to use as a guideline for the stretching exercises. Trismus is practically not correctable once it has developed but it may be prevented to some extent.

E. Neck

The neck region is included in the field of radiation when primary tumors of the upper aerodigestive tract or the neck lymph nodes that are the primary drainage site of head and neck malignancies are treated. Likewise, neck structures are radiated for the treatment of lymphomas which frequently involve nodes in this location. The supraclavicular regions are also frequently

treated for overt or subclinical metastatic disease from head and neck or intrathoracic malignancies or for lymphomas involving these nodes.

Irradiation of the soft tissues of the neck and supraclavicular areas is generally well tolerated. Erythema and dry desquamation are seen with doses of
4000-5000 rads. At these dose levels moist desquamation may be observed in
the base of the neck and superior aspect of the supraclavicular region where
the irradiation interacts with the tissues tangentially. This desquamation heals
spontaneously or with minimal care. When the treatment is given with lateral
portals or with anterior and posterior opposed portals, without midline blocking, the upper aerodigestive tract is affected. The hypopharynx and upper
portion of the esophagus, like the oral cavity, will begin to manifest signs of
reaction with doses of 2000-3000 rads. Between 3000-4000 rads most patients
will experience some degree of odynophagia. With doses in excess of 4000
rads, patients will experience significant discomfort and will be generally unable
to eat solid or semisolid food, or even take liquids. If the oral cavity has also
been included in the field, the reaction may be such that the patients may
have to have a feeding tube inserted or be maintained with parenteral nutrition.
This degree of reaction usually is not seen because the patients generally will
have had a rest period after a dose of 4000-5000 rads. To further avoid reactions at this dose level the fields are reduced and only portions of the
oropharynx are carried to higher doses.

The larynx is frequently included in the field of radiation not only because
laryngeal tumors are usually treated with radiation but also while treating
tumors in other structures of the neck. The acute effects of radiation on the
larynx parallel the effects seen in the oral cavity and hypopharynx in terms
of the degree and nature of mucosal reaction. The reaction is manifest as
hoarseness due to inflammation and edema of the larynx. Hoarseness, however, is almost always a symptom in patients with tumors of the larynx. As
with radiation reactions elsewhere in the head and neck area, the treatment is
purely symptomatic. During the period of acute reaction is is important that
the patients avoid further irritation to the larynx. They are strongly advised
to abstain from smoking and alcohol consumption and they should also avoid
dusty or polluted air environments. The use of air humidifiers may also be
helpful. Patients should avoid excessive use of their voice. In some cases,
although they otherwise may be able to work, it may be advisable to stop
working in order to minimize use of their voice (teachers, sales personnel, etc.).

The late effects of radiation on the larynx are primarily persistent edema of
the arytenoids, the false cords, and sometimes the true cords. This is not seen
unless doses of at least 5500 rads are delivered. The persistent edema causes
changes of the quality of the voice. In addition to the edema, the epiglottis
loses some of its mobility and often becomes rigid and rests against the
posterior pharyngeal wall. The edema and rigidity of the epiglottis make

post-treatment evaluation of these patients difficult. Necrosis of the mucosa and cartilage without persistence of tumor rarely occurs. The dose required to cause such necrosis is somewhere between 6500-7000 rads. Generally, the conservative treatment of necrosis is not successful and patients will require laryngectomy. Furthermore, the differential diagnosis between necrosis and persistent disease is quite difficult and the laryngectomy specimen may reveal persistent tumor when only necrosis had been clinically suspected.

III. THORAX

The thorax is commonly radiated for the treatment of lung or esophageal tumors, lymphomas, and, in recent years, primary treatment of breast cancer. From the point of view of the acute and late effects of radiation, the mediastinal structures and the lungs are the most important organs. Radiation sequelae in these organs can have serious consequences.

A. Esophagus

Radiation of the esophagus produces symptoms related to the gradual, progressive destruction of the mucosal lining in a pattern similar to that seen in the oral cavity. With doses as low as 2000 rads delivered in 2 weeks, patients begin to experience odynophagia. As the dose increases these symptoms get worse. At doses of about 4000-5000 rads, the patients are generally only able to take semisolid and liquid foods. When a dose of approximately 6000 rads is reached, depending upon the length of the esophagus radiated, the esophagitis may be so severe that parenteral nutrition may be necessary. Esophagitis persists for about 10 days after the radiation is discontinued. It then begins to heal rapidly and generally it is completely healed within four weeks after termination of treatment. Frequently, the esophagus is radiated to a dose of approximately 4000-4500 rads and then a rest period is allowed before delivering further therapy. This rest period usually prevents the development of severe esophagitis. During the course of radiation, patients are given instructions regarding semisolid, soft, and liquid diets and nutritional supplements. Patients are also advised against alcohol consumption and are given topical analgesics such as Viscous Lidocaine, ½ to 1 tsp in about ½ glass of water to swallow slowly 15 minutes before eating. Of help to some patients is to take 1 tbsp of vegetable oil about 15 minutes before eating or to put a piece of butter in the mouth and to allow it to dissolve. This provides lubrication to the esophageal mucosa and facilitates the passage of food. In some instances, systemic analgesics are needed. A nasogastric tube for feeding may be necessary. The tube, however, itself causes mechanical irritation. In some patients with carcinoma of the esophagus a feeding gastrostomy may be required as

the tumor obstructs the esophageal lumen. It is also important to rule out
infections of the oral cavity as well as the esophagus which can mimic and
aggravate the symptoms of radiation esophagitis.

The late effects of radiation of the esophagus are rarely encountered
because patients with esophageal tumors do not enjoy a long-term survival.
In a few instances, segmental narrowing of the esophagus may occur which
requires esophageal dilatation. This esophageal narrowing is more likely to
occur in patients who have had concomitant chemotherapy.

B. Heart

The heart had been considered a "radioresistant" structure when only
kilovoltage x-ray equipment was available. With this type of equipment, it
was not possible to deliver high doses to deep structures without causing damage to the superficial tissues. When supervoltage equipment became available
and higher doses of radiation could be given to the deep mediastinal structures,
it became apparent that the heart is moderately sensitive to radiation. The
basis for the injury to the heart is related to the sensitivity of small cardiac
vessels. Radiation may cause fibrosis of the pericardium, endocardium, and
myocardium.

The acute effects of radiation on the heart are generally not clinically overt
and may remain undiagnosed. Small radiation dose changes in the conduction
system of the heart have been described. These consist of inversion of the P
wave and prolongation of the S-T segment. Acute pericarditis manifested by
chest pain, fever, and pericardial rub, with or without pericardial effusion, can
occur at doses of radiation ranging from 1500-3000 rads (Ruckdeschel et al.,
1975). This acute pericarditis is more likely to happen when patients with
large, radiosensitive mediastinal tumor masses such as Hodgkin's disease are
treated (Applefield and Wiernik, 1983). The rapid regression of the mediastinal
mass may cause irritation of the pericardium which, coupled with tumor
necrosis, can lead to the effusion. If there is no pericardial effusion, then the
acute radiation pericarditis may be unrecognized. Treatment for the milder
forms of pericarditis is symptomatic with the use of salicylates. Acute radiation myocarditis is rarely observed clinically and the symptoms of it may be
overshadowed by the symptoms of radiation pericarditis.

The late effects of radiation on the heart are well recognized and can be
very serious (Cohn et al., 1967). The pathophysiology is similar to that of
the acute effects, namely small vessel injury within the myocardium and pericardium leading to fibrosis (Fajardo and Stewart, 1971; Stewart et al., 1967).
It is not clear whether and to what extent radiation can cause damage of the
main branches of the coronary arteries. Young patients have been reported to
have sustained myocardial infarcts after radiation of the mediastinum for
Hodgkin's disease (Applefield and Wiernik, 1983). When the mediastinum is

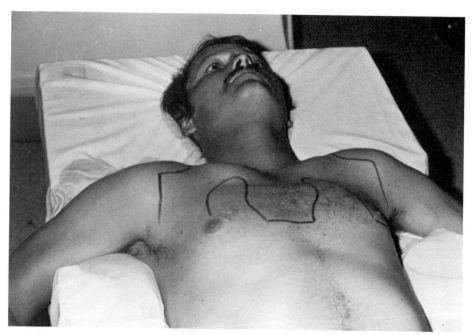

Figure 3a Patient being treated for Hodgkin's disease (mantle field). Patient is immobilized in an "alpha cradle" shaped for each individual patient. Note field drawn on patient's chest.

treated to a dose of 4000 rads delivered in 4 weeks, some degree of radiation pericarditis can be expected. This pericarditis is more likely to occur if a large portion of heart is included in the field and is manifest clinically in about 6% of patients (Figure 3). The frequency of radiation pericarditis can be higher with this dose (4000 rads) if all of the treatment to the mediastinum is given through an anterior portal only. The symptoms of chronic radiation-induced heart disease are primarily those of constrictive pericarditis. These may be progressive and severe in nature and may require pericardiectomy. The myocardium is also affected but the symptoms of myocardial disease generally appear about 2 years after the treatment has been given. The syndrome of chronic radiation myocarditis consists of symptoms of chronic heart failure, arrhythmias, and EKG waves of diminished amplitude. It should be kept in mind that in some instances patients receive anthracycline chemotherapy (doxorubicin and daunorubicin) which is intrinsically cardiotoxic. The combined use of these chemotherapeutic agents with radiation increases the frequency and severity of heart damage.

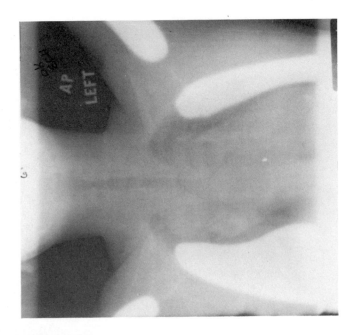

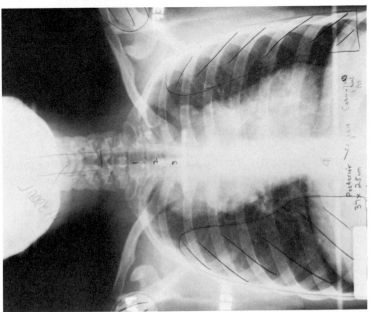

Figure 3b Simulator and port films show outline of field. The field is shaped by cerrobend blocks. Note the width of the mediastinal field needed to encompass the large mediastinal mass.

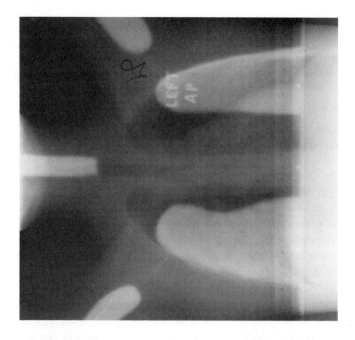

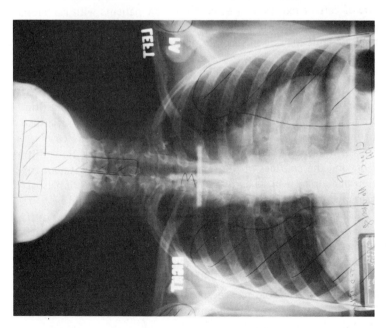

Figure 3c Simulator and port films after 2000 rads have been delivered. The mediastinal mass has shrunk. A new set of blocks is made. The width of the mediastinal field is reduced accordingly.

The management of radiation-induced heart disease is simply supportive, as it is with other forms of chronic heart disease. Depending upon the severity of the damage and the condition of the heart prior to the treatment, chronic radiation-induced heart disease may be disabling and may even cause death.

C. Lungs

Portions of the lungs are frequently radiated since one of the most common and lethal of all malignancies, carcinoma of the lung, is often treated with radiation therapy. Also, lymphomas, though less common, frequently involve the mediastinum and are generally treated with radiation. The acute and late effects of radiation in the lung are dose and volume related. Furthermore, these effects can be more severe or significant in patients with chronic bronchitis or tuberculosis. Foci of chronic tuberculosis included in the field of radiation are apt to become active and disseminate. In some instances the lung itself is not affected by the neoplastic process but it is radiated due to its proximity to tissues harboring tumor. The normal lung tissue in these cases may manifest more clearly the acute and late effects of radiation. However, the majority of patients who receive radiation to the lungs are patients with carcinoma of the lung who often have an associated inflammatory process along with the tumor, making it difficult to truly evaluate the extent of the acute and late effects of radiation. Furthermore, few patients with carcinoma of the lung will live long enough to manifest the late effects of radiation. However, some patients may be mistakenly diagnosed as having disease progression rather than post-radiation lung fibrosis.

Acute radiation pneumonitis is characterized by fever, nonproductive cough, chest pain and sometimes dyspnea but does not usually occur until 1-3 months after completion of the treatment. The chest x-ray usually shows an infiltrate which, unlike that of bacterial infections, does not follow an anatomical distribution but rather coincides with the radiation treatment portal (Roswit and White, 1977). In the cases where there is superimposed infection, this infiltrate may extend beyond the confines of the treatment portal. The treatment for acute radiation pneumonitis in its early and uncomplicated phase consists of supportive therapy. If there is productive cough, the sputum should be cultured so that appropriate antibiotic therapy may be given if necessary. If *Pneumocystis carinii* is suspected, a lung biopsy and silver stain are necessary to make this diagnosis. When the radiation pneumonitis is not complicated by infection, steroid therapy may be given, beginning with a dose of 60 mg of prednisone per day. Once there has been clinical improvement, the steroids should be tapered slowly to avoid reexacerbation of the symptoms (Pezner et al., 1984). In some instances a low, maintenance dose of steroids may have to be continued for several months. When the radiation pneumonitis encompasses substantial amounts of lung tissue, and particularly in patients

with compromised functional lung capacity or those who have received concomitant chemotherapy, the acute pneumonitis process can be very severe and
even fatal.

The late effects of radiation are manifested by chronic radiation pneumonitis which is likewise dependent upon volume and dose. Often this condition
is relatively asymptomatic and the diagnosis is made largely on the basis of a
dense infiltrate corresponding with the radiation treatment portal. This infiltrate represents fibrosis of the lung tissue caused by radiation. Whenever lung
tissue receives a dose of 3000-4000 rads or more with conventional fractionation, some degree of fibrosis will occur which may or may not be apparent in
the chest x-ray (Jennings and Arden, 1962). Typically this is observed in the
lung apices in patients having had treatment for carcinoma of the breast.
This is also frequently seen in the hilar regions and lung apices in lymphoma
patients treated with the "mantle" field. Also this is seen in patients treated
for carcinoma of the lung. In these patients, however, underlying residual
tumor can be partially responsible for the chest x-ray image. Patients may
complain of dry, hacking, nonproductive cough and sometimes they have a
low-grade fever. Dyspnea on exertion can occur but severe dyspnea is uncommon unless the patients have compromised pulmonary function, have
had surgery or have had a substantial portion of lung tissue included in the
field. If the process is not complicated by superimposed infection, the
symptoms will abate but the infiltrate on the chest x-ray will persist unchanged or may even be more dense with time. Post-radiation pulmonary
sequelae may be more prevalent now as a result of the greater utilization of
combined chemotherapy and radiotherapy. Some chemotherapeutic agents
such as methotrexate, busulfan, BCNU, and bleomycin are themselves associated with pulmonary toxicity (Glatstein and Carter, 1982).

The treatment of chronic radiation pneumonitis is supportive. Steroid
therapy is used, however, its value remains controversial. Undoubtedly steroid
therapy ameliorates the patient's symptoms, but they may reoccur when the
therapy is stopped. Nevertheless, some patients require long-term administration of steroids and sometimes oxygen therapy is needed as well. Chronic
radiation pneumonitis of clinical significance may be seen in patients who
have not had symptoms of acute radiation pneumonitis.

IV. ABDOMEN

Radiation of the entire abdomen is poorly tolerated and is rarely undertaken.
However, there is current interest in the administration of radiation in small,
multiple fractions per day (multifractionation) instead of the conventional
schemes of one relatively large fraction per day, as a means of achieving
greater antitumor effect and lesser normal tissue damage for some tumor and

normal tissue systems (Thames et al., 1983). It is therefore possible that radiation given in this way, which is very well tolerated, may be more effective for disseminated abdominal malignancies. If this is indeed the case, radiation to the whole abdomen for tumors such as carcinoma of the ovary may be used more often in the future. On the other hand, it is also possible that more effective chemotherapeutic agents may be developed for disseminated abdominal malignancies in which case radiation therapy may not be used routinely. Radiation is now utilized mainly in an adjuvant setting and is given to relatively localized areas. Frequently local control of the disease or cure is not the primary objective of radiation therapy given for abdominal malignancies but rather the goal is for relief of symptoms. It should be noted too that in recent years there has been a great deal of interest in the use of "intraoperative therapy" with high energy electron or low energy photon beams (Gunderson et al., 1984). Unfortunately, this is an approach that requires a substantial commitment of time and personnel and close cooperation with other services and this precludes wider application. Furthermore, the basic radiobiological principles of intraoperative therapy, such as tumor control doses and late effects on the normal tissues, have not been thoroughly investigated. Nevertheless, this is a promising approach that merits continuing investigation.

A. Liver

The liver is an organ that is rarely exposed to radiation in its entirety except when the whole abdomen is treated or when patients with multiple metastasis to the liver are treated for palliative purposes. Primary tumors in the liver are extremely rare and they are treated surgically, if possible. Other approaches, including hepatic infusion with chemotherapy, or the multidisciplinary approach of chemotherapy, external beam therapy, and radiolabeled antibodies, are also beginning to be used (Order et al., 1980). When a considerable amount of the liver is exposed to doses of 2400 rads or more, acute radiation hepatitis may occur (Ingold et al., 1965). The symptoms of radiation hepatitis are fever, nausea, malaise, rapid weight gain, and increased abdominal girth due to ascites. However, ascites is more likely to develop in cases of chronic radiation hepatitis. Perhaps more important for the diagnosis are the laboratory findings which include moderate elevation of the serum alkaline phosphatase and the SGOT and SGPT levels. The symptoms of radiation hepatitis may be obscured not only by the patient's general condition, but also by the symptoms associated with tumor involvement of the liver. Acute radiation hepatitis is, therefore, difficult to diagnose clinically and the definitive diagnosis rests on the histological picture (hyperemia, central lobular necrosis with fibrosis, and central vein thrombosis) (Reed and Cox, 1966), and for that reason this diagnosis is rarely established. The treatment of acute radiation hepatitis is purely symptomatic, but it is important to rule out viral or drug-induced hepatitis. Since there is no effective treatment for acute radiation hepatitis and the consequences can be quite serious, the maximum dose given to the entire liver should not exceed 2400 rads. Concurrent chemotherapy may sensitize the liver to radiation damage, however, the factor by which the radiation dose may have to be reduced when given concomitantly with chemotherapy is not known.

Chronic radiation hepatitis may occur a few months after completion of radiation therapy. As with the acute effects, unless a substantial amount of the liver is exposed to doses in excess of 2500-3000 rads with conventional fractionation, chronic radiation hepatitis should not occur. The patient may or may not have had manifestations of acute radiation hepatitis. Clinically the patient presents with hepatomegaly and ascites. The serum alkaline phosphatase may be elevated without significant elevation of the bilirubin and transaminase levels. Depending upon the total dose given and the portion of the liver radiated, liver failure may ensue. As for the acute radiation hepatitis, the histological diagnosis rests on the characteristic central vein thrombosis and fibrosis within the liver lobule. The treatment of chronic radiation hepatitis is purely supportive and there is nothing that can be done to revert this process. As in the case of acute radiation hepatitis, prevention of this condition by limiting the dose and volume of the liver radiated is essential, particularly in patients with a favorable long-term prognosis.

B. Gastrointestinal Tract

While the stomach, small intestine, and large intestine share some common features in terms of their response to radiation. These organs also differ to some extent with regard to their response to radiation and these factors warrant specific discussion. Because of the anatomy of the abdominal cavity, usually several organs or portions thereof are included in the field of radiation and thus the effects of the therapy are manifested in several organs. The long-term effects of radiation may be more sharply defined since they are associated with higher doses which are usually given only to limited volumes. The gastrointestinal tract occupies portions of the upper abdomen and pelvis and for the purpose of this discussion the stomach, small intestine, ascending, transverse, and descending colon will be discussed together. The effects of irradiation on the sigmoid and rectum will be discussed in the section dealing with the pelvic organs.

Exposure of the upper abdomen to radiation can produce anorexia, nausea, vomiting, and sometimes diarrhea. The severity of these symptoms depends largely on the time-dose-fractionation and volume parameters of radiation. Because of its proliferative kinetics, the epithelium of the gastrointestinal tract is quite sensitive to radiation. This has been thoroughly studied in the small bowel and it has been shown that within 24 hours following a single dose of 500-1000 rads, changes can be seen in the mucosa (Rubin and Casarett, 1966). Approximately 4 days after exposure to radiation, definite histological evidence of villous destruction is seen as a result of lack of replacement of cells that are normally shed into the intestinal lumen by new cells growing from the bottom of the crypts. Subendothelial edema, capillary congestion, and destruction of the lymphoid follicles are also noted. Even when a relatively small portion of the abdomen is exposed to radiation, the patients experience nausea and sometimes vomiting from the outset. These symptoms can be alleviated with antiemetics, avoidance of certain foods such as raw vegetables, fruit juices, fatty foods, and roughage. If necessary there can be a reduction of the daily radiation dose. Diarrhea, which is the main symptom of radiation enteritis, does not usually develop until a dose of at least 2000 rads has been given. If a significant portion of the small bowel has been included in the field of radiation, the diarrhea can be sufficiently severe to lead to fluid and electrolyte imbalances. This severe, radiation enteritis is not reached unless there is an associated predisposing condition or a substantial amount of small bowel receives at least 4000 rads. The more frequently seen mild to moderate enteritis is managed with low residue, low fat diet; antidiarrheal medications such as Iopenamide or Diphenoxylate Hydrochloride; reduction in the daily radiation dose; and if necessary a treatment interruption. Here again, limiting the treatment volume inasmuch as possible, using multiple fields, and careful treatment planning can reduce the frequency and severity of this side effect. The use of multifractionation treatment schemes will improve the tolerance to the treatment, however, it is not clear what impact this fractionation scheme has on tumor control.

When the stomach or a portion of it is exposed to radiation, the patients experience anorexia, nausea, and sometimes vomiting even at the outset. In addition to the effects on the mucosal lining, radiation interferes with function of the cells in the glands of the mucosa of the stomach. Acid and pepsin secretion decrease as a result of damage to the zymogenic and parietal cells (Rider et al., 1957). The acute effects of radiation on the stomach are rarely of any significant magnitude except for the nausea and anorexia, which may result in weight loss and malnutrition. Nausea can be managed with antiemetics and if necessary daily radiation dose reduction and ultimately a temporary treatment interruption may be needed.

C. Kidneys

Kidneys are relatively sensitive to radiation. It is generally accepted that a dose of 2500 rads given in 2.5-3 weeks constitutes the tolerance of the kidneys. If both kidneys are within the field of radiation, extreme care is given not to exceed their tolerance. On the other hand, in some instances, one kidney may have to be exposed to doses above tolerance. Acute, unilateral radiation nephritis is not detected clinically since the other kidney, if intact, can perform the necessary physiological functions.

The late radiation effects on the kidney are manifested by chronic renal failure. This is now very rarely seen since great care is given not to expose both kidneys to doses above tolerance. However, unilateral radiation nephropathy may cause hypertension in which case a unilateral nephrectomy is indicated. If both kidneys are exposed to doses in excess of 2500 rads given in 2.5-3 weeks, bilateral radiation nephropathy will likely develop. This is an insidious, progressive process for which medical management and dialysis are the only treatments available.

V. PELVIS

Radiation of the pelvis is generally given for gynecological or urological malignancies and more recently with increasing frequency for rectal and anal tumors. The acute and late effects of radiation on the small and large bowel have been described in the preceding section. The side effects of the treatment to this region pertain primarily to the bladder, the rectum, and also to the male and female reproductive organs. In dealing with this anatomical region, the side effects associated with the use of brachytherapy should be considered.

A. Bladder

The bladder is always included in the field of radiation in patients treated for gynecological, prostate, or bladder tumors. The effects of radiation on the bladder are dose and volume related like for all other organs, but also are influenced by the condition of the bladder prior to treatment. Acute radiation cystitis is manifested by frequency, urgency, dysuria, and sometimes hematuria. These symptoms are the result of denudation of the mucosal surface of the bladder. The symptoms of acute radiation cystitis can be aggravated by superimposed infection. The symptoms of cystitis do not develop until a dose of 3000 rads with conventional fractionation is reached and generally do not become severe unless the bladder receives at least 5000 rads. Urinary antispasmodics are helpful in controlling the frequency and dysuria. Medications such as Pyridium that combine antibacterial and analgesic agents can be very useful also. For cases refractory to these symptomatic measures, urinalysis with culture and sensitivity followed by specific antibiotic therapy are indicated. Frequently these symptoms of acute cystitis subside within about 2-4 weeks post-termination of the treatment.

After a variable period of well-being some patients may have reoccurrence of the symptoms of cystitis and thus manifest chronic radiation cystitis. The late effects of radiation on the bladder range from chronic radiation cystitis to fistulas. The latter is not seen unless the bladder has received doses in excess of 6500 rads, which can happen in patients treated for carcinoma of the cervix. In such patients the treatment often entails the combination of external beam and brachytherapy, and this can result in the delivery of high doses to small portions of the bladder. When patients have had treatment with external beam only, chronic radiation cystitis is much less likely to occur and fistulas are extremely rare (Montana et al., 1985). Chronic radiation cystitis is manifested by frequency, urgency, dysuria, and sometimes hematuria. If hematuria is present the patients should have examination of urinary cytologies and endoscopy to rule out other pathology. Biopsies of the bladder should be avoided unless there is a high index of suspicion of associated pathology. Severe hemorrhagic cystitis may require fulguration of localized bleeding sites. Allowing the bladder to "rest" by means of an indwelling catheter and using topical steroids may be necessary. After a variable period the process subsides, though sometimes resulting in a contracted bladder with reduced capacity. In cases of very severe, intractable radiation cystitis, urinary diversion with an ileoconduit, and even a cystectomy, may have to be performed. Vesicovaginal fistulas can develop as a result of radiation therapy, however, in the absence of initial tumor involvement of the bladder or of residual, uncontrolled tumor in the perivesical tissues, this is rarely seen. This complication occurs almost exclusively in patients who have had treatment for gynecological malignancies which, as noted before, entails the combined use of external beam and brachytherapy. The development of fistulas is always preceded by symptoms of cystitis. The diagnosis of a vesicovaginal fistula can be established easily on physical examination and by instillation of methylene blue in the bladder and the appearance of the dye in the vaginal cavity. The treatment of vesicovaginal fistula is surgical (Smith, 1980). Usually the surgical procedure required is urinary diversion with an ileoconduit but on rare instances a small fistula may be controlled with simple primary closure. Unfortunately, the fistula is sometimes associated with a rectovaginal fistula as well, in which case a much more extensive surgical procedure, including a colostomy, may be required.

B. Rectosigmoid

The acute effects of radiation on the rectosigmoid are manifested by tenesmus, diarrhea, and sometimes bleeding. Practically all of the patients who receive treatment to the pelvis to a dose of 3000 rads or more, develop some degree of radiation proctosigmoiditis. These symptoms can be managed well with a low residue bland diet, stool softeners, and anticholinergic medications. The symptoms usually subside 2-4 weeks after the completion of the course of radiation. Some patients continue to have sensitivity to greasy, spicy foods, fresh vegetables, and citrus fruits, which is manifest by episodes of diarrhea. During the course of treatment patients are advised to avoid certain foods and are encouraged to maintain a low residue, nonirritating bland diet. The symptoms of proctosigmoiditis are dose related and are more likely to be severe in patients who have received at least 5000 rads to the rectosigmoid. This is more apt to happen in patients being treated for gynecological malignancies. These patients usually receive treatment with a combination of external beam and brachytherapy and may receive 6500-7000 rads to a small area of the rectosigmoid. Even in severe cases the symptoms of proctosigmoiditis usually subside with conservative management within about 2 months post-completion of the treatment.

The late effects of radiation usually appear after a period of well-being. Some patients develop proctosigmoiditis as indicated by episodes of diarrhea, tenesmus, and sometimes rectal bleeding. If the proctosigmoiditis is of moderate severity, the patients can be managed symptomatically with low residue diet and stool softeners. As for the acute proctosigmoiditis, antispasmodics and sometimes intermittent, short courses of steroid enemas may be necessary. Generally the patients have a slight amount of rectal bleeding but in some patients the bleeding can be quite severe. Ultimately it may be necessary to perform a colostomy to allow the bowel to rest. The colostomy can be taken down after the process has resolved. The most severe proctosigmoid complications are the rectovaginal fistulas which are always preceded by symptoms of proctosigmoiditis. The diagnosis of rectovaginal fistula is easily established by the history of passage of gas or stool per vagina and by the physical examination. Some patients may have had biopsies of the rectum to rule out recurrent tumor. Biopsies of the rectum may precipitate the development of fistulae and are therefore discouraged. They should be performed only when recurrent tumor is strongly suspected. Once the diagnosis of rectovaginal fistula is made, the patient should have a colostomy (Smith, 1980). After the acute process has subsided, an attempt at primary closure of the fistula can be made, but if this is not successful the colostomy has to remain permanently. As in the case of vesicovaginal fistulas, this complication is rarely seen unless the patients have received treatment with the combination of external beam and brachytherapy, as is the case generally when gynecological malignancies are treated (Montana, 1985). This complication is also more likely to develop in patients with tumor involvement of the posterior vaginal wall and rectovaginal septum.

VI. GONADS

Although gonadal tissue is extremely sensitive to radiation, exposure of the testicles or the ovaries to radiation does not produce an acute reaction that can be detected clinically. In males transient aspermia can be seen even with small doses, but recovery has been documented even after relatively high doses (Lanshbaugh and Casasrett, 1976; Smithers, Wallace, and Anstern, 1973). Adequate radiation-dose-response studies of spermatogenesis are not available; therefore, it is not possible to counsel or advise patients regarding the potential for sterility or sublethal damage to the sperm cells which could lead to fetal malformations. It is always advisable to measure the gonadal exposure with thermoluminescent dosimeters in young males undergoing therapy to the lower pelvis or upper portions of the lower extremities. Whenever possible custom-made shields can be constructed to protect the testicles from direct exposure to radiation. Male patients who have received therapy to the abdomen, pelvis, or upper portion of the lower extremities are advised not to father children for at least 1 or preferably 2 years after completing the treatment to minimize the possibility of fetal malformations.

The reproductive function of the ovaries is also quite sensitive to radiation. Permanent sterility can be caused with relatively small doses of radiation. In young females with highly curable diseases such as Hodgkin's disease, the ovaries can be repositioned at the time of surgery so that they can be protected from direct radiation. Some of these patients have gone on to bear normal children (LeFloch, Donaldson, and Kaplan, 1976).

VII. EXTREMITIES

The extremities are usually radiated for sarcomas of the soft tissues or bones, and for primary tumors of the skin and skin appendages. In general, the treatment of skin tumors entails the use of limited fields and the acute and late effects are minimal. In rare instances extensive, squamous cell carcinomas of the skin, such as those that develop in scars of thermal burns (Novick et al., 1977), are treated and they require large fields carried to high doses. However, most of the effects that will be described in this section apply primarily to the use of radiation for soft tissue and bone sarcomas. Quite often the radiation therapy will be given in addition to surgery and chemotherapy though the sequence of these modalities and the extent to which it may be applied will vary considerably. The acute and the late effects of radiation will be directly related to the dose of radiation given but will also be determined by the magnitude of the surgery and chemotherapy given. It is assumed that the combined chemotherapeutic agents, drug reaction, dose and timing of administration (with respect to the radiation therapy) have an impact not only on the acute effects but more significantly on the late effects of radiation (Rubin, 1984).

The acute effects are primarily manifested by the skin reaction namely: erythema, dry desquamation, and ultimately denudation of the epidermis resulting in superficial ulceration. These changes are dose related and they do not begin to become clinically obvious until at least a dose of 3000 rads in 3 weeks or its equivalent has been given. Doses of approximatley 4000 rads in 4 weeks will produce dry desquamation but with doses in excess of 5000 rads areas of moist desquamation will be seen. This is particularly apparent in the natural creases, such as the inguinal, perineal, or the axillary folds which tend to accumulate moisture. This degree of reaction heals spontaneously. The acute effects of radiation on the muscles, bones, and joints are not clinically detectable with doses in the therapeutic range. If possible it is recommended that a strip of skin and subcutaneous tissue be spared from radiation to avoid venous and lymphatic capillary fibrosis that may be the cause, at least in part, for the development of edema in the distal radiated extremity.

The late effects of radiation on the extremities are also dose and volume related. They, too, bear relationship to the other therapeutic modalities employed, such as surgery and chemotherapy. The late effects of radiation have to do more with function than with esthetics. When high doses of radiation have been given to the mid or proximal segment of an extremity, even when a strip of tissue has been spared, lymphedema distal to the area of radiation generally develops. It begins to occur with doses of about 5000 rads delivered in 5 weeks. The edema begins to appear approximately 3-6 months after surgery and seems to level off at about 1-2 years post-treatment. The degree and extent of the lymphedema will depend upon the extent of the previous surgery as well as the dose and volume of tissue radiated. This can progress and cause incapacitation. A significant effect, but one more difficult to quantitate, is muscle fibrosis which can cause limitation of function of the extremity. In addition to muscle fibrosis there can be fibrosis of the tissues that surround the joints, leading to ankylosis. The effects of radiation on the articular surfaces and synovium are not well known and may be obscured by the effects on the regional muscle groups. These effects are progressive and are more marked in elderly patients. There are no preventive measures that can be taken aside from limiting the dose of radiation, leaving strips of tissue unirradiated if possible, and sparing the joints themselves, in as much as possible. Following the course of radiation, physical therapy of the involved extremity probably lessens the late effects of the treatment and the associated functional disability. Bone necrosis leading to fractures can also occur, particularly in bones that are effected by tumor or that have been weakened by partial surgical resection. It is not possible to determine the dose that causes bone necrosis because of the variety of circumstances that surround treatment in these patients, but it is estimated that doses in excess of 5000 rads delivered in 5 weeks would be necessary to cause necrosis

(Stokes and Walz, 1983). The significance and treatment of this complication would be largely related to the location of the affected bone.

VIII. HEMATOPOIETIC

The hematopoietic system is not confined to a limited anatomical area of
the body and therefore this system is not of great concern except when total
body radiation or large fields (hemibody or total nodal radiation) are contemplated. With limited fields bone marrow tolerance should present no
problems except in patients who have had marrow depression secondary to
intensive chemotherapy or to myelophthisic anemia. A single dose of 200-600
rads to the whole body in humans will cause marrow aplasia and death within
4-6 weeks unless the blood products are replaced and the patient is supported
with fluids, electrolytes, and antibiotics (Rubin and Casarett, 1968). Local
radiation destroys the bone marrow cells in the field; however, there is repopulation by migrating stem cells. After a dose of about 4000 rads the bone
marrow in the radiated area is hypocellular (Sacks et al., 1978). This is usually
of no significance even in patients who have had treatment with extended field
portals such as total nodal irradiation. Actively proliferating bone marrow in
the adult has primarily a truncal distribution and when a substantial portion
of the bone marrow, i.e., 25-50%, is included in the field, a gradual drop in
the peripheral leukocyte count is observed. The drop in peripheral granulocytes
is seen first since these cells have the shortest life span in circulation: 6-8 days.
A drop in platelet count is also seen early because of the short life span of
these cells—8-10 days—but a drop in the red cell count is not usually seen
since these cells have a long life span of about 120 days. If the granulocyte
count falls below $1,000/mm^3$ or the platelet count below 50,000 mm^3 the
treatment should be stopped temporarily to allow for bone marrow recovery.
The treatment, depending upon the volume of bone marrow included in the
field, may be restarted when the granulocyte count returns to about 2,000
$cells/mm^3$. A separate consideration in the hematopoietic effects of radiation
is the long-lasting depletion of bone marrow reserve thereby sometimes
comprising the ability of patients to receive chemotherapy. This is discussed
further in Chapter 5.

IX. CARCINOGENESIS

It is well known that radiation can induce neoplasia. Leukemia, thyroid
carcinomas, colon carcinomas, breast carcinomas, multiple myelomas, and
other tumors have been found to occur with a higher than expected frequency
among people exposed to radiation (Kohn and Fry, 1984). In addition to the
exposure to radiation there are other risk factors that predispose patients to

the development of radiation-induced tumors. The mechanism of induction of tumors is not clearly understood but it is believed to be related to chromosomal damage. At this time there is no known measure that can be taken to prevent this. It should be kept in mind that the number of patients who develop radiation-induced tumors is extremely small. Furthermore, the morbidity and mortality attributed to these radiation-induced tumors are vastly overshadowed by the benefits derived from the use of radiation for therapeutic purposes.

ACKNOWLEDGMENT

The author wishes to thank Ms. Renee Goodwin for typing this manuscript.

REFERENCES

Applefield, M. M., and Wiernik, M. D. (1983). Cardiac disease after radiation therapy for Hodgkin's disease: Analysis of 48 patients, *Am. J. Cardiol., 51*: 1679.

Cohn, K. E., Stewart, J. R., Fajardo, L. F., and Hancock, E. W. (1967). Heart disease following radiation, *Medicine, 46*:281.

Daly, T. E. (1980). Dental care in the irradiated patient, *Textbook of Radiotherapy* (G. H. Fletcher, ed.), Lea & Febiger, Philadelphia, p. 229.

Fajardo, L. F., and Stewart, J. R. (1971). Capillary endothelial cell injury preceding radiation-induced myocardial fibrosis in rabbits, *Radiology, 101*: 425.

Glatstein, E., and Carter, S. K. (1982). *The Chronic Toxicity of Cancer Treatment* (S. K. Carter, E. Glatstein, and R. B. Livingston, eds.), McGraw-Hill, New York, p. 221.

Gunderson, L. L., Martin, J. K., Earle, J. D., Byer, D. E., Voss, M., Fieck, J. M., Kvois, K., Dorie, D. K., Martinez, A., Nagorney, D. M., O'Connell, M. J., and Weber, F. C. (1984). Intra-operative and external beam irradiation with or without resection: Mayo pilot experience, *Proc. Mayo Clinic, 59*:691.

Ingold, J. A., Reed, G. B., Kaplan, H. S., and Bagshaw, M. A. (1965). Radiation hepatitis, *Am. J. Roentgenol., 93*:200.

Jennings, F. L., and Arden, A. (1962). Development of radiation pneumonitis: Time and dose factors, *Arch. Pathol., 74*:351.

Kohn, H. I., and Fry, R. J. (1984). Radiation carcinogenesis, *New Engl. J. Med., 310*:504.

Lanshbaugh, C. C., and Casarett, G. W. (1976). The effects of gonadal irradiation in clinical radiotherapy, *Cancer 37*:1111.

Larson, D. L., Lindberg, R. D., Lane, E., and Goeptert, H. (1983). Major complications of radiotherapy in cancer of the oral cavity and oropharynx: A ten-year retrospective study, *Am. J. Surg., 146(4)*:531.

Lederman, M. (1980). Radiotherapy in eye disease, *Textbook of Radiotherapy* (G. H. Fletcher, ed.), Lea & Febiger, Philadelphia, p. 509.

LeFloch, O., Donaldson, S. S., and Kaplan, H. S. (1976). Pregnancy following oophorectomy and total nodal irradiation in women with Hodgkin's disease, *Cancer, 38*:2263.

Merriam, G., Jr., and Focht, E. F. (1957). A clinical study of radiation cataracts and the relationship to dose, *Am. J. Roentgenol., 77*:759.

Montana, G. S., Fowler, W. C., Varia, M. A., Walton, L. A., Mack, Y., and Shemanski, L. (1986). Carcinoma of the cervix stage III, *Cancer, 57*:148.

Mosseman, K. L. (1983). Quantitative radiation dose-response relationships for normal tissues in man. II. Response of the salivary glands during radiotherapy, *Rad. Res., 95(2)*:392.

Nakissa, N., Rubin, P., Strohl, R., and Keys, H. (1983). Ocular and orbital complications following radiation therapy of paranasal sinus malignancies and review of literature, *Cancer, 51*:980.

Novick, M., Gard, D. A., Hardy, S. B., and Spira, M. (1977). Burn scar carcinoma: A review and analysis of 46 cases, *J. Trauma, 17(10)*:809.

Order, S. E., Klein, J. L., Ettinger, D., Alderson, P., Siegelman, S., and Leichner, P. (1980). Phase I-II study of radio-labeled antibody integrated in the treatment of primary hepatic malignancies, *Int. J. Rad. Oncol. Biol. Phys., 6*:703.

Parsons, J. T., Fitzgerald, C. R., Hood, C. I., Ellingwood, K. E., Bova, F. J., and Million, R. R. (1983). The effects of irradiation on the eye and optic nerve, *Int. J. Rad. Oncol. Biol. Phys., 9(5)*:609.

Pezner, R. D., Bertrand, M., Cecchi, G. R., Paladugu, R. R., and Kendregan, B. A. (1984). Steroid withdrawal radiation pneumonitis in cancer patients, *Chest, 85*:816.

Reed, G. B., Jr., and Cox, A. J., Jr. (1966). Human liver after radiation injury, *Am. J. Pathol., 48*:597.

Rider, J. A., Moelke, H. C., Alhausen, T. L., and Sheline, G. W. (1957). The effect of x-ray therapy on gastric acidity and on 17-hydrocortical and oropepsin secretion, *Am. Intern. Med., 47*:651.

Roswit, B., and White, D. C. (1977). Severe radiation injuries of the lung, *Am. J. Roentgenol., 129*:127.

Rubin, P. (1984). Late effects of chemotherapy and radiation therapy: A new hypothesis, *Int. J. Rad. Oncol. Biol. Phys., 10*:5.

Rubin, P., and Casarett, G. W. (1966). Alimentary tract: Small and large intestines and rectum, *Clinical Radiation Pathology*, W. B. Saunders, Philadelphia, p. 193.

Rubin, P., and Casarett, G. W. (1968). *Clinical Radiation Pathology*, Vols. I and II, W. B. Saunders, Philadelphia, p. 778.

Ruckdeschel, J. C., Chang, P., Martin, R. G., Byhart, R. W., O'Connell, M. J. Sutherland, J. C., and Wiernik, P. H. (1975). Radiation related pericardial effusions in patients with Hodgkin's disease, *Medicine, 54*:245.

Sacks, E. L., Goris, M. L., Glatstein, E., Gilbert, E., and Kaplan, H. S. (1978). Bone marrow regeneration following large field radiation. Influence of volume, age, dose, and time, *Cancer, 42*:1057.

Smith, J. P. (1980). Management of bowel and bladder complications from irradiation to pelvis and abdomen, *Textbook of Radiotherapy* (G. H. Fletcher, ed.) Lea & Febiger, Philadelphia, p. 809.

Smithers, D. W., Wallace, D. M., and Ansten, D. E. (1973). Fertility after unilateral orchidectomy and radiotherapy for patients with malignant tumors of the testis, *Brit. Med. J., 4:*77.

Stewart, J. R., Cohn, K. E., Fajardo, L. F., Hancock, E. W., and Kaplan, H. S. (1967). Radiation-induced heart disease: A study of twenty-five patients, *Radiology, 89:*302.

Stokes, S. H., and Walz, B. J. (1983). Pathologic fracture after radiation therapy for primary non-Hodgkin's malignant lymphoma of bone, *Int. J. Rad. Oncol. Biol. Phys., 9:*1153.

Thames, H. D., Peters, L. J., Withers, H. R., and Fletcher, G. H. (1983). Accelerated fractionation vs. hyperfractionation: Rationale for several treatments per day, *Int. J. Rad. Oncol. Biol. Phys., 9(2):*127.

Thompson, G. M., Migdal, C. S., and Whittle, R. J. (1983). Radiation retinopathy following treatment of posterior nasal space carcinoma, *Brit. J. Opthalmol., 67(9):*609.

Von Essen, C. F. (1980). Skin and lips, *Textbook of Radiotherapy* (G. H. Fletcher, ed.), Lea & Febiger, Philadelphia, p. 271.

William, C. (1983). Oral complications of cancer patients undergoing chemotherapy and radiation therapy (D. J. Higby, ed.), Martinus Nijhoff Publishers, Boston, p. 147.

7

Anticipation and Prevention of Neurological Complications of Cancer and Cancer Therapy

S. Clifford Schold, Jr.
Duke University Medical Center, Durham, North Carolina

I. INTRODUCTION

Many cancer patients suffer significant neurological disturbances during the course of their illness. These may be due either to the direct effects of the tumor itself, to secondary effects of the tumor, or to complications of treatment or procedures. Neurological symptoms are particularly frightening to patients and their families, and physicians not accustomed to dealing with these problems are often intimidated and perplexed. Since most neurological complications of cancer are treatable and many are preventable and since the central nervous system (CNS) heals slowly and incompletely after structural damage, early diagnosis is crucial to avoid permanent disability.

II. ANTICIPATION AND RECOGNITION OF DIRECT EFFECTS OF CANCER ON THE NERVOUS SYSTEM

A. CNS Metastases

Both the incidence and location of metastases affecting the nervous system vary with the underlying neoplasm. Melanoma, lung cancer, breast cancer, and testicular cancer frequently spread to the brain, whereas some relatively common neoplasms, such as those of the colon, pancreas, and cervix, uncommonly metastasize to the brain (Posner and Chernik, 1978). When renal cell carcinomas or germ cell tumors of the testis spread to the nervous system, they usually grow in the parenchyma of the brain. On the other hand, leukemias and lymphomas usually spread to the leptomeninges rather than to the brain parenchyma. Lung cancer, breast cancer, and melanoma can do either and frequently do both. There is no satisfactory explanation for these anatomical predilections, but the observations are important in anticipating sites of nervous system involvement in patients with these neoplasms.

In the great majority of cases, brain metastasis occurs in the setting of active systemic tumor. Specifically, pulmonary metastases are present in over 70% of patients with non-lung primary tumors who develop brain metastases (Cairncross, Kim, and Posner, 1980). In the absence of active non-CNS disease, one should be suspicious of the accuracy of the diagnosis of brain metastasis. On the other hand, the presence of pulmonary metastases should alert one to the possibility of CNS involvement.

Signs and symptoms of metastases affecting the nervous system vary with the location, the size, and the rate of growth of the lesion. Generalized neurological symptoms, such as headache, lethargy, and confusion, are caused by pressure of the tumor and surrounding edema on the intracranial contents. Localized symptoms, such as hemiparesis and aphasia, are more likely to be due to local compression, infiltration, and destruction of brain. Leptomeningeal metastasis can affect any level of the neuraxis and produces some combination of altered mental status, cranial nerve dysfunction, and spinal root dysfunction (Olson, Chernik, and Posner, 1974). Early recognition of any of these signs and symptoms, particularly in patients with appropriate underlying neoplasms, should lead to the relevant diagnostic test. Early diagnosis is critical to the success of therapy.

The most sensitive test for detecting metastasis to the brain is computerized cranial tomography (CT). The sensitivity of CT for detecting brain metastasis varies with the size of the lesion, its location (metastases near bone or in the posterior fossa are more difficult to visualize), and its permeability character- istics. However, most metastases over 0.5 cm in diameter will be detected by routine contrast-enhanced CT. The sensitivity of the test can be increased with a higher dose of the contrast agent and with a delay between contrast admin- istration and imaging ("double-dose delay"). CT is expensive, but its use is cost-effective in patients at high risk for brain metastasis who develop evidence of neurological dysfunction.

Leptomeningeal metastases are usually not detected by CT, and cerebrospinal fluid (CSF) analysis is required. The presence of neoplastic cells in a CSF preparation ("positive cytology") is diagnostic (Glass et al., 1979), but often several CSF examinations are necessary before the diagnosis is established. How- ever, patients with minimal symptomatology, who often have negative CSF cytology, are most important to diagnose because of the reversibility of the signs and symptoms at that stage. Detection of biochemical tumor markers in CSF may also aid in the early diagnosis of leptomeningeal tumor (Wasserstrom, Glass, and Posner, 1982).

This is not the appropriate forum for discussion of the treatment of central nervous system metastases. However, treatments are available, and they are generally safe and effective, at least in the short run. Corticosteroids and radiotherapy are the treatments of choice in most cases, and they are usually highly effective both in controlling symptoms and in reducing the tumor mass (Cairncross, Kim, and Posner, 1980). Best results occur in patients with only minor clinical disability and with relatively small tumors. Early diagnosis is therefore critical, and anticipation of this problem in the appropriate setting is crucial for prevention of neurological disability.

B. Spinal Cord Compression

Unlike brain metastases, spinal cord compression from epidural metastases reflects the propensity of the underlying neoplasm to spread to bone (Gilbert, Kim, and Posner, 1978). Neurological dysfunction is usually produced when the vertebral body metastasis expands and compresses, rather than invades, the nervous system. As in brain metastasis, the extent of residual disability after treatment is directly related to the degree of neurological deficit when treatment is instituted. Patients who are paraplegic from metastatic spinal cord compression are unlikely to walk again even if the offending tumor mass is effectively treated; on the other hand, patients who are ambulatory when treatment is instituted are likely to remain ambulatory and often do so for the duration of the illness. The most important early symptom of epidural metastasis is pain at the affected vertebra. Neurological symptoms, including weaknesses, sensory disturbances, and sphincter dysfunction, develop as the compression proceeds. In over 85% of patients with epidural spinal cord compression from metastatic solid tumor, there is radiographical evidence of vertebral involvement at the site of compression. The combination of an underlying neoplasm with a propensity to spread to bone (lung, breast, kidney, and prostate cancers, myeloma, Hodgkin's disease, etc.), back pain, and radiographical evidence of vertebral body metastasis should make one concerned about the possibility of impending spinal cord compression. Ideally, the diagnosis is made before neurological symptoms develop, but certainly at the first suggestion of a spinal cord disturbance myelography should be undertaken and treatment instituted to prevent further disability. Corticosteroids and radiotherapy are the treatments of choice in most cases. Surgery is indicated if the primary tumor is unknown, if the patient is deteriorating despite maximum medical treatment, or if the tumor recurs in a previously irradiated field.

C. Seizures

Patients with metastatic brain disease are susceptible to seizures. The incidence varies with the location and number of lesions and possibly with the
underlying tumor. Roughly 20% of patients have seizures as an initial manifestation of CNS metastasis, and once seizures have occurred, the use of anticonvulsants
is undisputed. However, in a patient with a brain metastasis who has not had
seizures, the indications for prophylactic anticonvulsants are unclear. In one series
of patients with metastatic melanoma, 21 of 63 patients with brain metastases who
had not previously had seizures developed a seizure disorder during the course of
their illness. The incidence was significantly lower in patients treated with prophylactic anticonvulsants (17%) than in patients not treated prophylactically (37%)
(Byrne, Cascino, and Posner, 1983). The authors concluded that prophylactic anticonvulsants were indicated in patients with brain metastasis from melanoma. However,
this was not a controlled series and peculiarities of melanoma in the brain might make
seizures more likely than with other tumors, so the applicability of these data to
patients with other primary tumors is uncertain.

It has recently been suggested that prophylactic diazepam in patients with
intracranial tumors may help prevent seizures related to contrast administration
for CT scans (Pagani et al., 1983). The data are convincing, but confirmatory
data from other centers and in other settings have not been reported.

D. Compression Neuropathies

Dysfunction of one or several peripheral nerves is also common in the cancer
patient. Neuropathies may be either treatment related (see below) or directly
caused by the tumor, but they are often unrelated to either and simply due to
nerve compression in a bedridden patient or during a surgical procedure. These
compression neuropathies can be anticipated and should be prevented by appropriate measures.

The classic compression neuropathy in the bedridden patient is a peroneal
nerve palsy. This occurs with pressure on the common peroneal nerve over
the lateral head of the fibula. It is often painless and can occur rapidly,
especially in a patient with altered mental status. "Foot-drop" with paresis of
ankle dorsiflexion and eversion is the most prominent finding. Inversion and
plantar flexion are unaffected. Sensory findings are highly variable, ranging
from essentially normal sensation to complete loss of sensation to loss of all
modalities on the dorsum of the foot. This variability is presumably related
to the anatomical relationship between the site of compression and division of
the nerve into superficial (sensory) and deep (motor) branches. Deep tendon
reflexes are preserved in a peroneal nerve palsy. This condition must be distinguished from L4-5 root lesions and from sciatic nerve palsy, both of which
overlap clinically with peroneal palsy. Less common compression neuropathies

Table 1 Common Compression Neuropathies in the Cancer Patient

Condition	Usual site	Neurological deficit	Differential diagnosis
Common peroneal nerve palsy	Lateral head of the fibula	Paresis of foot eversion and dorsi-flexion, variable sensory loss	L_{45} root
Sciatic nerve palsy	Sciatic notch	Paresis of all foot muscles, depressed Achilles reflex	L_5-S_1 root
Ulnar nerve palsy	Epicondylar groove	Weakness and wasting of intrinsic hand muscles, loss of sensation in an ulnar distribution	C_8-T_1 root
Radial nerve palsy	Lower third of the humerus	Wrist drop, variable sensory loss on the dorsum of the hand	C_{5-6} root

in the inactive patient are sciatic, ulnar, and radial nerve palsies (Table 1). All should be anticipated, regular brief examinations should be performed, and preventive measures (change of position, protective devices) should be employed.

E. Pain

Pain is a pervasive and feared symptom in the cancer patient. Although it is by no means always present in the face of cancer, it is common (Cleland, 1984) and many dread pain in the terminal stages of their illness as much as they fear death itself. In dealing with pain as a potentially disabling complication of cancer, the physician should interact with the patient at three stages: anticipation, diagnosis, and treatment.

First, the possibility of pain developing during the course of the illness should be discussed openly at an early stage. Pain is a common complication in certain neoplasms, particularly those that metastasize to bone, whereas it is uncommon in others, such as the leukemias. This concern should be anticipated early so the patient will be confident that the physician will attend to this problem and manage it effectively. The patient should be assured that his/her questions about pain are appropriate and that they will be handled maturely. He/she should also realize that should pain develop, it would be treated aggressively and adequately.

Second, the accurate diagnosis of a pain syndrome in the cancer patient will aid in directing its management and in preventing secondary disability. Pain in the presence of cancer is most often caused by the tumor itself. However, in 20-30% of cases pain is due either to cancer therapy or to conditions that are independent of the neoplasm (Payne and Foley, 1984). Whatever the cause of pain, preexisting personality factors, the coexistence of depression or anxiety, and individual tolerance all contribute to the total syndrome.

Third, pain in the cancer patient should be treated aggressively. The most common cause of failure to control pain in cancer patients is undertreatment. Several means of treatment are available:

1. Treat the offending tumor. Effective surgery, radiotherapy, or chemotherapy is the best way of controlling pain due to cancer.
2. Use nonnarcotic analgesics. These drugs are often not adequately utilized because the physician believes that stronger measures will be required. However, the patient should first demonstrate this by failing to respond to appropriate doses of aspirin, acetaminophen, and nonsteroidal anti-inflammatory agents.
3. Use analgesic "adjuvant" drugs. These include several nonanalgesic drugs that can be of great relief in the appropriate setting. Worthy of particular note are corticosteroids (highly effective in controlling pain from bone metastasis), amitryptiline (useful in "neuropathic" pain syndromes), and phenothiazines.
4. If narcotics are used, use them in adequate doses (see Table 2). There is no strong argument for choosing one narcotic analgesic over another, but the physician should be aware of the equianalgesic doses of these drugs (Moertel et al., 1974) as well as their appropriate dosing intervals. Round-the-clock doses may be more effective than giving the drug on an "as needed" basis, although some of the narcotics (e.g., methadone) have long plasma half-lives, and repeated dosing at regular intervals may enhance toxicity. Tolerance and physical dependence develop with all narcotic analgesics. Addiction is also possible, although it is quite uncommon in the cancer patient. Methadone, levorphanol, hydromorphone, and codeine have low p.o./I.M. dosage ratios and are useful for oral administration. Pentazocine is a mixed agonist-antagonist and may cause withdrawal symptoms in narcotic-dependent patients. All have a mean duration of action of 4-6 hours, although there is considerable variability among patients. Alternative means of administration (slow release subcutaneous pumps, epidural infusion, etc.) may improve pain control in selected patients.

Table 2 Equivalent Doses of Common Narcotic Analgesics

Drug	Equianalgesic dose[a]
Morphine	10 mg I.M.
Meperidine	75 mg I.M.
Methadone	20 mg p.o.
Levorphanol	2 mg I.M.
	4 mg p.o.
Hydromorphine	1.5 mg I.M.
	7.5 mg p.o.
Codeine	130 mg I.M.
	200 mg p.o.
Pentazocine	60 mg I.M.

[a]Equivalent in efficacy to 10 mg morphine I.M. (taken from various sources).

5. Use surgical procedures in carefully selected patients. Anterolateral cordotomy, dorsal root entry zone radiofrequency lesions, and hypophysectomy are all useful procedures in the right setting (Payne and Foley, 1984).

Pain in the cancer patient should be anticipated, recognized, and treated aggressively. With a systematic, rational approach adequate pain control with undesirable toxicity should be achieved in most patients.

III. NONMETASTATIC EFFECTS OF CANCER ON THE NERVOUS SYSTEM

A. Metabolic Disturbances

A common cause of altered mental status in the cancer patient is a "metabolic encephalopathy." This can be produced by a variety of metabolic disturbances, including hypercalcemia, hyponatremia, hypoxemia, and hepatic failure, among others. Many of these syndromes have characteristic clinical appearances (Plum and Posner, 1980). Not uncommonly, more than one metabolic abnormality that affects cognitive function is present, and although none alone would be likely to produce a clinically significant encephalopathy, their combination can do so. Furthermore, altered mental status often persists beyond the laboratory evidence of a metabolic disturbance. For example, one can incorrectly conclude that a persistent encephalopathy in a patient whose serum calcium has been corrected from 16 to 12 in a 48-hour period is due to another cause. In this situation, one is better off waiting another 24-72 hours before embarking on

Table 3 Common CNS Infections in Cancer Patients

Host defense abnormality	Common underlying conditions	Common infections
Altered cellular immune system	Lymphoma Corticosteroid drugs Organ transplantation	*Listeria meningitis* Cryptococcal meningitis *Toxoplasma* abscess *Nocardia* abscess
Altered neutrophil function	Acute leukemia Myelosuppressive chemotherapy	Gram-negative meningitis *Aspergillus* abscess *Candida* meningitis Mucormycosis
Immunoglobulin deficiency	Multiple myeloma Chronic lymphocytic leukemia	Pneumococcal meningitis
Splenectomy	Hodgkin's disease/ lymphomas	Pneumococcal meningitis
Altered anatomic barriers	Ventricular shunts or reservoirs Neurosurgical procedures Head and neck tumors extending into cranium or spine	Staphylococcal meningitis

a search for an alternative explanation. One should also remember that cancer patients are often nutritionally compromised for a variety of reasons and therefore susceptible to vitamin deficiencies and their consequences. Thiamine should be used liberally as it is in other situations.

The differential diagnosis of a metabolic encephalopathy in the cancer patient is primarily metastatic central nervous system disease. In purely metabolic disturbances, usually no focal signs are present, the CT is normal, and the electroencephalogram (EEG) shows diffuse slowing of a mild to moderate degree. The spinal fluid examination may be nonspecifically abnormal with an elevated protein concentration, but the fluid should not contain an excessive number of leukocytes nor should the glucose concentration be depressed. Usually in the presence of CNS metastases, focal findings are present, the EEG shows localized abnormalities, and either the CT shows a mass lesion or neoplastic cells are present in the CSF.

B. Infections

CNS infections are important and often treatable causes of neurological disability in cancer patients (Chernik, Armstrong, and Posner, 1977). They should be anticipated in certain specific clinical situations. For example, in patients whose neoplasm is associated with selective immunodeficiencies, such as disorders of cell-mediated immunity, opportunistic infections, such as cryptococcal meningitis, should be suspected in the presence of CNS findings. On the other hand, patients who have had physical barriers to the CNS disrupted by cancer or its treatment (e.g., insertion of an indwelling ventricular reservoir) are susceptible to common, usually nonpathogenic organisms (e.g., *Staphylococcus aureus*) that are "opportunistic" only because of their artificial introduction into a normally protected area. Common CNS infections and the corresponding setting in which they are most likely to occur are listed in Table 3.

A variety of CNS viral infections also occur with increased frequency in the cancer patient. Herpes zoster, herpes simplex, and cytomegalovirus infections all either occur more often or are more severe in the immunocompromised patient. The herpes infections are particularly important to recognize since effective treatments are now available, and to be most effective treatment should be instituted early in the course of the illness.

IV. NEUROTOXICITY OF CANCER TREATMENT

A. Sedatives

A common, if not the most common, cause of altered mental status in the cancer patient is the use of drugs with sedative properties. This includes not only drugs used for their sedative effects, most commonly benzodiazepines, but also drugs that when used for other purposes produce sedation or confusion as a side effect. Examples include phenothiazines, analgesics, diphenhydramine, cimetidine, metoclopramide, tricyclic antidepressants, and barbiturates. Cancer patients are often more susceptible to the sedating properties of these drugs for several reasons: (1) they may have organ failure, especially hepatic, which interferes with drug metabolism; (2) they may have multiple mild metabolic disturbances none of which would alone be sufficient to produce an encephalopathy but which predispose to drug-induced confusion; (3) they are often on multiple medications and again additive side effects of these drugs may produce an encephalopathy that would not have been produced by any of them alone; and (4) they may be cachectic, depressed, and sufficiently lacking in external stimuli to make them excessively sensitive to side effects of these medications. The physician's first priority in evaluating a cancer patient with altered mental status is to determine what drugs the patient has been receiving.

Even if another cause of an encephalopathy is discovered it would be wise to discontinue possibly sedating drugs so the condition is not compounded.

B. Corticosteroids

Corticosteroids are commonly used in patients with cancer and most side effects of these drugs are dose and time related. The most frequent neurological side effects are muscle weakness, hyperglycemic/hyperosmolar coma, anxiety/insomnia, and a "steroid psychosis." Steroid myopathy is quite common if patients are carefully examined, and it may be incapacitating in the vulnerable patient. It preferentially affects proximal muscles of both the upper and lower extremities, mimicking polymyositis and other acquired myopathies. However, muscle enzymes are usually normal or only mildly elevated. Mild psychiatric symptoms (insomnia, anxiety) are also quite common in patients on corticosteroids. More severe disturbances (acute psychosis, hypomania, depression) are unusual but dramatic. Curiously, risk factors, such as a previous psychiatric history, have been difficult to identify (Ling, Perry, and Tsuang, 1981). Detailed discussion of these syndromes is not pertinent here, but in principle each is best avoided by the use of the lowest possible corticosteroid dose for the shortest period of time, and sensitivity of the physician to early manifestations of any of these conditions is important.

C. Antineoplastic Agents

The potential for nervous system toxicity produced by antineoplastic drugs complicates the differential diagnosis of neurological changes in the patient with cancer. Table 4 lists antitumor drugs that are associated with neurological side effects. The list changes continuously as schedules and dosages of available drugs are modified and as new drugs are introduced.

Vinca Alkaloids

The vinca alkaloids (vincristine, vinblastine, etc.) are commonly associated with a polyneuropathy that is dose and time related (Kaplan and Wiernik, 1982). The neuropathy is usually the dose-limiting factor in the use of the drug. The patient's first complaint is numbness in the tips of the fingers and toes, and an early objective physical finding is symmetrical suppression of the Achilles tendon reflex. Loss of the tendon reflex, when it occurs without other neurotoxicity, is not an indication to stop the drug. On continued drug administration, one must inquire about loss of feeling in the hands and feet, muscle weakness, and gait disturbances, because if the drug is continued the problems may progress to the point of incapacitation. Patients with preexisting neuropathies are probably more susceptible to the neurotoxic effects of the drugs. Autonomic nervous system effects are occasionally the

Table 4 Neurotoxicity of Commonly Used Antineoplastic Agents

Drug	Neurological complication
Vincristine (and other vinca alkaloids)	Polyneuropathy
	Jaw pain
	Autonomic neuropathy
Cis-platinum	Polyneuropathy
	Neurogenic hearing loss
	Optic neuritis
Interferon	Polyneuropathy
	Encephalopathy
Cytosine arabinoside	Encephalopathy, ataxia, dysarthria
Procarbazine	Encephalopathy
Asparaginase	Encephalopathy
Misonidazole	Neuropathy
Fluorouracil	Cerebellar syndrome

first signs of toxicity, especially with vinblastine; the usual manifestations are colicky abdominal pain and constipation. Unless treated with stool softeners, mild laxatives or dosage adjustments, the constipation can progress to fecal impaction and adynamic ileus. Bladder atony is another autonomic nerve toxicity that should be considered when patients receiving vinca alkaloids experience difficulty voiding.

Severe jaw pain and pain at sites of tumor have also been associated with administration of vincristine and especially vinblastine (Lucas and Huang, 1977). Both autonomic symptoms and jaw pain are more common in children. These symptoms are not as clearly dose related as the polyneuropathy. In fact, the jaw pain usually occurs with the first dose of the drug and does not recur with subsequent treatments. It is not an indication for discontinuing therapy.

When drug is discontinued the neuropathy is partially or completely reversible, but recovery is often slow, requiring several months. Nonetheless, because of the proven efficacy of the vinca alkaloids it is inadvisable to discontinue therapy at the first sign of a neuropathy. Clinical judgment is important in determining when the degree of incapacitation should interrupt therapy.

Cis-Platinum

Cisplatin has been associated with various forms of central and peripheral neurotoxicity that may be the dose-limiting toxicity in its use (Loehrer and Einhorn, 1984). The neuropathy differs from the vincristine neuropathy in that large diameter fibers, conducting proprioception and vibratory sensibility, are preferentially affected. It is frequently painless, the primary complaint being that of a gait disturbance. Central and ophthalmological effects (papilledema, retrobulbar neuritis) similar to heavy metal intoxication have also been reported. Damage to the organ of Corti has been described in up to 50% of patients tested (Reddel et al., 1982). Tinnitus and high-frequency hearing loss are the most common symptoms. Patients with preexisting high-frequency hearing loss are more susceptible to the ototoxic effects of the drug, and previous cranial radiation may also increase the risk (Granowetter, Rosenstock, and Packer, 1983; Melamed, Selim, and Schuchman, 1985). Otometric abnormalities precede clinical toxicity, and laboratory evidence of high-frequency defects without clinical symptoms usually does not mandate alteration of cisplatin dosage. However, both the neuropathy and the hearing loss may become disturbing enough to the patient to require cessation of the drug.

Interferon

Neurological toxicity has occasionally been a dose-limiting side effect of alpha interferon (Kirkwood and Ernstoff, 1984). Somnolence, lethargy, memory loss, and other cognitive defects may occur, and EEG changes consistent with metabolic encephalopathy have been seen (Adams, Quesada, and Gutterman, 1984). Curiously, these complications do not appear to be more common after intrathecal administration of the drug. Peripheral neuropathy characterized by paresthesias in hands and feet and loss of tendon reflexes have also been reported.

Cytosine Arabinoside

In conventional systemic doses, cytosine arabinoside (Ara-C) rarely, if ever, produces neurological side effects. The recent use of high-dose Ara-C infusions has essentially created a new neurological disorder that is characterized clinically by marked ataxia and dysarthria and mild confusion (Lazarus et al., 1981). It occurs toward the end of, or shortly after, the infusion and, curiously, is almost always transient, requiring no other investigations or interventions. Its incidence is directly related to the total dose of the drug. The condition can be fatal, and neuropathological studies have demonstrated profound and selective loss of Purkinje cells in the cerebellum. Direct ocular toxicity and transient cortical blindness have also been described in patients receiving high-dose Ara-C. The mechanism of this damage is not known.

Other Drugs

Procarbazine inhibits monamine oxidase and other enzymes and may predispose patients to a variety of drug interactions including synergistic sedative effects with phenothiazines, hypertensive headaches when tyramine-containing foods are eaten, and alcohol intolerance. Patients who are being treated with daily oral procarbazine may develop disorders of consciousness or a mild peripheral neuropathy, but in only about 10% of cases are the symptoms severe enough to interfere with therapy. On the other hand, neurotoxicity was usually the dose-limiting factor in clinical trials of high-dose intravenous procarbazine (Chabner et al., 1973).

Very high doses of alkylating agents that are being used in autologous bone marrow transplantation and certain aggressive chemotherapy programs can cause a variety of major neurological side effects, some of which are associated with multifocal lesions of the nervous system (Burger at al., 1981). Neurological toxicity may be dose limiting in several of the high-dose programs.

It has been reported that 25-50% of patients receiving L-asparaginase will experience a disorder of consciousness (Haskell et al., 1969). This "asparaginase encephalopathy" usually begins within a day or so of therapy and clears rapidly after treatment is discontinued. Less commonly, as organic brain syndrome may develop one or more weeks after therapy. The absence of a clear dose-toxicity relationship makes it imperative that all patients be observed closely. Although the severity of cerebral dysfunction is highly variable, it is usually not the cause for discontinuing therapy.

Misonidazole may produce either peripheral neuropathy or central nervous system depression. The antimetabolite 5-fluorouracil may produce an acute cerebellar syndrome characterized by dysmetria, ataxia, and dizziness. These effects are usually seen at high dosages, such as 4-day continuous infusion of therapy of 1 $g/M^2/day$. Several other compounds, including hexamethylmelamine, have occasionally produced neurotoxicity.

Intrathecal Chemotherapy

Intrathecal (IT) administration of antineoplastic drugs to treat or prevent CNS metastasis can cause several types of undesirable reactions. Methotrexate, the most commonly used intrathecal drug, may produce meningeal irritation, arachnoiditis, and rarely, paraplegia (Weiss, Walker, and Wiernik, 1974). This occurs exclusively after spinal subarachnoid injection, and it is unclear how often the solvent for the drug has contributed to the problem. The drug should not be injected if the flow of CSF is irregular or if the patient experiences pain during its administration. Methotrexate is also linked to chronic leukoencephalopathy, particularly when it is combined with cranial irradiation (Rubinstein et al., 1975). In most of these cases, the drug has been given intraventricularly, but some cases have been associated with high-dose intravenous administration (Allen and Rosen, 1978; Allen et al., 1980). The encephalopathy usually begins insidiously and may cause confusion (progressing to dementia), ataxia, and spasticity. Seizures are not infrequent and EEGs often demonstrate diffuse slow waves. The CT scan is usually the best diagnostic tool, revealing low density, nonenhancing areas in several regions, hydrocephalus, and occasionally calcifications in the central white matter. The presence of myelin basic protein in the CSF may be a marker of white matter damage from the drug (Mahoney et al., 1984). Although the syndrome may be fatal, some patients survive for months or years with chronic deficits and some have shown varying degrees of recovery.

Risk factors for the development of methotrexate-induced leukoencephalopathy are incompletely understood. Clearly radiation, improper drug instillation, and total dose of methotrexate are important. The presence of active CNS leukemia may alter drug disposition and predispose the patient to the development of an encephalopathy (Morse et al., 1985). Elevated subarachnoid drug levels have been related to this condition (Bleyer, Drake, and Chabner, 1973), and it is recommended that CSF levels be obtained at least once in patients receiving intrathecal treatment (Bleyer, 1977).

D. Radiotherapy

Brain

Nontherapeutic effects of radiation on the brain take several forms. At one extreme, patients undergoing radiotherapy for brain neoplasms may experience transient deterioration of their neurological status after the first few treatments. This is presumably due to worsening of the edema surrounding the radiated neoplasm, and it responds to a temporary increase in the dose of corticosteroids. At the other extreme, delayed radionecrosis of brain tissue is a serious, although infrequent, complication of therapeutic radiation, and the possiblity of its occurrence is dose limiting for the radiation treatment of most forms of primary and metastatic brain tumors. It is related to dosage in that it rarely occurs at doses below 5500 rads (Sheline, 1980), fractionation, and volume irradiated, as well as other incompletely understood factors (Marks et al., 1981; Glass et al., 1984). Radiation necrosis acts as a mass lesion, producing signs, symptoms, and radiographical appearances that are indistinguishable from recurrent tumor. The diagnosis can only be made surgically, and excision is the only available treatment. Between these two extremes, patients experience a variety of sometimes transient and often ill-defined symptoms related to radiotherapy. These include excessive somnolence which occurs 2-3 months after whole brain radiotherapy of children ("the somnolence syndrome") (Freeman, Johnston, and Voke, 1973), hydrocephalus and radiographical white matter attenuation that may or may not be clinically apparent (Riccardi et al., 1985), and subtle loss of intellectual function, again usually most notable in children. The details of these intermediate syndromes have not yet been established, nor has the influence of other factors such as the concomitant administration of chemotherapy, corticosteroids, or other drugs.

Spinal Cord

Radiotherapy that encompasses the spinal cord can also produce a spectrum of neurological dysfunction. Many patients being treated for spinal cord compression from epidural metastases will experience varying degrees of deterioration following the first one to two treatments. As in the treatment of brain metastases, this is presumably due to increased swelling around the tumor and will respond to higher doses of corticosteroids. A transient, reversible myelopathy occurs several months after radiotherapy and is characterized by "Lhermitte's phenomenon," or an electrical sensation down the spine that occurs with neck flexion. It is unaccompanied by abnormalities on neurological examination. It is frightening to the patient and may be confusing to the physician, but it is a benign condition and requires neither investigation nor therapy. Of greater concern is that late occurrence of radiation myelopathy, or radionecrosis of the spinal cord (Reagan, Thomas, and Colby, 1968). This generally occurs 12 months or more following radiotherapy and clinically presents as a subacute transverse myelopathy affecting multiple systems below the level of the lesion. The principal differential diagnostic consideration is neoplasm compressing the spinal cord, but myelography is generally normal and the CSF shows only an elevated protein concentration. The course is usually progressive and irreversible, although some patients stabilize with fixed neurological deficits. When the myelopathy is incomplete, the posterior columns are usually spared. The reason for this selectivity is unknown, although the pattern suggests a vascular etiology. An occasional patient has apparently responded to corticosteroids, but this has not clearly been demonstrated to be effective therapy. Details of risk factors for the development of radiation myelopathy are unknown, although clearly dose, fractionation, and volume are important. For example, radiation myelopathy rarely occurs at doses below 4500-5000 rads (Wara et al., 1975).

E. Surgery

Common neurosurgical procedures in the cancer patient include excision of a brain metastasis, insertion of an intraventricular ("Ommaya") reservoir, laminectomy for epidural spinal cord compression, and cordotomy for pain control. Each of these carries risks that must be considered in recommending therapy for individual patients. Patients undergoing excision of a metastasis may develop increased neurological deficit, they may develop intracerebral hemorrhage or postoperative infection, or they may die. The occasional instance of the surgeon being unable to find the lesion visualized on CT should also be considered a complication. The most important complications of insertion of an intraventricular reservoir are hemorrhage and misplacement of the catheter tip. The position of the tip should always be checked with a contrast material (such as air) before terminating the procedure. In addition to the usual risks of hemorrhage and infection, extensive laminectomy may require secondary stabilization of the spinal column. After successful cordotomy there is of course anesthesia in the affected areas. Cordotomy at a cervical level carries with it the risk of serious, although transient, hypotension postoperatively. However, each of these complications of surgical procedures in the cancer patient is uncommon. With skilled hands and with proper judgment, surgery plays an important role in the management of the neuro-oncologic patient.

V. CONCLUSION

Neurological disorders in patients with cancer are frequent, frightening, and often profoundly disabling. However, most can be anticipated and should be recognized at a stage when they are reversible. With early and appropriate treatment, most neurological complications of systemic cancer can be successfully managed.

REFERENCES

Adams, F., Quesada, J. R., and Gutterman, J. U. (1984). Neuropsychiatric manifestations of human leukocyte interferon therapy in patients with cancer, *J.A.M.A., 252*:938-941.

Allen, J. C., and Rosen, G. (1978). Transient cerebral dysfunction following chemotherapy for osteogenic sarcoma, *Ann. Neurol., 3*:441-444.

Allen, J. C., Rosen, G., Mehta, B. M., and Horten, B. (1980). Leucoencephalopathy following high dose IV methotrexate chemotherapy with leucovorin rescue, *Cancer Treat. Rep., 64*:1261-1273.

Bleyer, W. A. (1977). Clinical pharmacology of intrathecal methotrexate. II. An improved dosage regimen derived from age-related pharmacokinetics, *Cancer Treat. Rep., 61*:1419-1425.

Bleyer, W. A., Drake, J. C., and Chabner, B. A. (1973). Neurotoxicity and elevated cerebrospinal fluid methotrexate concentration in meningeal leukemia, *New Engl. J. Med., 289*:770-773.

Burger, P. C., Kamenar, E., Schold, S. C., Fay, J. W., Phillips, G. L., and Herzig, G. P. (1981). Encephalomyelopathy following high-dose BCNU therapy, *Cancer, 48*:1318-1327.

Byrne, T. N., Cascino, T. L., and Posner, J. B. (1983). Brain metastasis from melanoma, *J. Neuro-Oncol., 1*:313-317.

Cairncross, J. G., Kim, J.-H., and Posner, J. B. (1980). Radiation therapy for brain metastases, *Ann. Neurol., 7*:529-541.

Chabner, B. A., Sponzo, R., Hubbard, S., Canellos, G. P., Young, R. C., Schein, P. S., and DeVita, V. T. (1973). High-dose intermittent intravenous infusion of procarbazine (NSC-77213), *Cancer Chemother. Rep., 57*:361-363.

Chernik, N. L., Armstrong, D., and Posner, J. B. (1977). Central nervous system infections in patients with cancer: Changing patterns, *Cancer, 40*:268-274.

Cleland, C. S. (1984). The impact of pain on the patient with cancer, *Cancer* 54:2635-2641.

Freeman, J. E., Johnston, P. G. B., and Voke, J. M. (1973). Somnolence after prophylactic cranial irradiation in children with acute lymphoblastic leukemia, *Brit. Med. J., 4*:523-525.

Gilbert, R. W., Kim, J.-H., and Posner, J. B. (1978). Epidural spinal cord compression from metastatic tumor, *Ann. Neurol., 3*:40-51.

Glass, J. P., Melamed, M., Chernik, N. L., and Posner, J. B. (1979). Malignant cells in cerebrospinal fluid (CSF): The meaning of a positive CSF cytology, *Neurology, 29*:1369-1375.

Glass, J. P., Hwang, T.-L., Leavens, M. E., and Libshitz, H. I. (1984). Cerebral radiation necrosis following treatment of extracranial malignancies, *Cancer, 54*:1966-1972.

Granowetter, L., Rosenstock, J. G., and Packer, R. J. (1983). Enhanced cis-platinum neurotoxicity in pediatric patients with brain tumors, *J. Neuro-Oncol., 1*:293-297.

Haskell, C. M., Canellos, G. P., Leventhal, B. G., Carbone, P. P., Block, J. B., Serpick, A. A., and Selawry, O. S. (1969). L-asparaginase: Therapeutic and toxic effects in patients with neoplastic disease, *New Engl. J. Med., 281*: 1028-1034.

Kaplan, R. S., and Wiernik, P. H. (1982). Neurotoxicity of antineoplastic drugs, *Semin. Oncol., 9*:103-130.

Kirkwood, J. M., and Ernstoff, M. S. (1984). Interferons in the treatment of human cancer, *J. Clin. Oncol., 2*:336-352.

Lazarus, H. M., Herzig, R. H., Herzig, G. P., Phillips, G. L., Roessmann, U., and Fishman, D. J. (1981). Central nervous system toxicity of high-dose systemic cytosine arabinoside, *Cancer, 48*:2577-2582.

Ling, M. H. M., Perry, P. J., and Tsuang, M. T. (1981). Side effects of corticosteroid therapy: Psychiatric aspects, *Arch. Gen. Psych., 38*:471-477.

Loehrer, P. J., and Einhorn, L. H. (1984). Cisplatin, *Ann. Intern. Med., 100*: 704-713.

Lucas, V. S., and Huang, A. T. (1977). Vinblastine-related pain in tumors, *Cancer Treat. Rep., 61*:1735-1736.

Mahoney, D. H., Jr., Fernbach, D. J., Glaze, D. G., and Cohen, S. R. (1984). Elevated myelin basic protein levels in the cerebrospinal fluid of children with acute lymphoblastic leukemia, *J. Clin. Oncol., 2*:58-61.

Marks, J. E., Baglan, R. J., Prassad, S. C., and Blank, W. F. (1981). Cerebral radionecrosis: Incidence and risk in relation to dose, time, fractionation, and volume, *Int. J. Radiat. Oncol. Biol. Phys., 7*:243-252.

Melamed, L. B., Selim, M. A., and Schuchman, D. (1985). Cisplatin ototoxicity in gynecologic cancer patients, *Cancer, 55*:41-43.

Moertel, C. G., Ahmann, D. L., Taylor, W. F., and Schwartan, B. S. (1972). A comparative evaluation of marketed analgesic drugs, *New Engl. J. Med., 286*:813-815.

Morse, M., Savitch, J., Balis, F., Miser, J., Feusner, J., Reaman, G., Poplack, D., and Bleyer, A. (1985). Altered central nervous system pharmacology of methotrexate in childhood leukemia: Another sign of meningeal relapse, *J. Clin. Oncol., 3*:19-24.

Olson, M. E., Chernik, N. L., and Posner, J. B. (1974). Infiltration of the leptomeninges by systemic cancer: A clinical and pathologic study, *Arch. Neurol., 30*:122-137.

Pagani, J. J., Hayman, L. A., Bigelow, R. H., Libshitz, H. I., Lepke, R. A., and Wallace, S. (1983). Diazepam prophylaxis of contrast media-induced seizures during computed tomography of patients with brain metastases, *Am. J. Neuroad., 4*:67-72.

Payne, R., and Foley, K. M. (1984). Advances in the management of cancer pain, *Cancer Treat. Rep., 68*:173-183.

Plum, F., and Posner, J. B. (1980). *The Diagnosis of Stupor and Coma,* F. A. Davis, Philadelphia.

Posner, J. B., and Chernik, N. L. (1978). Intracranial metastases from systemic cancer, *Adv. Neurol., 19*:579-592.

Reagan, T. J., Thomas, J. E., and Colby, M. Y., Jr. (1968). Chronic progressive radiation myelopathy, *J.A.M.A., 203*:128-132.

Reddel, R. R., Kefford, R. F., Grant, J. M., Coates, A. S. Fox, R. M., and Tatesall, M. H. N. (1982). Ototoxicity in patients receiving cisplatin: Importance of dose and methods of administration, *Cancer Treat. Rep., 66*: 19-23.

Riccardi, R., Brouwers, P., Di Chiro, G., and Poplack, D. G. (1985). Abnormal computed tomography brain scans in children with acute lymphoblastic leukemia: Serial long-term follow-up, *J. Clin. Oncol., 3*:12-18.

Rubinstein, L. J., Herman, M. M., Long, T. F., and Wilbur, J. R. (1975). Disseminated necrotizing leukoencephalopathy: A complication of treated central nervous system leukemia and lymphoma, *Cancer, 35*:291-305.

Sheline, G. E. (1980). Irradiation injury of the human brain: A review of clinical experience, *Radiation Damage to the Nervous System* (H. A. Gilbert and A. R. Kagan, eds.), Raven Press, New York, pp. 39-58.

Wara, W. M., Phillips, T. L., Sheline, G. E., and Schwade, J. G. (1975). Radiation tolerance of the spinal cord, *Cancer, 35*:1558-1562.

Wasserstrom, W. R., Glass, J. P., and Posner, J. B. (1982). Diagnosis and treatment of leptomeningeal metastases from solid tumors: Experience with 90 patients, *Cancer, 49*:759-772.

Weiss, H. D., Walker, M. D., and Wiernik, P. H. (1974). Neurotoxicity of commonly used antineoplastic agents, *New Engl. J. Med., 291*:75-81, 127-133.

8

Depression and Other Psychiatric Disorders Associated with Cancer

Allan A. Maltbie
Duke University Medical Center, Durham, North Carolina

Patricia Cotanch
Duke University School of Nursing, Durham, North Carolina

I. INTRODUCTION

A common and pervasive fear people have is that they may develop cancer and, if so, of the dreaded certainty that they will inevitably experience a slow and agonizing death. There are many vivid stories in the newspaper and lay press describing the horrors of cancer. Few people have not been personally touched by the loss of a neighbor, friend, or relative with cancer. Consequently, the diagnosis of cancer is a potent stress factor which strongly challenges the afflicted individual's adaptive capabilities. Under these circumstances, maladaptive and frankly psychopathological responses may result.

The purpose of this chapter is to describe the common psychiatric disorders associated with cancer. Attention will be given to depression both as a coexistent primary disorder and also as a secondary reaction. Together, depression remains the most commonly encountered psychiatric complication observed with cancer patients. Some of the psychotherapy and pharmacotherapeutic interventions that have been shown to be clinically useful will be explained. Finally, attention will be given to the problems of differential diagnosis and preventative management.

II. DEPRESSION

The most common psychiatric disorder experienced by cancer patients is depression. Depression is defined as a disorder of the mood [*Diagnostic and*

Statistical Manual of Mental Disorder (DSM-III, 1980)]. Characteristically, the depressed individual experiences a dysphoria with a loss of interest or pleasure in practically all of the usual pastimes and interests of life that were previously enjoyable. Persistent feelings of sadness and hopelessness are observed; at times there is also irritability. Spells of crying are common as are feelings of worthlessness, inadequacy and guilt. Loss of appetite is often associated with significant weight loss. There may also be disturbed sleep, characterized by insomnia, which may involve difficulty falling asleep (initial insomnia), fitful sleep with frequent awakenings throughout the night (middle insomnia), or, commonly, early morning awakening (terminal insomnia). Changes in psychomotor function are characteristic. Psychomotor retardation, characterized by marked slowing of movement as well as thought, is most common. On occasion, psychomotor agitation characterized by restlessness and irritability is encountered. Fatigue and loss of energy are frequent complaints as is loss of interest in such life pursuits as work, recreational, social, religious, marital, and sexual activities. At times there is difficulty in concentrating or thinking, and thinking may be perceived as slowed or confused. Lastly, suicidal thoughts and attempts are common in patients who suffer from depression. These preoccupations are often associated with themes of guilt for past wrongs, and perceptions of self as a burden on others where suicide is rationalized as an outlet or release from this untenable situation.

  Depression is a clinical syndrome that has been recognized since antiquity. The term "melancholia" was introduced by Hippocrates to describe this syndrome, the symptoms of which he believed were the result of an excessive accumulation of black bile. "Melancholia" continues to be used in the literature and the term is currently being resurrected by some psychiatrists to describe the profound depression observed in the genetically vulnerable bipolar and unipolar affective syndromes. It has been suggested (DSM-III, 1980) that the use of the term melancholia be reserved for those depressions characterized by a profound loss of pleasure in practically all activities which previously had been pleasurable. This is coupled with a significantly depressed mood that is characteristically worse in the morning. Accompanying symptoms of melancholia include early morning awakening, marked psychomotor retardation or agitation, significant weight loss, and at times excessive and inappropriate guilt.

  Critical to the assessment of depression is careful attention to past history of previous depressions. If previous depressions have occurred then one needs to know the specific circumstances surrounding those depressions, precipitating stresses, duration of illnesses, suicidal attempts, treatments, and response to those treatments. Likewise, a strong family history of depression is consistent with the diagnosis of a primary affective syndrome.

In recent years various nomenclatures have been applied to depression in an effort to subdivide clinical syndromes for research purposes and for making therapeutic decisions (Klerman, 1978). Unipolar and bipolar groups of patients with recurrent depressions were distinguished by the existence of manic episodes for the bipolar subgroup with no manic episodes in the unipolar subgroup. Considerable evidence has been established to support differences in genetic, biochemical, familial, physiological, and pharmacological response characteristics with which to distinguish these two groups. Additionally, depressions have been divided in terms of endogenous and reactive forms where the endogenous group was believed to manifest depression as a product of a biological disorder while the reactive group was felt to be a stress-sensitive vulnerable personality type. Klerman points out that in clinical practice, the endogenous reactive division arranges patients in a continuum commonly presenting various admixtures of reactive and endogenous features rather than confirming the existence of two pure subgroups. He notes that the presence or absence of stressful life events has not been found to distinguish the two groups where major life stresses may or may not be found clinically in either. He observes finally that the usefulness of the endogenous concept has been to draw attention to the symptom cluster as it is composed of the vegetative signs of depression: namely, early morning awakening, psychomotor retardation, and weight loss. When found together these features are statistically associated with a favorable response to tricyclic antidepressant drugs and electroconvulsive therapy.

Finally, a distinction between primary and secondary forms of affective disorder has been suggested (Robins et al., 1972). A primary affective disorder would occur in the situation where pure depression or mania exists in the absence of another preexisting psychiatric or medical condition. Secondary affective disorders are those associated with or related to various psychiatric or medical illness (including cancer) or which may be precipitated by pharmacological agents such as reserpine. The concept of secondary affective conditions complicating primary medical illnesses, metabolic states, or pharmacological therapy is particularly useful for our purposes in this chapter. Obviously, individuals with primary affective syndromes may also present with neoplastic disorders. The past history of a depression or manic episode should be established.

III. ASSOCIATION OF DEPRESSION TO CANCER

Levine et al. (1978) in a review of psychiatric consultations performed on 100 cancer patients referred from a university hospital noted that 56% were diagnosed as depressed. They further noted that psychiatric referrals represented 2% of cancer patients admitted to the hospital with the result that in their population, depression was the leading psychiatric referral problem and occurred in about 1% of the hospitalized population. In a 1979 report, Massie and associates noted that depression was the most frequent reason given for requesting psychiatric consultation in a cancer center. In their series of 334 consultations, which represented 5% of admissions to the hospital, they reported that 49% were diagnosed as depressed. They added that two-thirds of these depressed cancer patients were believed to have reactive depressions. The most severe depressive symptomatology was observed in those patients who were more severely ill and more advanced in age. Both of these studies noted that the second most common diagnosis in psychiatric referral of cancer patients were the organic brain syndromes (delirium and dementia).

Inpatient cancer populations have been studied in recent years in an effort to define the prevalence of depression. In a 1981 report, Petty and Noyes review five separate studies (Bukberg and Holland, 1980; Craig and Abeloff, 1974; Hinton, 1980; Koenig, Levin, and Brennon, 1967; Plumb and Holland, 1977) from 1963-1980 which dealt with this topic and they noted that from 17-25% of all their patients were identified as suffering from moderate to severe depression. They observed that the studies are flawed by problems of definition of depression in the cancer population, and are therefore difficult to compare.

In a recent study by Bukberg and Holland (1980), 62 randomly selected oncology admissions were interviewed for the presence of depression. The diagnosis of depression was based on modified DSM-III criteria which excluded somatic symptoms. This was in conjunction with a Beck depression inventory assessment. In this study, 24% of patients were considered sufficiently depressed to require psychiatric management (scored 6-16 on the Beck rating). An additional 18% had Beck scores from 3-5 and were believed to have significant depressive symptomatology. Depression was more frequently encountered in cancer patients with a history of depression and in those who were severely ill.

IV. SUICIDE AMONG CANCER PATIENTS

Despite the frequency of depression in patients with cancer, suicide is surprisingly uncommon. Indeed, there is a paucity of written information regarding the incidence of suicide and cancer patients. One author gives the following reasons for the lack of information on the topic: both cancer and suicide are socially taboo areas; investigation of taboo areas are laden with methodological problems; ethical questions regarding "suicide" as an appropriate intervention; and the inability to accurately assess the frequency of passive suicide (Forman, 1979).

There is wide variation in studies reporting the incidence of suicide in cancer patients. In Finland, there was no greater incidence of cancer among "completed" suicides than was found in the general population (Holland, 1973). By contrast, another study shows that cancer patients are 50-100% more likely than nonpatients to commit suicide (Marshall, Burnett, and Brasure, 1983).

Many of the common types of cancer are closely related to the consumption of alcohol and tobacco. Holland (1973) stated that excessive emotional problems may lead to excessive use of alcohol and tobacco, a point with which most people would agree. Therefore alcohol and tobacco use are the intervening variables that lead to cancer. Consequently, suicide might be expected to be higher in these patients, not because they have cancer, but due to their underlying emotional problems.

Most, if not all, oncologists would agree that the incidence of suicide among hospitalized cancer patients is rare. A goal of suicide research is to investigate and document the incidence and precipitating factors producing the risk of suicide. In summary, the definitive studies of the incidence and determination of cancer as causal to suicide have not been done. Supportive care of the cancer patient expressing suicidal ideation is important. For example, common themes in suicidal ideation may be the patients' desire for control when feeling helpless; an escape from pain; being a burden to family; a desire for peace; or perhaps that patients conceive the idea of abandoning before being abandoned (Forman, 1979).

V. SPECIAL DIAGNOSTIC PROBLEMS IN CANCER PATIENTS

The accurate diagnosis of depression in patients suffering from serious illnesses such as cancer can be difficult. Since the "vegetative symptoms" of depression are also commonly encountered in cancer patients, the use of these symptoms as diagnostic criteria for depression is clearly less reliable and ambiguous. Anorexia, weight loss, and fatigue are expected somatic complaints of patients with cancer which may be intensified by cancer treatments. Psychomotor changes and alterations in sleep patterns, particularly early morning awakening, would be less likely somatic symptoms directly explainable as cancer effects and, hence, more reliable for making the diagnosis of depression.

Because somatic symptoms are confounding variables, most investigators studying depression in the cancer patient focus on its psychological symptomatology in order to reach a diagnosis (Petty and Noyes, 1981). Diagnosis of depression in a cancer population is more commonly made on the clear presence of dysphoric depressive mood with loss of interest, loss of self-esteem, feelings of hopelessness and helplessness, complaints of worthless-ness or guilt, problems concentrating, irritability, lack of initiative, crying spells, and thoughts of suicide (Stewart, Drake, and Winokur, 1965; Schwab, Bialow, and Brown, 1967). In a recent paper addressing the topic of measurement of depression in patients with cancer, Endicott (1984) suggests a substitution of alternative diagnostic criteria from those used in making the diagnosis of major depression for use with medically ill patients. In place of weight loss and poor appetite, she suggests fearfulness or depressed appearance in face or body posture. For insomnia or hypersomnia, she suggests social withdrawal or decreased talkativeness and for loss of energy or fatigue she suggests that substitution of brooding, self-pity, or pessimism. Cavanaugh, Clark, and Gibbons (1983) present evidence to suggest that feelings of failure, loss of social interest, feeling of being punished, suicidal thoughts, severe in-decisiveness, and frequent episodes of crying are useful discriminators for severity of depression in the medically ill population.

VI. NORMAL EXPECTED REACTIONS TO CANCER OR OTHER SERIOUS ILLNESSES

Development of a life-threatening illness such as cancer is a major life stress and as such presents a crisis for the patient and family; a crisis is defined as an insoluble problem brought on by stressful events, causing loss of equilibrium in an individual. Such an intrusion generates profound feelings of anxiety or loss. Because the crisis differs from previously encountered problems, previously established problem-solving strategies are ineffective. The person finds him/herself in a state of helplessness. The crisis points that occur with cancer patients tend to be at the time of diagnosis, during treatment, completion of therapy, at relapse, and at end stage disease.

Reiser and Schroder (1980) suggest that a useful way of conceptualizing the reaction to illness (which is readily applicable to cancer patients) is as a developmental crisis occurring within the overall context in the life of the individual. They suggest that this developmental crisis evolves over the three identifiable stages of awareness, disorganization, and reorganization. They ob-serve that awareness is best understood in terms of an internal ambivalent struggle between knowing and not knowing the truth. They note that denial is a defense commonly seen during this stage, but feel that focus on denial represents only half of the patient's conflict, as they wish to know the truth even as they fight against it. During this struggle, procrastination in accepting the need for help or seeking help may occur which, when protracted, can markedly alter survival. Thus, this ambivalent struggle for awareness in a setting where denial is a primary defense may account in large measure for the problem of delay in seeking medical attention for early signs of cancer

(Henderson, Wittkower, and Longheed, 1958; Henderson, 1966; Greer, 1974; Hinton, 1980).

Reiser and Rosen (1984) describe the second stage of the developmental crisis precipitated by major illness as that of disorganization. Here, the individual experiences a highly traumatic process often characterized by tense confusion, despair, and anxiety that emerges as the individual realizes that there really is something seriously wrong that cannot be denied or rationalized. This challenges the person's sense of omnipotence and invulnerability, the "it could never happen to me." Additionally, during the crisis the individual frequently is hospitalized with attendant separation from friends, family, job and social pursuits. This is further compounded by an array of complex and frightening examinations and tests which may further serve to confuse, isolate, and demoralize. The outcome is often a sense of profound threat to self and a powerful stress to the individual's psychological defense structure and coping abilities. Not only is there a real threat to physical survival, but the demise of integrity of self which may result in lasting psychological injury.

Reiser and Rosen's (1984) final stage of developmental crisis associated with serious illness is the reorganization phase. During this period, coping mechanisms and defenses are reinstituted and the stricken individual begins to accept the reality of the disease, including the attendant life changes and the necessary tasks that must be faced in the future. This is an integration process where the illness is accepted as a reality and is associated with such comments as "You've got to go on" and "You can't keep lying around feeling sorry for youself." Thus, both recognition and acceptance of the reality of the illness are accomplished and the task becomes one of coping or "making the best of it." The authors note that several factors determine whether a patient copes well or fails to adapt to a major illness including the following: individual personality; previous experience with illness and doctors; meaning of the illness to the patient; quality of patient support systems; specific environments; severity and nature of the disease itself; and effectiveness of the medical care.

In order to provide improved care for cancer patients who are enduring the concomitant stress of the disease and related treatment, the subspecialty of psychiatric oncology has developed. Oncology specialists work closely with the primary physicians to plan interventions that assist patients in decreasing emotional distress and increase their coping ability. In assisting patients to successfully deal with emotional trauma of cancer, it is possible to offer patients a sense of well-being and improved quality of life. To achieve such a goal both patients and physicians have to be open to a change in treatment practices. One noticeable change in recent years has been greater attention to supportive care. Another change is the appreciation of early recognition and early intervention to ward off potential complications.

VII. DIFFERENTIAL DIAGNOSIS

Various conditions may mimic or approximate the symptoms of depression in a cancer population and should be considered as possible causes for apparent depressive symptomatology. Included would be bereavement, anxiety disorders, organic brain disorders, psychosis, and various personality disorders. Critical to understanding coexistent psychopathology in a cancer patient is to take a careful and thorough past history. Special attention to previous episodes of depression or psychiatric treatment, as well as a careful history of emotional reactions at times of major losses, may be particularly helpful in understanding the patient's present problems. Determining a history of recent personality changes, presence or absence of distorted reality testing such as visual or auditory hallucinations or delusional thinking, and recent changes in memory function or impulse control are additional important information. Lastly, a picture of a person's pre-illness life adaptation is useful including information about marital status, sexual adjustment, employment history, church involvement, social activity, and educational accomplishments. Has the individual matured to a reasonably independent and productive life or, conversely, does the individual show patterns of overdependency on others? Is there a pattern of inability to maintain consistency and continuity in a marital relationship, jobs, friendships, or social activities? Such data can help define the coping ability and areas of vulnerability of the patient. We will further discuss the alternative diagnoses.

A. Bereavement

The coexistence of grief or bereavement with cancer has been discussed often. The mortality rate of widows or widowers has been reported to be two- to tenfold that of nonbereaved age-matched controls (Jacobs and Ostfeld, 1977). This increase was higher for widowers than widows. In another prospective study of bereavement (Helsing and Szklo, 1981) comparing 4032 adults widowed over a 12-year period in Washington County, Maryland to an equal number of married persons matched for sex, race, age, and residence it was demonstrated that significantly higher mortality rates existed among widowers compared to married males. However, this relationship was not found to hold for women. Cancer was second only to arteriosclerotic cardiovascular disease as the leading cause of death in the widowed men, accounting for 17% of deaths (Helsing, Comstock, and Szklo, 1982). Other authors argue that there is no compelling evidence to support an increased risk of cancer in a bereaved population (Bieliauskas and Garron, 1982).

Regardless of whether bereavement should be considered as a risk factor for cancer, there is no question that the presence of bereavement in a patient with cancer may lead to clinical complications and difficulties in the management of the patient, particularly if unrecognized. Engle (1961) suggested that grief be considered a disease as a result of its massive impact on normal function with its predicted symptomatology and the inherent suffering that is involved. Symptoms may occur in bereaved people that are the same as those seen in depression, including poor appetite, weight loss, and insomnia, but such symptoms are generally not enduring and would be unlikely to persist beyond a few weeks. Additionally, morbid preoccupation with worthlessness, marked psychomotor retardation, and significant decrease in function would be uncommon with bereavement and their presence would tend to suggest a depressive disorder. Guilt, if present, generally is related to compulsive rehashing of details surrounding the death of a loved one characterized by various "if only" themes. If the bereaved has thoughts of dying, the content of those thoughts is usually in terms of joining the lost person rather than feelings of worthlessness or badness. Management of simple bereavement is usually through supportive reassurance or at times with psychotherapy. Where bereavement is protracted and complicated by persistent symptoms of depression (page 2), treatment for acute depression is appropriate (Section VII.H).

B. Anxiety States

Mild anxiety commonly accompanies the cancer patient: it is often manifest at critical points in the course of the illness. Exacerbated states of anxiety may be encountered when a patient first experiences symptoms and suspects cancer. At the time of diagnostic assessment, when the patient is informed of the diagnosis or treatment plan, at the time of learning of the presence of a recurrence, or when learning that a treatment effort has been unsuccessful. Anxiety symptoms may include problems concentrating, feelings of restlessness, and sleep disruption often characterized by initial insomnia with fretful preoccupations of mind or with "worry." Other symptoms are shortness of breath, "racing" or "skipping" heart (sinus tachycardia and PVCs), and elevated blood pressure. Anxiety may appear in the form of panic attacks characterized by episodes of extreme apprehension or fear in which shortness of breath, palpitations, chest pain, choking or smothering sensations, dizziness, feelings of unreality, paresthesias in the hands or feet, hot or cold flashes, sweating, faintness, or trembling or shaking may occur. Such attacks generally have sudden onset and are intense with a feeling of impending doom, fear of dying, fear of losing one's mind, or fear of losing control. Attacks are generally brief, lasting only a few minutes but may occasionally be protracted for several hours (DSM-III, 1980). Treatment of anxiety, as with bereavement, is generally best handled psychotherapeutically. At times when symptoms are severe, anxiolytic medications (benzodiazapines) are useful as may be tricyclic antidepressants or beta blockers in some situations.

C. Organic Brain Disorders

The second most common diagnosis found in cancer patients referred for psychiatric assessment is that of organic brain disease. Levine, Silberfarb, and Lipowski (1978) report data on 100 consecutive hospitalized cancer patients who were referred for psychiatric consultation. These patients were seen over a 5-year period during which time a total of 5321 patients were hospitalized with cancer, accounting for a referral rate of approximately 1.9% per year of total cancer admissions referred for psychiatric assessment. Of the psychiatric referrals, 56% were diagnosed as depressed and 40% as having organic brain disease. The authors note that 26 of the 100 referred patients had been misdiagnosed by the referring physician as being depressed, when, in fact, they were found to be suffering from an organic brain syndrome. The authors make a special point of emphasizing the importance of the assessment of mental status, especially of cognitive and intellectual functioning (Jacobs et al., 1977).

Cancer patients are particularly prone to delirious states which may be induced by systemic infections, metabolic instability, hypoxia, electrolyte imbalance, hepatic or renal dysfunction, fever, direct or indirect effects of cancer itself, medication side effects, or direct complications of therapeutic management (radiation therapy, chemotherapy, postoperative instability, etc.). Diagnostic criteria of delirium include clouding of consciousness with disorientation and memory impairment and at times perceptual disturbance characterized by hallucinations (most commonly visual, but can involve all senses) or misinterpretations of environmental stimuli. Speech may be confused or incoherent, sleep is disturbed, often with insomnia or daytime drowsiness, and psychomotor activity may be increased or decreased. Additionally, the clarity of thought and consciousness tends to fluctuate over the course of the day, such that there will be intervals of relative clarity interspersed with intervals of clouding.

Cancer patients may also have symptoms of dementia. Dementia is typically characterized by a clear consciousness with a marked loss of intellectual ability such that the individual is impaired in social or occupational activity. Memory impairment is typical where the capacity for new learning is impaired. This results in failure of recent memory whereas distant memory is commonly preserved. Additionally, impairment of abstract thinking, judgmental impairment, personality change, and other disturbances of cortical function may be observed. Symptoms of dementia in cancer patients may reflect an exacerbation of a preexisting dementing illness such as Alzheimer's disease or other primary brain disease or may represent the influence of central nervous system mass lesions. Often, dementia is complicated by superimposed delirium.

Treatment of organic brain syndromes entail correction of the primary cause of delirium where possible and treatment of the cancer itself. Efforts to minimize the use of psychotropic medications in the presence of delirium or dementia are well advised since psychoactive agents may markedly increase organic symptomatology. Treatment of delirium includes simple efforts to provide increased human contact and sensory stimulation to the patients. Simple things such as a night light, having a family member present, or a roommate or sitter, use of a television or radio, and frequent nurse contact can keep these patients mildly stimulated and enhance orientation and control. With agitation or psychotic distortions, the patient may require a restraint. Such behavior often can be controlled with an antipsychotic agent such as haloperidol. Benzodiazapines and sedative hypnotics are best avoided in delirious and demented patients as they often promote a confusional syndrome.

D. Psychosis

Psychotic symptoms may occur in patients with cancer. Psychosis is a term used to describe a person who is shown to have a gross impairment in awareness of reality. In this situation, the psychotic individual incorrectly interprets external reality, even when given clear evidence to the contrary. For such a distortion to be considered psychotic it must not be shared by others in the family or culture. A psychosis is commonly associated with hallucinations or delusions. Hallucinations may occur in any sensory modality, and commonly occur in the form of voices, visions, smells, or strange feelings about the body. Hallucinated experience is only psychotic if it is believed to be real. Delusions are psychotic by definition in that these are misbeliefs based on incorrect inference about external reality which is unshakable despite obvious evidence or proof to the contrary. Common delusions encountered in cancer patients are those of paranoid suspiciousness, with a belief of being persecuted, poisoned, controlled, or plotted against (sometimes by the medical staff). Somatic delusions occasionally occur in a setting wherein physical complaints are based on delusional misbeliefs that are usually bizarre enough to be obvious. Such complaints may involve gross distortions of body image or absurd beliefs to explain symptoms which are not in keeping with observation or perception. Examples would include ideas of being inhabited by insects or parasites, the presence of implanted transmitters in the body, a snake in the abdomen, and the like.

Psychotic distortions can occur as symptoms of a wide variety of mental disorders affecting cancer patients. Unless there is a past history of schizophrenia, it is unlikely that schizophrenia would be the explanation of such symptoms. More commonly, psychotic symptoms would be complicating features of depression or organic brain syndromes. Management of psychotic distortions is best accomplished by means of careful attention to differential diagnosis of the underlying disorder that has led to the psychosis. Effective treatment of that primary condition will usually correct the problem. Symptoms may require antipsychotic management with haloperidol or other antipsychotic agents and may necessitate management on a psychiatric inpatient unit. Usually psychotic patients are responsive to calming and reassuring attention where an effort is made to understand the worries of the patient while avoiding any direct challenge of the psychotic distortions. Such a challenge might alienate and excite the patient. It is important to remember that the presence of psychotic material is not diagnostic of any single disorder but rather provides evidence of extreme mental impairment which may be the product of depression, mania, delirium, dementia, schizophrenia, or other less common conditions.

E. Personality Factors

In the differential diagnosis of depressive disorders, there are patients who have chronic behavioral patterns characterized by persistent dissatisfaction and unhappiness often with feelings of inadequacy, low self-esteem, and inability to find pleasure in their lives. Such personality patterns are usually longstanding, dating back to childhood or adolescence and may be associated with occasional bouts of depressive illness. Often, a clear pattern of chronic discontent, sadness, and unhappiness is apparent that has been present for years. Such personality patterns may be associated with depressive disorders, but should not in and of themselves be confused diagnostically with depression.

The dysthymic disorder (DSM-III, 1980) is a condition characterized by chronic depressive affect often associated with problems experiencing pleasure in all or many life activities. Other features of depressive disorder may be noted but of lesser degree than found in major depression. Such features may be interspersed from time to time with periods of normal function, but the typical pattern is one of chronic sadness and dissatisfaction. Vegetative symptoms of depression may be observed but are inconsistent. Common to these character types are superimposed somatic preoccupations sometimes with a history of hypochondriasis and persistent preoccupation with physical ills. Such patients frequently have problems functioning independently and interpersonally. Excessive alcohol consumption, obesity, and heavy smoking habits are often encountered as additional evidence of conflicts and frustrated dependency issues. Individuals with dependent personality structures are often less adaptive with stressful situations than less dependent people and may well be more vulnerable to the development of secondary depression with the stress of a diagnosis of cancer.

The approach to treatment of patients who have a dependent personality is primarily supportive in nature and often enhanced via involvement with other family members who are usually deeply involved in the care and maintenance of these individuals. Essentially, the problem encountered with patients having dependent personalities of this sort is one of a deficiency or paucity of adaptive coping skills. Since this is a lifelong character pattern, treatment is targeted toward correction of depression or anxiety symptoms with specific help in coping with identified problems. Psychotropic medications are generally ineffective unless there are clear superimposed symptoms of depressive disorder or anxiety. An additional problem often seen with dependent patients of this type is a tendency to substance abuse, where alcohol or drugs may be seen as a source of gratification or fulfillment. If a history exists of street drug abuse, misuse of prescribed medications, or alcohol excess, care should be exercised with the use of narcotics, sedative hypnotics, or anxiolytics where such medications are needed. Direct family involvement in the management and dispensing of medication may be warranted.

F. Problem of Misdiagnosis and Undertreatment

Derogatis et al. (1979) reported on a survey of psychotropic drugs prescribed for approximately 1600 cancer patients who were being treated in five separate centers. At least half of the population received some form of psychotropic drug; hypnotics were the most frequently prescribed and accounted for 48% of all prescriptions. Of interest, only 1% of the patients were given antidepressant medications, and of that 1%, a third were prescribed antidepressants for pain rather than depression. The infrequent use of tricyclic antidepressants suggests a failure to recognize depression as a treatable disorder in the practice of oncology. Where depression is perceived as a normal reaction rather than a treatable disorder in the practice of oncology. Where depression is perceived as a normal reaction rather than a treatable condition, undertreatment and attendant suffering would be expected (Schacter, 1983). This problem seems to be one of failure to distinguish between the normal grief reaction to cancer which should be relatively brief and not incapacitating from a full-blown depressive disorder. Such confusion leads to underrecognition with undertreatment of depression (Derogatis, Abeloff, and McBeth, 1976; Petty and Noyes, 1981). Optimal care of a cancer patient focuses both on quality and quantity of life, therefore careful attention to the treatment of depression should be a primary treatment concern.

Effective pharmacotherapy can produce many positive results for the depressed cancer patient. For example, sleep can be substantially improved,
often alleviating the need for sedative hypnotics. Mood and the capacity
for experiencing pleasure can improve considerably in spite of the reality of
the illness. A substantial enhancement of vigor and vitality is possible for
many patients. The patient's appetite may improve together with increased
enjoyment in eating as well as potential weight gain. Although the so-called
vegetative symptoms of depression and the symptoms of cancer are often
hard to distinguish and the symptoms are usually attributed to the cancer
itself, the reverse may be true on occasion whereby these symptoms are, in
fact, depressive in etiology. Consequently, dramatic change may occasionally
be observed when tricyclic antidepressants are used in the depressed patient
with cancer.

G. Association of Pain and Depression

Pain, a problem common to the cancer population described elsewhere in this
book, may have attendant depressive features. The association between pain
and depression has long been recognized and has recently been discussed in the
literature (Maltbie, 1983; Blumer and Heilbronn, 1982; Schaffer, Doulon, and
Bittle, 1980).

Tricyclic antidepressants have been reported to be useful in the treatment
of various types of chronic pain including that associated with cancer (Maltbie,
1983; Shimm et al., 1979; Kocher, 1976; Ward, Bloom, and Friedel, 1979).
Tricyclic antidepressants are now in common use in pain clinics, throughout
the country. While there is mixed opinion regarding which antidepressants
are more desirable in the treatment of chronic pain, those antidepressants that
are more active in blocking reuptake of serotonin are believed, by most authors,
to be more efficacious. Amitriptyline and doxepin are usually used for this
purpose. There is evidence that there may be three different ways in which
tricyclic antidepressants are useful in the treatment of pain: through antidepressant effects, through direct analgesic effects, and through synergistic
effects with narcotics (Ward, Bloom, and Friedel, 1979; Lee and Spencer, 1977;
Maltbie, 1984).

Clinically, a trial of doxepin or amitriptyline should be considered for any
cancer pain patient where sleep is significantly disturbed by pain or where
pain control is inadequate with the use of mild analgesics. The dosage of
these drugs is comparable for pain as for depression.

H. Treatment of Depression with Cancer

The treatment of choice for depressed cancer patients is to use the tricyclic
antidepressants. Common tricyclic antidepressants include amitriptyline,

imipramine, doxepin, nortriptyline, and desipramine. Selection of an antidepressant depends in large measure on the specific depressive symptoms of
the patient as well as potential side effects of the antidepressant drug selected.
Where the depression is characterized by insomnia and agitation, one of the
more sedating antidepressants should be chosen. Here amitriptyline and
doxepin would be most commonly selected. Where psychomotor retardation
and low energy levels are the major symptoms and sleep is not seriously impaired, desipramine or nortriptyline would be the more likely choice. Where
symptoms are mixed, imipramine is often a good choice. Amitriptyline,
doxepin, and imipramine can often be given in single nightly dosage to enhance sleep, minimize side effects, and simplify administration. Conversely,
desipramine and nortriptyline, having little sedative effect, can be given in
divided dosage without sedating the patient and still achieve some reduction in
side effects where side effects are a problem. Where hepatic function is impaired,
tricyclines should be administered with caution, monitoring hepatic enzymes.
Generally, tricyclines are well tolerated without compromise of hepatic status.

The principal side effects of tricyclic antidepressants are anticholinergic in
type including dry mouth, blurred vision, constipation, and urinary retention.
Of the antidepressants, amitriptyline is the most anticholinergic, with doxepin
and imipramine somewhat less potent as anticholinergic agents, and nortriptyline
and desipramine the least anticholinergic in their effects. While less common,
anticholinergic effects can lead to delirium, particularly if the patient has
underlying organic brain syndrome. This complication is even more likely
when combinations of anticholinergic drugs are used since these effects are
additive. Thus, when delirium is present, tricyclic antidepressant should be
discontinued. Cardiovascular side effects include prolongation of conduction
time and direct suppression of myocardial contractility. Consequently, there
may be some risk of an increased frequency of congestive heart failure,
cardiac arrythmias, and left ventricular hypertrophy (Walker and Covington,
1984; Baldessarini, 1977). This is of some concern in patients who have received large amounts of anthracyclines (doxorubicin) because of their
cardiotoxicity. Orthostatic hypotension is an additional side effect that can
be clinically distressing and should be watched for by monitoring postural
changes in blood pressure and pulse. Lastly, tricyclic antidepressants are
contraindicated in the presence of monoamine-oxidase inhibitors. Consequently, the use of the chemotherapeutic agent procarbazine is incompatible
with tricyclic antidepressants. The combination of these two agents could
result in a hypertensive crisis.

Dosage of antidepressants in a cancer population is comparable to that
suggested for elderly patients. An initial (25 mg) regular nightly dose of
imipramine, amitriptyline, or doxepin is suggested with gradual titration upward

in 25 mg increments every second or third night to a nightly maintenance dose
of from 75-100 mg, depending on tolerance of the drug and therapeutic result.
Nortriptyline and desipramine can be given by divided dose starting with
desipramine at 25 mg once or twice a day and nortriptyline, 10 mg 2-3 times
a day. The usual maintenance dosage of desipramine is from 75-150 mg/day
and nortriptyline between 50 and 75 mg/day.

An adequate trial of a tricyclic antidepressant usually requires 3-4 weeks.
Where depression is clearly a problem and a given antidepressant is not effective,
then a trial with a different type of drug may be indicated. Likewise, should
troublesome side effects occur with one antidepressant, another can be substituted at equipotent dosage without losing antidepressant gains and yet often
altering the side effects such that the second drug is tolerated. New antidepressants have been introduced to the market including such agents as
amoxapine, maprotiline and trazodone. When the previously listed older
agents are not tolerated by a patient, one of the newer ones may be tried; the
latter have not been proven to have a better therapeutic ratio. One author
states that trazadone and maprotiline have a faster onset of action and fewer
anticholinergic side effects and therefore may be better tolerated by cancer
patients (Massie, 1983). Psychostimulants such as dextroamphetamine and
methylphenidate are sometimes used in cancer patients who are depressed or
in patients who are in the terminal phase of illness. Starting dosages are often
2.5 mg of dextroamphetamine given twice a day, with increases made in
dosages as patients become tolerant to the effects. It is also important to
remember that amphetamines can potentiate the analgesic effect of opiates.

In addition to pharmacological approaches, effective treatment of profound
depression can be accomplished with electroconvulsive therapy (ECT). When
patients are severely withdrawn and rapidly failing physically as a complication
of their depression, treatment with electroconvulsive therapy can be lifesaving.
Modern ECT is both safe and effective for severe depressions and may, in fact,
be more consistently effective than antidepressant pharmacotherapy (Baldessarini,
1977). Modern technique combined with use of effective anesthesia and
neuromuscular blockade has dramatically reduced complications to the point
that very little risk exists. The only established contraindication to ECT is
found in the presence of intracranial mass lesion (Maltbie et al., 1980) where
a high risk of serious morbidity or even mortality exists.

Seriously depressed cancer patients should be referred for psychiatric
assessment and, when indicated, hospitalized for psychiatric care where more
intensive combined therapies would be appropriate. Most secondary depressions
will not require extensive psychiatric involvement and will generally respond to
tricyclic antidepressants and supportive medical care by the oncology staff.

Treatment of the dying patient, whether depressed or not, includes several salient features of considerable importance to the patient. Cassem and Stuart (1975) delineated eight such factors, which are as follows:

1. Competence. Skill and a sense of competence are reassuring to the patient whose life and care are dependent upon the training and talent of the caretakers.
2. Concern. Compassion and genuine concern are factors that are evident to patients in their relationship with their caretakers. Honest empathy is meaningful and supportive to the patient. Personal avoidance or contrived involvement can serve to distance the relationship and increase the discomfort of the patient.
3. Comfort. Detailed attention to comfort needs is of considerable importance to the dying patient. Pain relief, management of constipation, oral and skin care, and care of nausea and vomiting are essential.
4. Communication. Here the capacity to listen is the essential quality. Listening coupled with taking the necessary time to get to know something special about the patient as a unique person is central. Effective communication requires that the caretaker take time to let the person talk and pay attention to his/her worries or concerns.
5. Children. Visits from children are very helpful in bringing relief and consolation to the terminally ill. Cassem notes that a useful rule of thumb in choosing whether a particular child should visit a terminal patient is simply asking the child whether he/she wants to.
6. Family. Family support can be very helpful to the terminal patient. Conversely, this is a critical time for the family in preparation for the work of bereavement. This is a time for flexibility where the wishes of family and patient are of primary importance.
7. Cheerfulness. Terminal patients and their families may be uplifted by a pleasant cheerful disposition. Gentle and appropriate humor, likewise, can be very helpful provided that the patient is receptive. Cassem cautions that the listener should take the cue from the patient regarding appropriateness of humor to the situation.
8. Consistency. Regular and consistent visits, even when brief, can be very useful to the patient. Such regular and predictable contact is evidence of continuation of support and concern.

Quality treatment that includes the essentials suggested by Cassem and Stuart should have prophylactic effects on the development of secondary depression and will go a long way in identifying depression early in its development and initiating appropriate treatment.

I. Depression and Progression of Cancer

There is evidence that the presence of depression may be associated with a more rapid progression of neoplastic diseases. Greater psychological distress, including depression, has been identified in several studies as being present among patients who have more rapid advancing illness and shortened survival time (Miller and Spratt, 1979; Davies et al., 1973). Apathy and hopelessness were significantly related to shortened survival time among patients with advanced disease. Derogatis, Abeloff, and McBeth (1976) noted that cancer patients with high depression scores were among the shortest in survival time. Petty and Noyes (1981) note that the relationship may go both ways, where rapidly progressive cancer may contribute to the development of depression, and depression, when present, may speed the process of decline thus shortening survival.

A recent study by Cassileth et al. (1984) compared patients with six different diseases in an effort to determine whether significant differences in mental health status existed between these illnesses: these included arthritis, diabetes, cancer, end-stage renal disease, and dermatological disorders. No significant differences could be found between these populations and the general public on a mental health index score, but all were found to have significantly higher mental health index function than a group of patients under treatment for depression. The authors noted that one of the remarkable findings was the quality of psychological adaptation among most patients with chronic illnesses which seemed fundamentally independent of primary diagnosis. They argue that psychological stereotyping occurs with a natural tendency to infer psychological status from the presence of a specific diagnosis. A common example is that "all cancer patients are depressed." Their work does not support that supposition.

In conclusion, the prompt diagnosis and appropriate treatment of depression can significantly alter the quality of life and may even have an influence on the progression of the cancer itself; they certainly influence the way in which patients can tolerate these treatments. The assumption that depression is normal in cancer patients is not supported by recent studies and such an assumption can only interfere with effective diagnosis and proper treatment. Insofar as our task is one of maximizing function and comfort and minimizing suffering in our patients with cancer, it becomes essential that we not deny them adequate and proper antidepressant treatment.

REFERENCES

Baldessarini, R. J. (1977). *Chemotherapy in Psychiatry*, Harvard University Press, Cambridge.

Bieliauskas, L. A., and Garron, D. G. (1982). Psychological depression and cancer, *Gen. Hosp. Psychiat., 4*:187-195.

Blumer, D., and Heilbronn, M. (1982). Chronic pain as a variant of depressive disease: The pain prone disorder, *J. Nerv. Men. Dis., 170*:381-406.

Bukberg, J. B., and Holland, J. C. (1980). A prevalence study of depression in a cancer hospital population, *Proc. A.S.C.O., 21*:382 (C-251).

Cassem, N. H., and Stewart, R. S. (1975). Management and care of the dying patient, *Int. J. Psychiat. Med., 6*:574-585.

Cassileth, B. R., Lusk, E. J., Strouse, T. B., Miller, D. S., Brown, L. L., Cross, P. A., and Tenaglia, A. N. (1984). Psychosocial status and chronic illness: A comparative analysis of six diagnostic groups, *New Engl. J. Med., 311*: 506-511.

Cavanaugh, S., Clark, D. C., and Gibbons, R. D. (1983). Diagnosing depression in the hospitalized medically ill using the Beck depression inventory, *Psychosomatics, 24*:809-815.

Craig, T. J., and Abeloff, M. D. (1974). Psychiatric symptomatology among hospitalized cancer patients, *Am. J. Psychiat., 131*:1323-1327.

Davies, R. K., Quinlan, D. M., McKegney, F. P., and Kimball, C. P. (1973). Organic factors and psychological adjustment in advanced cancer patients, *Psychosomat. Med., 35*:464-471.

Derogatis, L. R., Abeloff, M. D., and McBeth, C. D. (1976). Cancer patients and their physicians in the perception of psychological symptoms, *Psychosomatics, 17*:197-201.

Derogatis, L. R., Feldstein, M., Morrow, G., Schmale, A., Schmitt, M., Gates, C., Murawski, B., Holland, J., Penman, D., Melisaratos, N., Enelow, A. J., and Adler, L. M. (1979). A survey of psychotropic drug prescriptions in an oncology population, *Cancer, 44*:1919-1929.

Diagnostic and Statistical Manual of Mental Disorders, 3rd Ed. (1980). American Psychiatric Association, Washington, D.C.

Endicott, J. (1984). Measurement of depression in patients with cancer, *Cancer, 53(10)*:2243-2248.

Engle, G. L. (1961). Is grief a disease?, *Psychosomat. Med., 23*:18-22.

Foreman, B. F. (1979). Cancer and suicide, *Gen. Hosp. Psychiat., 1*:108-114.

Greer, S. (1974). Psychological aspects: Delay in the treatment of breast cancer, *Proc. R. Soc. Med., 67*:470-473.

Helsing, K. J., Comstock, G. W., and Szklo, M. (1982). Causes of death in a widowed population, *Am. J. Epid., 116*:524-532.

Helsing, K. J., and Szklo, M. (1981). Mortality after bereavement, *Am. J. Epid., 114*:41-52.

Henderson, J. G. (1966). Denial and repression as factors in the delay of patients with cancer presenting themselves to the physician, *Ann. N.Y. Acad. Sci., 125*:856-864.

Henderson, J. G., Wittkower, E. D., and Longheed, M. N. (1958). A psychiatric investigation of the delay factor in patient to doctor presentation in cancer, *J. Psychosomat. Res., 3*:27-41.

Hinton, J. (1980). The cancer ward, *Adv. Psychosomat. Med., 10*:78-98.

Holland, J. (1973). Psychologic aspects of cancer, *Cancer Medicine* (J. F. Holland and E. Frei, III, eds.), Lea & Febiger, Philadelphia, pp. 991-1021.

Jacobs, J. W., Bernhard, M. R., Delgado, A., and Strain, J. J. (1977). Screening for organic mental syndromes in the medically ill, *Ann. Intern. Med.,* *86*:40-55.

Jacobs, S., and Ostfeld, A. (1977). An epidemiological review of the mortality of bereavement, *Psychosomat. Med., 39*:344-357.

Klerman, G. L. (1978). Affective disorders, *Harvard Guide to Modern Psychiatry* (A. M. Nicholi, Jr., ed.), The Belknap Press of Harvard University Press, Cambridge, pp. 253-281.

Kocher, R. (1976). The use of psychotropic drugs in treatment of chronic severe pains, *Eur. Neurol., 14*:458-464.

Koenig, R., Levin, S. M., and Brennan, M. J. (1967). The emotional status of cancer patients as measured by a psychological test, *J. Chron. Dis., 20*: 923-930.

Lee, R., and Spencer, P. S. J. (1977). Antidepressants and pain: A review of the pharmacological data supporting the use of certain tricyclics in chronic pain, *J. Int. Med. Res., 5(1)*:146-156.

Levine, P. M., Silberfarb, P. M., and Lipowski, Z. J. (1978). Mental disorders in cancer patients: A study of 100 psychiatric referrals, *Cancer, 42*:1385-1391.

Maltbie, A. A. (1984). Chronic pain, *Biomedical Psychiatric Therapeutics* (J. L. Sullivan and P. D. Sullivan, eds.), Butterworth Publishers, Boston, pp. 169-190.

Maltbie, A. A. (1984). Pain management, *Current Geriatric Therapy* (T. R. Covington and J. I. Walker, eds.), W. B. Saunders, Philadelphia, pp. 422-434.

Maltbie, A. A., Wingfield, M. S., Volow, M. R., Weiner, R. D., Sullivan, J. L., and Cavenar, J. O. (1980). Electroconvulsive therapy in the presence of brain tumor: Case reports and an evaluation of risk, *J. Nerv. Men. Dis., 168*:400-411.

Marshall, J. R., Burnett, W., and Brasure, J. (1983). On precipitating factors: Cancer as a cause of suicide, *Suicide Life-Threaten. Behav., 13*:15-27.

Massie, M. J. (1983). Psychopharmacologic management of psychiatric syndrome in cancer patients, *Supportive Care of the Cancer Patient* (R. Gralla, ed.), Biomedical Information Corporation, New York, pp. 40-43.

Massie, M. J., Gorzynski, G., Mastrovito, R., Theis, D., and Holland, J. (1979). The diagnosis of depression in hospitalized patients with cancer, *Proc. A.S.C.O., 20*:432 (C-587).

Miller, T., and Spratt, J. S., Jr. (1979). Critical review of reported psychological correlates of cancer prognosis and growth, *Mind and Cancer Prognosis* (E. A. Stoll, ed.), John Wiley & Sons, New York, pp. 31-37.

Petty, F., and Noyes, R., Jr. (1981). Depression secondary to cancer, *Biol. Psychiat., 16*:1203-1220.

Plumb, M. M., and Holland, J. (1977). Comparative studies of psychological function in patients with advanced cancer. I. Self-reported depressive symptoms, *Psychosomat. Med., 39*:264-276.

Reisner, D. E., and Rosen, D. H. (1984). The experience of illness in hospital-ization, *Medicine as a Human Experience* (D. E. Reisner and D. H. Rosen, eds.), University Park Press, Baltimore, pp. 113-135.

Reiser, D. E., and Schroder, A. K. (1980). *Patient Interviewing: The Human Dimension*, Williams & Wilkins, Baltimore.

Robins, E., Munoz, R. A., Martin, S., and Gentry, K. A. (1972). Primary and secondary affective disorders, *Disorders of Mood* (J. Zubin and F. A. Freyhan, eds.), The Johns Hopkins Press, Baltimore, pp. 33-49.

Schacter, L. (1983). Depression and anxiety in cancer patients, with a reply by Derogatis, *J.A.M.A., 250*:728-729.

Schaffer, C. B., Doulon, P. T., and Bittle, R. M. (1980). Chronic pain and depression: A clinical and family history survey, *Am. J. Psychiat., 137*: 118-120.

Schwab, J. J., Bialow, M., Brown, J. M., and Holzer, C. E. (1967). Diagnosing depression in medical inpatients, *Ann. Intern. Med., 67*:695-707.

Shimm, D. S., Logue, G. L., Maltbie, A. A., and Dugan, S. (1979). Medical management of chronic cancer pain, *J.A.M.A., 241*:2408-2412.

Stewart, M. A., Drake, F., and Winokur, G. (1965). Depression among med-ically ill patients, *Dis. Nerv. Syst., 26*:479-485.

Walker, J. I., and Covington, T. R. (1984). Psychiatric disorders, *Current Geriatric Therapy* (T. R. Covington and J. I. Walker, eds.), W. B. Saunders, Philadelphia, pp. 75-103.

Ward, N. G., Bloom, V. L., and Friedel, R. O. (1979). The effectiveness of tricyclic antidepressants in the treatment of coexisting pain and depression, *Pain, 7*: 331-341.

9

Special Considerations for Children

William H. Schultz, Marilyn J. Hockenberry, and John M. Falletta
Duke University Medical Center, Durham, North Carolina

I. INTRODUCTION

When cancer occurs in a child it is an especially tragic event. The life of the child is threatened, as are the hopes and aspirations of the parents for the child. Family and friends grieve, the health care team tries to initiate successful therapy and rally support for the child and family, and everyone hopes for the best.

These events are in common with people at any age who develop a life-threatening illness. But the child with cancer is different from the adult because the illness occurs while the child is growing and developing and remains largely dependent on others for nurture and support. Also, the illness in the child creates an illness in the family which must be treated. The child with cancer differs from most other children, even those with a chronic illness, because successful cancer therapy itself may threaten the life of the child and frequently creates major organ dysfunction that may interfere with growth and development. The child cured of cancer may have 60 or 70 years to develop late complications of the therapy.

For these reasons, a special focus on the child is necessary when one considers complications of cancer care. If the goal of cancer treatment is to provide curative therapy with the fewest early and late complications, then identifying these complications permits a clear statement of the shortcomings of current care. Only with this focus will the true cost of care be defined and better care developed.

II. PARENT-CHILD COMMUNICATION

Successful treatment of children with cancer is no longer measured only by
how often the disease is eradicated, but also by how little the treatment affects
the child's opportunity for continued growth and development. The family
must provide an environment in which the child evolves into a unique human
being. Families differ, but all share unique characteristics in providing nurture
to their members (Schuster and Ashburn, 1980). Stability of a family, as
well as experiences within the family, greatly affect the development of each
child's self-esteem (Stanwyck, 1983). Families who value each member as a
special person and who are open to change are more likely to foster individuals
with a positive self-image. Growth and development as a family unit are
essential to promote self-realization of all family members (Schuster and
Ashburn, 1980).

The behavior of an ill child affects the entire family. A child who is secure,
independent, and who has a positive sense of self will adjust more easily to
the onset of cancer than one who is not comfortable with his/her world
(Hughes, 1976). It is essential to explore the child's personality in order to
provide support to the parents in dealing with the child. Play therapy is helpful in allowing the younger child to explore fears regarding cancer and its
treatment. By means of stories and drawings one can evaluate the child's perceptions of cancer. While the younger child may be totally unaware of the
severity of cancer, the teenager usually has an acute awareness of what the
diagnosis means. This awareness requires that the parents deal with their
fears and concerns not only between themselves, but directly with the child.
Fostering a child's efforts to grow and develop within a treatment environment is a complex and important task for the health care team. Failure to
succeed, even while curing the child's cancer, leaves the child emotionally
crippled and unable to achieve his/her potential.

Cancer in a child imposes an acute threat to the psychological and physical
well-being of parents (Krouse and Krouse, 1982). Parents perceive the development of cancer in their child as a personal loss. They no longer have complete
control and authority over the child. Realization that the child's total care is
being placed in the hands of others may lead to guilt and anguish. Parents
often see themselves as failures, as having let the child down. They frequently
have difficulty in fulfilling their responsibilities at work and in the home
(Kaplan, 1973). To deal with their guilt, the parents must accept the diagnosis,
have confidence in the plan of therapy, and recognize the importance of their
mental and physical health in helping the child to recover (Hughes, 1976).
They often need to be assisted in making provisions in the home environment
for those restrictions placed upon the child by the illness. They must seek
out ways to carry out the family lifestyle in the framework of changes brought

on by the child's illness (Spinetta and Deasy-Spinetta, 1981). Positive parental attitudes convey acceptance to the child and support self-esteem. Health care personnel can facilitate this adjustment by providing a safe environment in which the parents can gain trust in those involved with their child. The parents must feel that the child is safe within the health care system.

The outcome of parental stress brought on by the onset of cancer in a child is dependent upon a variety of factors (Kaplan, 1973). Parents must first comprehend the nature of the illness and be able to communicate its seriousness to immediate family members, while also maintaining a positive attitude about the curability of the illness. This is often difficult for parents who want to protect siblings and other family members from grief but must enlist their realistic support and tolerance of disruptions. Without realizing it, parents may ignore siblings and other family members and appear no longer to care about them. Parents who share appropriate feelings of grief and sadness with all family members are able to deal with the stress of cancer more effectively (Krouse and Krouse, 1982). Sharing feelings allows for participation by all family members in the adjustment period. Professionals can help parents identify and build upon their strengths, allowing for the development of positive methods for coping early in the illness (Hughes, 1976). With the identification of these strengths, parents are able to accept cancer in the child and develop ways in which to carry out much of their previous lifestyle. This may not occur without drastic change, but the parent who utilizes strengths and coping skills developed through previous experiences will be able to contribute to a lifestyle for all family members similar to that prior to the onset of cancer in the child.

III. IMPLICATIONS OF INFORMED CONSENT: PARENTS SPEAKING FOR CHILDREN

Children have a constitutionally protected right to privacy but often cannot exercise this right since they are considered legally incompetent. They also have a commonly accepted right to give an informed assent to medical treatment. Parents usually exercise their children's rights, maintaining a degree of control over the child's upbringing. Parental authority is limited, however, by virtue of the state's power as *parens patriae,* which establishes the court's interest in the health and welfare of children (Horwitz, 1979).

A complicating feature of pediatric cancer care is the issue of parents and children entering the informed consent process. Parents and physicians share a responsibility to provide the child with the best cancer therapy available. Parents must keep themselves informed as fully as possible regarding the treatment, its side effects, and possible alternatives. The child, too, must be involved in the process of informed consent, although the degree to which the child is involved is a controversial matter. Most would agree that children with cancer should be informed about their disease at diagnosis. However, the informed consent procedures for investigational cancer therapy are laden with controversy. Some clinicians have cautioned against full disclosure, believing that a flood of information compounds the anxiety children and parents feel at diagnosis. Others have observed minimal anxiety during consent discussions with adults and point out that the main reason endorsed by patients for accepting treatment is "trust in the physician" (Penman et al., 1984). The degree to which the child trusts the physician is initially a reflection of parental attitude. Independent of this is the relationship that develops between the physician and child during treatment.

If therapeutic options are openly discussed at the time of diagnosis, then the discussions with the child and family are more likely to be open and supportive if the child's medical condition deteriorates. Some investigators have reported that children older than 5 years have the capacity to make decisions about further therapy when standard therapy has failed (Nitschke et al., 1982). Others take issue with this position, believing that it is the physician who should assume responsibility for making decisive recommendations regarding care without asking the child's opinion about the options (Shumway, Grossman, and Sarles, 1983). We believe that the physician's responsibility should be aligned with the child's right to be fully informed. The reality of worsening disease and the therapeutic options should be openly discussed. The parents and child should be helped to understand that the effectiveness of phase II drugs against malignancy has not been established. It is the uncertainty surrounding the outcome of treatment with phase II agents which allows the clinician to deviate from the traditional physician's duty to select and recommend a particular treatment in favor of leaving the choice of therapy to chance. The child and parents should also be given support and reassurance in their decision, and if asked, the physician should be prepared to recommend a therapeutic approach if the parents and child are unable to decide.

A special problem encountered in the pediatric setting involves parents who choose unorthodox medical treatment for children with life-threatening conditions. All pediatric cancer types have well-defined conventional medical treatments that offer a substantial chance of cure or remission. Parents may turn to unconventional therapy due to the pain and side effects associated with standard treatments, and due to their desire to maintain a larger measure of control over their child's therapy. Or it may be a decision based on religious belief. State agencies are empowered to protect children from parental actions that threaten children's well-being. Physicians can ask the court to intervene under the *parens patriae* point of law and petition for legal custody of the child in order to administer lifesaving treatment.

Transfusion therapy to Jehovah's Witness patients requires this kind of intervention when parents refuse to consent to the administration of blood products to their child. Parents have no right to prevent lifesaving treatment for their child although they may assert the child's right to privacy and refuse treatment if it is only life prolonging (Monaco, 1983).

IV. THERAPEUTIC ORPHANS

The application of investigational drugs to the treatment of cancer in children has a rich heritage, dating back to the first successful induction of remission of a patient with acute lymphocytic leukemia, which occurred in a child in 1948. Indeed the dramatic improvement that has occurred in the outlook for children with cancer is a result of the orderly trial of investigational drugs to patients with resistant malignancies. Yet this orderly process has been challenged by an attitude, fortunately not dominant as yet, which would require that only those drugs that have demonstrated efficacy in adults would be available for use in children. Even though the malignancies that occur commonly in adults differ dramatically from those in children, this proposal would seek to restrict the application of potentially promising drugs from children because the drugs were ineffective in adult malignancies. These children with cancer could then become "therapeutic orphans."

Many examples exist of new drugs that became commercially available and were approved for use in adults but not in children, in part because investigation of the drug in children was given low priority by funding agencies and pharmaceutical corporations. One complication of the success associated with children's cancer care may be the development of a casual attitude about the importance of new drug development for childhood malignancies. Fortunately the National Cancer Institute is once again targeting new phase I trials in pediatric malignancies, with limited funding for the near future. In order to avoid complacency and subsequent lack of progress in children's cancer therapy, such vigorous investigation must proceed uninterrupted if the most serious complication of cancer care is to be avoided —the continued use of toxic but inadequate therapy.

V. PROBLEM OF UNDERTREATMENT

By today's standards, many children treated for cancer even 5 years ago received inappropriate therapy. Some received too little therapy [high-risk acute lymphocytic leukemia (ALL), advanced non-Hodgkin's lymphoma (NHL)], some too much (early Wilms' tumor or NHL), and some received qualitatively wrong therapy (cranial radiation in low-risk ALL patients). Presumably a critical review of this subject 10 years hence will describe additional current practices which in retrospect were inappropriate. If the major complication of cancer care is the use of ineffective but toxic therapy, then the next most serious complication is using too little or too much of what is actually effective therapy.

The complication of too little effective therapy is recurrent or progressive disease. Fortunately few U.S. children with cancer receive too little therapy by today's standards because the vast majority receive care from recently trained expert pediatric oncologists. However, as the competition for patients intensifies, or as medical cost containment dictates restricted or delayed referral of patients to pediatric oncologists, the problem of patients failing therapy because it was too little or too late will predictably increase.

VI. PROBLEM OF OVERTREATMENT

Present day treatment programs are rescuing most children with cancer. The "cost" of these apparent cures may not be fully realized, but the body of literature devoted to the late effects of childhood cancer therapy is growing rapidly. Knowledge concerning the risks of treatment-related morbidity is being applied to design of treatment protocols that seek to minimize damaging side effects without compromising curative therapy. Virtually all tissues and organs are susceptible to the toxicity of cancer treatment. Many of the problems seen in the treatment of children relate to effects on developing tissues. As a general principal it is known that cytotoxic therapy is far more harmful to growing tissue than to static or slowly renewing tissue. Therefore, children with cancer are at high risk for disturbances in physical as well as psychological growth and development. Acute toxicities in children are similar to those affecting adults as described elsewhere in this book, particularly regarding the pulmonary, cardiovascular, and genitourinary systems. Special problems of children are the focus of this chapter and are presented system by system.

A. Central Nervous System

A major contribution to the improved survival of children with acute lymphocytic leukemia has been the prophylactic treatment of the central nervous system (CNS) with cranial irradiation and intrathecal chemotherapy. The long-term toxicity of this essential treatment is now well recognized. Both intellectual and perceptual motor function may be impaired due to interference with neural development before maturation of the brain is complete (Moss, Nannis, and Poplack, 1981). Abilities of younger children are more compromised than those of older children since development of many skills is age dependent. Significant CNS injury and reduction in overall I.Q. scores have been reported

in some children treated with CNS prophylaxis consisting of 2400 rads of
cranial irradiation and 6 doses of intrathecal methotrexate (Meadows et al.,
1981). The extreme result is the syndrome of leukoencephalopathy, characterized by ataxia, spasticity, somnolence, seizures, and dementia and with
histological evidence of white matter necrosis and intracerebral calcifications
(Rubinstein et al., 1975; Flament-Durand et al., 1975). Focal leukoencephalopathy develops in about 10% of children with acute leukemia receiving
CNS radiation therapy. This syndrome of somnolence, irritability, tremors,
and forgetfulness is usually transient and occurs 3-8 weeks after treatment.
It is often referred to as the post-irradiation somnolence syndrome and resolves spontaneously without therapy weeks to months after its onset
(Freeman, Johnston, and Voke, 1973). Griffin and associates described
the effect of radiation on the blood-brain barrier in mice, demonstrating
an increased permeability to methotrexate (Griffin, Rasey, and Bleyer, 1977).
Indeed, the combined use of intrathecal methotrexate and cranial radiation
has an enhancing effect on the degree of neurological toxicity, and abnormalities in the computed tomographic (CT) brain scans have been
described in patients treated with such combined therapy (Peylan-Ramu
et al., 1978). (See Figure 1.)

Chemotherapeutic agents alone can produce significant neurological abnormalities (Weiss, Walker, and Wiernik, 1974). Methotrexate has been
implicated as a neurotoxic drug when given intrathecally or intravenously
(Bleyer, Drake, and Chabner, 1973; Meadows and Evans, 1976). There is
little doubt that the neurotoxic effect of methotrexate may be predicted
by excessive levels of the drug in the CSF (Bleyer, 1977). Meadows and
Evans (1976), evaluating 23 children surviving lymphoma or leukemia who
received high doses of intravenous methotrexate, found 4 who had severe
brain damage while 10 others had either major EEG changes or clinical abnormalities. Eight patients who had received primarily oral methotrexate
had no recognizable neurological abnormalities.

Overt radiation-induced injury to the CNS is not common when the
dose is limited to less than 2400 rads, but the late effects of higher doses
of radiation on the CNS can create significant morbidity. Radiation to the
spinal cord can induce permanent transverse myelitis resulting ultimately in
flaccid paralysis (Wara et al., 1975).

While many children are treated with cranial radiation and intrathecal
chemotherapy without developing measurable adverse neurological effects,
catastrophic neurological complications as well as mild transient neurological
symptoms are incentives to alter therapeutic regimens in an effort to decrease neurotoxicity. Currently the Pediatric Oncology Group is utilizing
a regimen of prophylactic central nervous system chemotherapy for acute
leukemia patients who have non-T-cell ALL, one that avoids cranial irradiation,

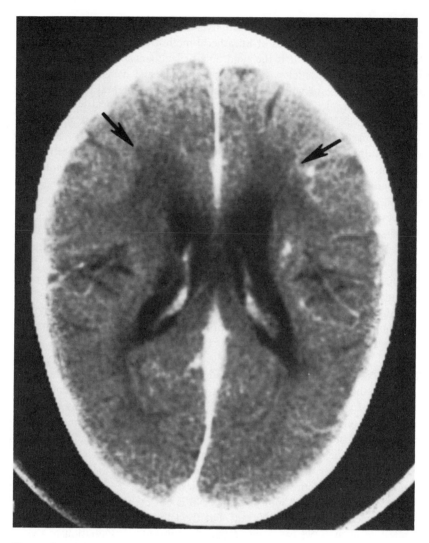

Figure 1 Brain CT scan of a child with severe disseminated leukoencephalopathy
following radiation therapy and intrathecal chemotherapy. Decreased density of
white matter in the centrum semiovale (arrows) is secondary to leukoencephalopathy.

in an attempt to minimize neurological sequelae. Concomitant use of cranial irradiation and intrathecal chemotherapy is limited to high-risk T-cell patients whose risk of CNS relapse exceeds 25% without the use of cranial irradiation.

B. Endocrine System

The developing tissues of the child's neuroendocrine system place the pediatric cancer patient particularly at risk for development of abnormalities of hypothalamic pituitary axis function. Panhypopituitarism, growth disturbance, infertility, delayed or absent pubertal development, and hypothyroidism are several of the adverse effects associated with cancer therapy in children (Shalet, 1983).

Hypothalamic Pituitary Axis

Short stature has been observed in children treated with cranial irradiation (Shalet et al., 1975) and found to be associated with growth hormone deficiency. Shalet and others suggested that the dose of irradiation to the hypothalamic pituitary axis could have direct effect on the growth hormone response to the insulin tolerance test (Shalet et al., 1976).

In one group of 18 children with ALL treated with 2400 rads of prophylactic cranial irradiation, 9 had deficiency of growth hormone (GH) (Oliff et al., 1979). Most patients receiving greater doses of radiation for nasopharyngeal carcinoma develop endocrine deficiencies (Samaan et al., 1975). Not all children with documented abnormal GH responses secondary to cranial irradiation have short stature (Shalet et al., 1979). The recognition of endocrine system abnormalities can be difficult since abnormal laboratory tests do not necessarily correlate with clinical endocrine deficiencies. Replacement therapy can be instituted to reverse the clinical manifestations of hormone deficiencies.

Thyroid

Radiation therapy for Hodgkin's disease often encompasses the thyroid gland. In children with this disease who have had prior lymphangiography there is a higher incidence of thyroid dysfunction secondary to radiation therapy. There is an apparent enhancement by the low levels of circulating iodine to account for this phenomena (Shalet, et al., 1977; Fuks et al., 1976). Others have reported relatively few clinically apparent thyroid complications following treatment of childhood Hodgkin's disease. One group noted elevated thyroid-stimulating hormone (TSH) levels in 21 of 37 children evaluated but only 1 who developed clinical hypothyroidism (Mauch et al., 1983). The use of a larynx block and a posterior spine block in addition to thyroid replacement may prevent this complication. Hormonal therapy is recommended for patients with elevated TSH levels following radiation to prevent overt hypothyroidism. Such supplemental therapy can also reduce the risk of radiation-induced thyroid carcinoma (Schimpft et al., 1980). It is imperative that periodic clinical and laboratory assessment of thyroid function be done to minimize the late effects of radiation to the thyroid gland.

C. Reproductive System

Gonadal irradiation may lead to hormonal dysfunction, reduced fertility, or sterility. The degree of gonadal dysfunction depends on the patient's age and sex and the specific program of radiotherapy employed (Lushbaugh and Casarett, 1976). Direct damage to the gonad by either radiation or chemotherapy is the leading cause of gonadal dysfunction in children (Shalet, 1982).

Alkylating agents such as cyclophosphamide and chlorambucil may damage germinal epithelium in children. Testicular histology is clearly altered in boys receiving combination chemotherapeutic agents for ALL. One group of investigators reported dramatic reductions in spermatogonia in this population of patients compared to age-matched controls (Lendon et al., 1978).

Infertility or hormonal dysfunction may occur as a result of gonadal injury from cancer therapy (Chapman, 1982). The adverse effect of radiation on the adult testis is well known (Rowley et al., 1974). The degree of long-term damage to the ovaries or testes in children as a consequence of a given dose of radiation is not fully appreciated. It has been demonstrated that boys with leukemia who had testicular relapse and were treated with testicular irradiation (2400 rads) had no testosterone response to human chorionic gonadotropin and were permanently sterile (Oakhill et al., 1980; Shalet, 1982). Rarely, surviving prepubescent boys who receive this therapy need hormone replacement to stimulate normal pubertal development. Prepubertal girls whose ovaries are exposed to 2000 rads may not develop secondary sexual characteristics. They may also have elevated levels of follicle-stimulating hormone and luteinizing hormone and may fail to menstruate. Other reports indicate that the ovaries of some patients can withstand high doses of radiation with little permanent diminution of ovarian function (D'Angio, 1980).

In a recent report, three children who received cranial irradiation before seven years of age had precocious puberty combined with growth retardation due to untreated growth hormone deficiency (Brauner, Czernichow, and Rappaport, 1984). The reported cases of asymptomatic increases in plasma luteinizing hormone and follicle-stimulating hormone in prepubertal children receiving cancer therapy were considered to be associated with primary ovarian injury due to chemotherapy or spinal irradiation. However, hypothalamic or pituitary dysfunction similar to that seen in true precocious puberty may also occur in children receiving cranial irradiation. Prevention of ovarian dysfunction in females receiving pelvic irradiation can be accomplished by oophoropexy (LeFloch, Donaldson, and Kaplan, 1976). Adolescent girls scheduled to have radiotherapy for Hodgkin's disease commonly have this procedure done at the time of staging laparotomy. The ovaries are moved out of the treatment field with wide lateral or medial displacement behind the uterus (Barber, 1982). Preservation of fertility and normal endocrine function are apparently more likely using wide lateral displacement. Pregnancies have occurred in women after oophoropexy and below the diaphragm irradiation (Thomas et al., 1976).

The adverse effects of drug therapy on the gonads of children are less well-defined. Prepubertal females appear to have less gonadal damage as a consequence of chemotherapy than do prepubertal males or adults in general (Stillman et al., 1981). Alkylating agents are most commonly associated with gonadal injury (Kumar et al., 1972). Spermatogenesis is reported to resume in many boys treated with single antineoplastic agents. But permanent azoospermia has also been reported following certain combinations of chemotherapeutic agents in men (Chapman et al., 1979). Azoospermia has also been documented in boys treated with combination chemotherapy for Hodgkin's disease (Whitehead et al., 1982). Alternative approaches to the treatment of childhood Hodgkin's disease have been formulated to reduce the risk of infertility. Early stage patients may require radiation therapy alone and still have a high probability of cure while avoiding the risk of sterility associated with combined chemotherapy and radiation therapy.

D. Skeletal System

Developing bone and cartilage are adversely affected by radiation. Epiphyseal injury results in arrested chondrogenesis, while metaphyseal injury results in deficient absorptive processes in calcified bone and cartilage. Diaphyseal injury results in altered periosteal activity with consequent disturbance in bone modeling (Parker and Berry, 1976). The degree of skeletal injury is related to the total dosage of radiation used, the area treated, and the age of the child.

Kyphoscoliosis is commonly seen in children who receive spinal irradiation in the treatment of Wilms' tumor or neuroblastoma (see Figure 2). In other diseases, such as leukemia and lymphoma, the entire length of the spine may be irradiated. These children will often develop growth retardation with reduction in their sitting height. This abnormality has been seen in children with Hodgkin's disease who have received mantle irradiation or those with posterior fossa tumors who have received neuraxis radiotherapy. The spine and other bones are most susceptible to radiation injury when the therapy is administered to children less than 6 years of age or during puberty, both periods of rapid bone growth. Greater damage occurs to bone at higher doses of radiation. The joint spaces of long bones can be widened and the development

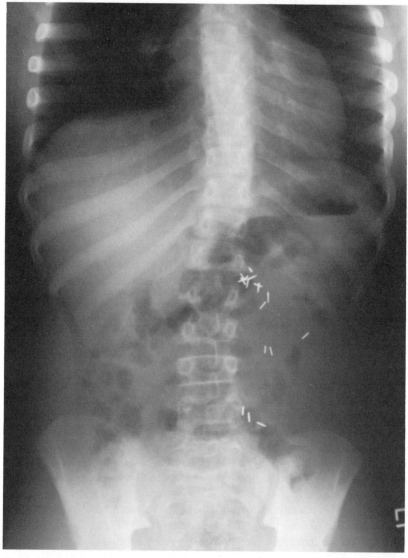

Figure 2 Scoliosis of the dorsolumbar spine of a 9-year-old girl with left Wilms'
tumor 7 years following surgery and radiation therapy.

of osteoporosis has been observed. When the radiation field includes the femoral neck, slipped capital femoral epiphysis can occur. Tooth buds may fail to develop and erupt when irradiated (Lines et al., 1979).

VII. PSYCHOLOGICAL ADAPTATION TO CHILDHOOD CANCER

A major coping task for children with cancer involves maintaining self-esteem. Physical changes caused by the disease and its therapy may cause a major change in the child's body image. The child may be unable to develop a satisfactory self-image due to the effects of the disease and its therapy. The illness creates a whole new world to which the child must adjust.

Symptoms of the disease may occur suddenly, or they may even be absent at the time of diagnosis. A previously well child may develop a slight fever and a few days later be diagnosed as having leukemia. The child, who may have never been ill before, is immediately placed on a treatment program to control the disease. The child's world has suddenly changed, and there is no choice but to comply with a treatment plan that the child does not understand. The therapy may cause nausea, vomiting, malaise, mouth sores, fever, weight gain or loss, or loss of hair. The child observes other children, siblings, and friends who have not experienced the effects of disease upon their body. The child does not understand what is happening, and to make matters worse, has no control over the situation. This profound change in the child's life causes great confusion.

The intensity of treatment causes fear of injury which, in turn, may intensify the perception of pain (Katz, Kellerman, and Siegal, 1980). Children, due to their great imagination, may consciously or unconsciously misinterpret the cause of their cancer and perceive it as a punishment or persecution. Younger children may tend to attribute the development of cancer to their parents. Older children and adolescents may think the cancer was caused by their own misdeeds or unacceptable feelings.

Apathy or withdrawal indicate depression in the child (Lazarus, 1976). Young children may display feeding, sleeping, and motor disturbances as depressive equivalents. Older children and adolescents may show mood changes. Adolescents may express their anxiety and depression by severe withdrawal or acting out.

Middle to late adolescents may develop problems with identity and self-image (Zeltzer, 1978). Adolescents are distressed with the thought of establishing long-term goals, career choice, sexual identity, morals, and their sense of self. Their confusion regarding who they are and what will happen to them may lead to impaired academic, job, or social functioning (Zeltzer, 1978). Hospitalization magnifies fears and adjustment difficulties (Spinetta

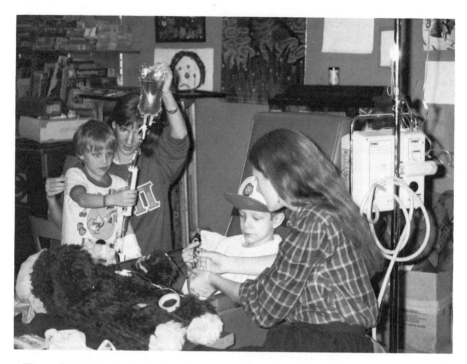

Figure 3 Highly trained play therapists observe and facilitate the child's play with medical gear. The therapist assesses the child's level of understanding, encourages the expression of feelings, and addresses misconceptions that may have developed.

and Deasy-Spinetta, 1981). Children less than 4 years of age may demonstrate separation anxiety with protest and despair in response to any separation from their parents. Fears regarding bodily injury in children may result in attacks upon hospital personnel. Surgery, when necessary, not only serves as a focus for fears of mutilation, but also brings about fears of loss of control from anesthesia, a common anxiety in early adolescents.

Poor adaptation to cancer can result in a wide spectrum of personality disturbances from an overdependent, overanxious, passive, withdrawn, and overprotected child, to an overindependent, aggressive, risk-taking child who utilizes excessive denial (Zeltzer, Ellenberg, and Rigler, 1980). Children and adolescents adapting poorly to their illness or treatment may require psychiatric evaluation and intervention. Diagnostically, it is important to determine whether the disturbance is in response to the stress of cancer and is therefore probably transient, or represents an exacerbation of more fundamental psychological difficulties.

Successful adaptation to cancer is dependent upon the child's coping techniques and upon the quality of the parent-child relationship. Adaptation is enhanced by a family that masters its fear and guilt, overcomes the tendency to overprotect, and learns to accept the child's limitations through grief and mourning (Lazarus, 1976).

Successful intervention requires a multidisciplinary team approach to formulate an understanding of the child's behavioral responses and develop treatment approaches. A cohesive team is also important to help families of terminally ill children work through the process of loss and mourning. Although children cannot fully conceptualize the meaning of death until early adolescence, they are able to deal with the emotional aspects of loss and death at their own level of development.

Trauma of hospitalization and treatment can be minimized by careful preparation of the family and child. Separation anxieties in infants and preschoolers can be avoided by parental rooming-in. Education about the cancer and treatment procedures is crucial in alleviating anxiety-provoking misunderstandings and uncertainties. Special play opportunities can help children understand their illness and upcoming procedures as well as encourage them to play out and actively master their anxieties (see Figure 3). Adolescents often benefit from patient groups. Such groups not only offer support, but can provide positive models for identification (peers, older patients) and help strengthen their adolescent self-image. Parent therapy helps the parents work through their guilt and misunderstandings. Active participation in treatment and hospital ward activities also minimizes threatening passivity and regression. When indicated, supportive psychotherapy can help promote successful coping mechanisms and facilitate adaptive functioning.

REFERENCES

Barber, H. R. K. (1982). The effect of cancer and its therapy upon fertility, *Int. J. Fertil.*, *26*(4):250-259.

Bleyer, W. A. (1977). Clinical pharmacology of intrathecal methotrexate. II: An improved dosage regimen derived from age-related pharmacokinetics, *Cancer Treat. Rep.*, *61*:1419-1425.

Bleyer, W. A., Drake, J. C., and Chabner, B. A. (1973). Neurotoxicity and elevated cerebrospinal-fluid methotrexate concentration in meningeal leukemia, *New Engl. J. Med.*, *289*:770-773.

Brauner, R., Czernichow, P., and Rappaport, R. (1984). Precocious puberty after hypothalamic and pituitary irradiation in young children (letter), *New Engl. J. Med.*, *311*:920.

Chapman, R. M. (1982). Effect of cytotoxic therapy on sexuality and gonadal function, *Semin. Oncol.*, *9*:84-94.

Chapman, R. M., Sutcliffe, S. B., Rees, L. H., Edwards, C. R. W., and Malpas, J. S. (1979). Cyclical combination chemotherapy and gonadal function, *Lancet, 1*:285-289.

D'Angio, G. J. (1980). Late sequelae after cure of childhood cancer. *Hospital Practice, 15*:109-121.

Flament-Durand, J., Ketelbant-Balasse, P., Maurus, R., Regnier, R., and Spehl, M. (1975). Intracerebral calcifications appearing during the course of acute lymphocytic leukemia treated with methotrexate and x-rays, *Cancer, 35*:319-325.

Freeman, J. E., Johnston, P. G. B., and Voke, J. M. (1973). Somnolence after prophylactic cranial irradiation in children with acute lymphoblastic leukaemia, *Brit. Med. J., 4*:523-525.

Fuks, Z., Glatstein, E., Marsa, G. W., Bagshaw, M. A., and Kaplan, H. S. (1976). Long-term effects of external radiation on the pituitary and the thyroid glands, *Cancer, 37*:1152-1161.

Griffin, T. W., Rasey, J. S., and Bleyer, W. S. (1977). The effect of photon irradiation on blood-brain barrier permeability to methotrexate in mice, *Cancer, 40*:1109-1111.

Horwitz, E. T. (1979). Of love and laetrile: Medical decision making in a child's best interests, *Am. J. Law Med., 5*(3):271-294.

Hughes, J. G. (1976). The emotional impact of chronic disease, *Am. J. Dis. Child., 130*:1199.

Kaplan, D. M. (1973). Family mediation of stress, *Soc. Work, 18*:60.

Katz, E. R., Kellerman, J., and Siegal, S. E. (1980). Behavioral distress in children with cancer undergoing medical procedures: Developmental considerations, *J. Consult. Clin. Psychol. 48*(3):356-365.

Krouse, H. J., and Krouse, J. H. (1982). Cancer as crises: The critical elements of adjustment, *Nurs. Res., 31*(2):96.

Kumar, R., Biggart, J. D., McEvoy, J., and McGeown, M. G. (1972). Cyclophosphamide and reproductive function, *Lancet, 1*:1212-1214.

Lazarus, R. S. (1976). *Patterns of Adjustment,* McGraw-Hill, New York.

LeFloch, O., Donaldson, S. S., and Kaplan, H. S. (1976). Pregnancy following oophoropexy and total nodal irradiation in women with Hodgkin's disease, *Cancer, 38*:2263-2268.

Lendon, M., Hann, I. M., Palmer, M. K., Shalet, S. M., and Morris-Jones, P. H. (1978). Testicular histology after combination chemotherapy in childhood for acute lymphocytic leukaemia, *Lancet, 2*:439-441.

Lines, L. G., Hazra, T. A., Howells, R., and Shipman, B. (1979). Altered growth and development of lower teeth in children receiving mantle therapy, *Radiology, 132*:447-449.

Lushbaugh, C. C., and Casarett, G. W. (1976). The effects of gonadal irradiation in clinical radiation therapy: A review, *Cancer, 37*:1111-1120.

Mauch, P. M., Weinstein, H., Botnick, L., Belli, J., and Cassady, J. R. (1983). An evaluation of long-term survival and treatment complications in children with Hodgkin's disease, *Cancer, 51*:925-932.

Meadows, A. T., and Evans, A. E. (1976). Effects of chemotherapy on the central nervous system: A study of parenteral methotrexate in long-term survivors of leukemia and lymphoma in childhood, *Cancer, 37*:1079-1085.

Meadows, A. T., Gordon, J., Massari, D. J., Littman, P., Fergusson, J., and Moss, K. (1981). Declines in IQ scores and cognitive dysfunctions in children with acute lymphocytic leukaemia treated with cranial irradiation, *Lancet, 2*:1015-1018.

Monaco, G. P. (1983). Informed consents: Does the consent process reflect the realities of current treatment, procedures, and side effects?, *The Am. J. Pediatr. Hematol./Oncol., 5*:401-407.

Moss, H. A., Nannis, E. D., and Poplack, D. G. (1981). The effects of prophylactic treatment of the central nervous system on the intellectual functioning of children with acute lymphocytic leukemia, *Am. J. Med., 71*:47-52.

Nitschke, R., Humphrey, G. B., Sexauer, C. L., Catron, B., Wunder, S., and Jay, S. (1982). Therapeutic choices made by patients with end-stage cancer, *J. Pediatr., 101*:471-476.

Oakhill, A., Mainwaring, D., Hill, F. G. H., Gornall, P., Cudmore, R. E., Banks, A. J., Brock, J. E. S., Martin, J., and Mann, J. R. (1980). Management of leukaemic infiltration of the testis, *Arch. Dis. Child., 55*:564-566.

Oliff, A., Bode, U., Bercu, B., DiChiro, G., Graves, V., and Poplack, D. G. (1979). Hypothalamic pituitary dysfunction following CNS prophylaxis in ALL: Correlation with CT scan abnormalities, *Med. Pediatr. Oncol., 7*: 141-151.

Parker, R. G., and Berry, H. C. (1976). Late effects of therapeutic irradiation on the skeleton and bone marrow, *Cancer, 37*:1162-1171.

Penman, D. T., Holland, J. C., Bahna, G. F., Morrow, G., Schmale, A. H., Derogatis, L. R., Carnrike, C. L., Jr., and Cherry, R. (1984). Informed consent for investigational chemotherapy: Patients' and physicians' perceptions, *J. Clin. Oncol., 2(7)*:849-855.

Peylan-Ramu, N., Poplack, D. G., Pizzo, P. A., Adornato, B. T., and DiChiro, G. (1978). Abnormal CT scans of the brian in asymptomatic children with acute lymphocytic leukemia after prophylactic treatment of the central nervous system with irradiation and intrathecal chemotherapy, *New Engl. J. Med., 298*:815-818.

Rowley, M. J., Leach, D. R., Warner, G. A., and Heller, C. G. (1974). Effect of graded doses of ionizing radiation on the human testis, *Radiat. Res., 59*: 665-678.

Rubinstein, L. J., Herman, M. M., Long, T. F., and Wilbur, J. R. (1975). Disseminated necrotizing leukoencephalopathy: A complication of treated central nervous system leukemia and lymphoma, *Cancer, 35*:291-305.

Samaan, N. A., Bakdash, M. D., Caderao, J. B., Cangir, A., Jesse, R. H., and Ballantyne, A. J. (1975). Hypopituitarism after external irradiation—evidence for both hypothalamic and pituitary origin, *Ann. Intern. Med., 83*:771-777.

Schimpff, S. C. Diggs, C. H., Wiswell, J. G., Salvatore, P. C., and Wiernik, P. H. (1980). Radiation-related thyroid dysfunction: Implications for the treatment of Hodgkin's disease, *Ann. Intern. Med., 92*:91-98.

Schuster, C. S., and Ashburn, S. S. (1980). *The Process of Human Development*, Little, Brown & Co., Boston.

Shalet, S. M. (1982). Abnormalities of growth and gonadal function in children treated for malignant disease: A review, *J. R. Soc. Med., 75*:641-647.

Shalet, S. M. (1983). Disorders of the endocrine system due to radiation and cytotoxic chemotherapy, *Clin. Endocrinol., 18*:637-659.

Shalet, S. M., Beardwell, C. G., Jones, M., and Pearson, D. (1975). Pituitary function after treatment of intracranial tumours in children, *Lancet, 2*:104-107.

Shalet, S. M., Beardwell, C. G., Pearson, D., and Morris-Jones, P. (1976). The effect of varying doses of cerebral irradiation on growth hormone production in childhood, *Clin. Endocrinol., 5*:287-290.

Shalet, S. M., Price, D. A., Beardwell, C. G., Morris-Jones, P. H., and Pearson, D. (1979). Normal growth despite abnormalities of growth hormone secretion in children treated for acute leukemia, *J. Pediatr., 94*:719-722.

Shalet, S. M., Rosenstock, J. D., Beardwell, C. G., Pearson, D., and Morris-Jones, P. H. (1977). Thyroid dysfunction following external irradiation to the neck for Hodgkin's disease in childhood, *Clin. Radiol., 28*:511-515.

Shumway, C., Grossman, L. S., and Sarles, R. M. (1983). Therapeutic choices by children with cancer, *J. Pediatr., 103*:168.

Spinetta, J. J., and Deasy-Spinetta, P. (1981). *Living with Childhood Cancer*, C. V. Mosby, St. Louis.

Stanwyck, D. J. (1983). Self-esteem through the lifespan, *Fam. Community Health, 6(2)*:11-28.

Stillman, R. J., Schinfeld, J. S., Schiff, I., Gelber, R. D., Greenberger, J., Larson, M., Jaffe, N., and Li , F. P. (1981). Ovarian failure in long-term survivors of childhood malignancy, *Am. J. Obstet. Gynecol., 139*:62-66.

Thomas, P. R. M., Winstanly, D., Peckhan, M. J., Austin, D. E., Murray, M. A. F., and Jacobs, H. S. (1976). Reproductive and endocrine function in patients with Hodgkin's disease: Effects of oophoropexy and irradiation, *Brit. J. Cancer, 33*:226-231.

Wara, W. M., Phillips, T. L., Sheline G. E., and Schwade, J. G. (1975). Radiation tolerance of the spinal cord, *Cancer, 35*:1558-1562.

Weiss, H., Walker, M., and Wiernik, P. (1974). Neurotoxicity of commonly used antineoplastic agents. I, *New Engl. J. Med., 291*:127-133.

Whitehead, E., Shalet, S. M., Morris-Jones, P. H., and Deakin, D. P. (1982). Gonadal function after combination chemotherapy for Hodgkin's disease in childhood, *Arch. Dis. Child., 57*:287-291.

Zeltzer, L. (1978). Chronic illness in the adolescent, *Topics in Adolescent Medicine* (I. R. Shenker, ed.), Stratton Intercontinental Medical Book Corp., New York, pp. 226-253.

Zeltzer, L., Ellenberg, L., and Rigler, D. (1980). Psychologic effects of illness in adolescence. II. Impact of illness in adolescents—crucial issues and coping styles, *J. Pediatr., 97*:132-138.

10

Comprehensive Cancer Care: Special Problems of the Elderly

Harvey J. Cohen
Duke University Medical Center and Veterans Administration Medical Center, Durham, North Carolina

Louis C. DeMaria
Duke University Medical Center, Durham, North Carolina

I. INTRODUCTION

The management of biomedical problems of elderly patients is readily recognized as a complex task. The treatment, rehabilitation, and follow-up care for geriatric stroke victims, e.g., involves a multitude of adjustments on the part of the practitioner. Changing physiology and organ system function requires attention. Supportive services for rehabilitation and for home care need to be planned, coordinated, and implemented. However, most of these considerations deal with the individual's organized hierarchy and biopsychosocial profile (Engel, 1980). When cancer is anticipated as a diagnosis, the new implication is that a process or intervention will be brought into the patient's biopsychosocial sphere from sources external to the patient, which carries with it a new scope of effects and countereffects. These interventions and their impact on elderly cancer patients will be discussed in terms of surgery, radiation therapy, hormonal therapy, and chemotherapy. Reciprocal effects between the patient as the host and the intervention modality will be noted where appropriate or where the impact is significant for these elderly patients.

The elderly population in the United States (approximately 11% of the total) will experience over one-half of all cancers (Butler, 1979). The probability of developing cancer within 5 years, which is 1 in 700 at age 25, increases to 1 in 14 by age 65 (Lancet, 1976). There are clearly rising age-specific incidence rates and mortality rates, when adjusted for decreasing population size (Cohen et al., 1983), supporting the fact that cancer is the second leading cause of death in those over 65 (Libow and Sherman, 1981). These age-specific mortality rates for elderly patients rise at a rate that is actually higher than the rate of increase of cancer incidence. This segment of the population is subjected to the cumulative effect of a lifetime of carcinogenic influences, and immune senescence (Weksler, 1981).

The elderly patient with cancer presents a special set of needs that require the clinician's attention when one treats the cancer and manages the elderly host. The elderly host has a number of aging organ systems that require functional assessment. This assessment further assists the clinician in anticipating toxicity and responses to therapy while expanding the knowledge of selection criteria for elderly patients and tumor susceptibility to particular kinds of treatment. Thus, the appropriate treatment of elderly cancer patients contributes a challenge that has been described as the management of two basic elements at the cellular level: the cancer cell population and the complex arrangement of the aging cell population (Holland, 1981). The further integration of declining organ function with the psychosocial elements of the person and one's support system defines the functional status of the elderly patient. This can become a potential predictor of outcome (Becker and Cohen, 1984).

A. Cellular Elements of Aging

As mentioned above, the elderly patient with cancer exhibits a multifaceted arrangement of aging cell populations which comprises the aging host. This arrangement of cells as they are organized into physiological systems defines part of the challenge that is inherent in the care of these patients. The study of cellular aging provides clues not only for evaluation and alteration of these cells, but also demonstrates a curious overlap with many characteristics of neoplastic cell lines. Although aging is a universal process, the morphological and physiological manifestations of this process vary to such a degree that a definition by any one process or theory is virtually impossible. All species demonstrate a cumulative effect of biological changes that result in a decreasing ability to function in and adapt to the environment and a greater increase in mortality with advancing age (Rockstein, Chesky, and Sussman, 1977). Physical and biological factors in the environment, in conjunction with one's genetically determined longevity, ultimately dictate the life span of a given organism. Gerontological studies, carefully planned to investigate the effect of heredity and environment on aging, have utilized inbred animals that have short life spans in order to compare the cellular effects occurring not only in aging but also in neoplastic processes. A remarkable number of similarities have been pointed out in the literature for aging and neoplastic cellular processes, regarding increasing prevalence rates, decrease by antioxidants, effects of fasting, effects of unsaturated fats in the diet, altered enzyme responses, effect of hormonal status, change in DNA repair, altered mRNA template stability, and decreased capacity for drug metabolism (Pitot, 1977). One must recognize that differences between the processes of aging and neoplasia at the cellular level define the true characters of these cell lines: finite versus immortal life span, stable versus unstable karyotypes, and the presence of inactive enzyme molecules versus no evidence of altered protein molecules in aged versus neoplastic cells, respectively.

This comparative analysis of aging and neoplastic cells may be helpful in understanding the current model of cellular aging. This model is based on the observation that normal human fibroblasts have a limited doubling potential in cell culture (Hayflick and Moorhead, 1961). Whether or not this phenomenon is related to biological aging is debatable because experimental designs cannot exclude other biological phenomenon leaving age as an association. In addition, biological phenomena are not consistently acknowledged to be age associated. Certainly, in vitro events cannot be directly extrapolated to in vivo events (Hayflick, 1977). Nevertheless, Hayflick's model has generated a new series of approaches to cellular aging by studying the life cycle of cells maintained in cell culture.

Medical models for premature aging in children (progeria) and young adults (Werner's syndrome) are currently being studied utilizing fibroblasts from patients with these disorders. The population doubling potential of these cells in culture seems to be reduced uniformly. However, the significance of these syndromes in relation to aging is uncertain since patients with other disorders, including diabetes mellitus, also demonstrate fibroblasts with reduced population doubling potential (Hayflick, 1977).

B. The Aging Host and the Organization of Systems

The management of clinical problems for elderly patients with cancer requires the acknowledgment that these patients are extremely complex in their description and heterogeneous by their nature. A model is proposed (Figure 1) which will assist the clinician in conceptualizing this complex situation by modifying a previously described framework (Becker and Cohen, 1984). The basis for this model is Engel's description of a hierarchy of organization within the individual's personal domain (Engel, 1980). This comprehensive geriatric model (CGM) (Figure 1) graphically presents a number of concepts that are critical to the care of the elderly: functional reserve status, effects of aging organ systems, and the interrelationships between biological function and one's psychological and social performance.

The aging host is comprised of an ascending hierarchy of complex systems all of which are influenced by the cancer cell mass and its respective treatment. The hosts's hierarchy begins at the cellular level, ascends to the system of the

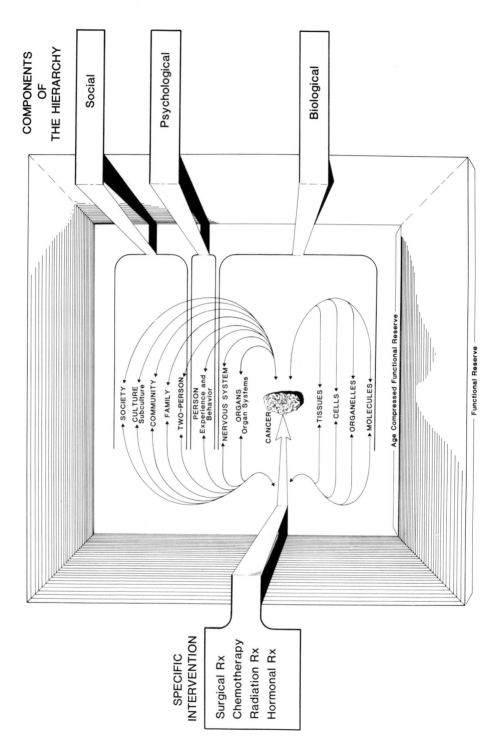

COMPONENTS
OF
THE HIERARCHY

Social

Psychological

Biological

SOCIETY
CULTURE
Subculture
COMMUNITY
FAMILY
TWO-PERSON
PERSON
Experience and
Behavior
NERVOUS SYSTEM
ORGANS
Organ Systems
CANCER
TISSUES
CELLS
ORGANELLES
MOLECULES

Age Compressed Functional Reserve

Functional Reserve

SPECIFIC
INTERVENTION

Surgical Rx
Chemotherapy
Radiation Rx
Hormonal Rx

Figure 1 The comprehensive geriatric model (CGM) is presented as a reminder of the many competing forces involved in the treatment of elderly patients; in this case, the interventions for cancer treatment are described. The patient exists in a setting that is composed of a hierarchy of levels beginning with the molecular and cellular, and continuing through to complex, interpersonal, social, and cultural influences. These levels can be subdivided into the biomedical, psychological, and social components shown on the right, as proposed by Engel (1980). In the aged patient, the functional reserve for the variety of the components involved may be diminished as shown by the compressed frame of the model. A disease, i.e., cancer, may develop within this host, which may affect any or all of the aging organ systems or components, or in turn be affected by them. Likewise, the treatments for the disease (as shown in the left panel) can affect or be affected by any of these components. This model can provide an organized conceptualization that the health care provider can utilize when considering the variety of potential interactions that may be demonstrated in the aging cancer patient.

person, i.e., experience and behavior, and culminates in the social systems of family and community. A brief description of the effects of aging upon this CGM, especially at the organ system level, will assist in the comprehension of the problems manifested at the clinical level.

A central theme needs to be kept in mind when one is confronted with management issues in elderly cancer patients. This theme acknowledges the decrease in the homeostatic reserves that exist in all elderly patients, as well as the effect of co-morbid diseases that predate or coexist with cancer cell populations. One way to measure an effect on the host has been to characterize the functional status of the patient—an integration of biomedical and psychosocial parameters (Becker and Cohen, 1984). Previously, the Karnofsky scale was developed to assess functional levels, and assist in medical decision making. Its value in the integration of biomedical and psychosocial status, and its utilization in the measurement of outcome by oncologists need to be reaffirmed (Schag, Heinrich, and Ganz, 1984). The inclusion criteria for treatment protocols involving elderly cancer patients should not use chronological age alone because patients who develop cancer in the seventh, eighth or ninth decades are in effect "survivors" and demonstrate a substantial life expectancy. The average life expectancy for a 70-year-old man is 11 years and for a 70-year-old woman it is 15 years (American Association of Retired Persons, 1984). At age 85, the figure is 5.3 years for men and 7 years for women. The measure of functional status is a tool that can provide highly valuable information regarding inclusion criteria for treatment protocols, clinical course assessment, and measurement of outcome. A discussion of these functional status measures is certainly beyond the scope of this discussion. Nevertheless, when these appraisals are defined, tested, or evaluated, they could become the standards for future use in decisions to admit and assignments of level of care within institutional settings.

C. Functional Status as a Measure of Co-Morbid Disease

Before selective problems in cancer care for the elderly can be addressed, the concept of functional assessment requires explanation and discussion. The comprehensive geriatric model defines the hierarchial organization of the host and his/her environment, the effects of aging on vital organ systems, and a certain level of functional status. Before interventions with modalities outside of the hierararchical organization can be described, some appraisal of the summation effects of aging and co-morbid disease is required. Chronological age alone does not give a clear perspective of the host's ability to withstand certain treatment modalities. There is no simple practical way to measure physiological age at the tissue level. In order to define "margins of safety" for selected organ systems (Kark and Wardle, 1980), newer models and

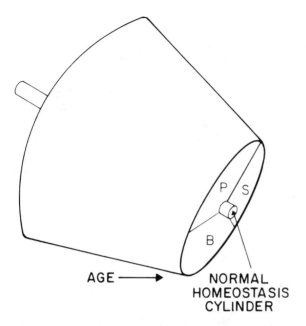

AGE ⟶   NORMAL
HOMEOSTASIS
CYLINDER

Figure 2   The concept of diminishing functional reserve with increasing age is described by this narrowing life cycle cylinder (Becker and Cohen, 1984). The central core of homeostasis is maintained throughout life despite these decreasing reserves. The maintenance of the physical and instrumental activities of daily living exemplify a basic level of functioning that is represented by the central homeostasis core. A cross-sectional view of the cylinder at a specific point in time reveals the integration of psychological (P), social (S), and biomedical (B) components of the patient's overall functional reserve. Acute stresses, such as cancer and its therapeutic interventions, require compensations in one or all of these components in order for the system to reestablish homeostasis in the face of decreasing functional reserve.

abstractions are being developed which are able to conceptualize the issues involved (Wiliams, 1984; Becker, 1984). As demonstrated in Figure 2, the homeostatic core of functional status, including instrumental and physical activities of daily living (ADLs), are maintained as the area of reserve diminishes with age. ADLs that are instrumental include such activities as using a telephone, traveling, shopping, preparing meals, performing housework, taking one's medicine, or managing money. ADLs that are physical or basic include such activities as bathing, dressing, grooming, toileting, transferring, walking, eating, and maintaining continence (Becker and Cohen, 1984). The maintenance of this functional reserve requires the management of co-morbid disease, homeostatic compensation of the host, and supportive services from family and environment. Williams (1984) describes this concept in a two-dimensional graph that also acknowledges the rate of atrophy when the system is never stressed, a disuse syndrome.

Biomedical therapy and social support systems help to restore the homeostatic core of functional status in cancer patients regardless of age. However, the psychosocial supports for a middle-aged woman may be taken for granted because of the assistance of spouse, family, and friends. The elderly female has unique needs that are compromised by fixed income, loss of social status, loneliness through widowhood, and loss of self-esteem through chronic dysphoria.

D. Aging Changes in Selected Organ Systems

The measure of physiological age at the tissue level is a critical issue to consider when patients, e.g., are enrolled in surgical treatment programs or chemotherapy protocols. Complication rates, drug side effects, and other consequences of cancer treatment impact greatly on exclusionary guidelines. The age of the patient is certainly a basic issue to be contemplated. However, what determines the significance of a given age vis-a-vis a specific intervention? Physiological reserve of selected organ systems, i.e., the physiological "age" of those systems characterize the significant parameters to consider.

Cardiovascular System

Circulatory function is a crucial issue when surgery is contemplated for an elderly patient. The ability of a given individual to withstand the stresses of general anesthesia and an operative procedure determines the exclusionary guidelines for these patients.

The cardiovascular system by virtue of its rich supply of connective tissue demonstrates a number of effects based on the aging of this connective tissue. These effects induce loss of elasticity and subsequent stiffening (Kohn, 1977). On the other hand, an intrinsic, degenerative process within individual cellular elements of the myocardium or vascular system cannot be conclusively ruled out. Functionally, decreases are recognized in heart rate as a response to stress, in pump efficiency of the heart itself, velocity of contraction and relaxation of heart muscle, and in the rate of cardiac hypertrophy (Kohn, 1977). Peripheral vascular resistance increases and organ perfusion decreases. Collagen accumulates focally within the heart and in the intima and media of arteries. The aorta loses its elasticity and increases in mean circumference (Caird and Dall, 1980). This results in an increase in pulse pressure and systolic pressure with little effect on diastolic pressure. These changes are further minimized by the dilatation of the aorta, which increases the size of the compression chamber into which the stroke volume is ejected. Cardiac assessment is vitally important when the clinician considers certain cardiotoxic chemotherapeutic agents, e.g., Adriamycin. Although these effects will be discussed in detail later, it should be noted that the effects of aging need to be separated from other causes of cardiac dysfunction before drug effects can be evaluated. Cardiac output decreases with age as a result of a fall in stroke volume, with pulse rate remaining unchanged. The usual risk factors for ischemic heart disease (smoking, obesity, hypercholesterolemia, type A personality) demonstrate a decreased effect on mortality in elderly patients (Rodstein, 1981). Systolic and diastolic hypertension and electrocardiographical evidence of left ventricular hypertrophy and strain (in the absence of hypertension) still remain as significant risk factors for these patients.

Pulmonary System

Co-morbid disease may produce changes in the lungs that are indistinguishable from the effects of aging. These changes influence the net, functional capacity manifested by an elderly cancer patient. In addition to pulmonary complications in intraoperative and postoperative care, chemotherapeutic agents (e.g., bleomycin) produce fibrotic changes in the lung which may limit the inclusion of elderly patients in treatment protocols. Studies designed to investigate aging changes in the lung contain a high degree of sampling bias, thus limiting the amount of usable data for functional alterations at the organ system level). When studied in male populations, aging exerts the following changes in lung volumes: total lung capacity, inspiratory capacity and functional residual capacity remain *constant*; residual volume *increases*; and vital capacity and expiratory reserve volume *decrease* (Boren, Kory, and Syner, 1966).

Although etiological factors have yet to be elucidated for the decrease in flow rates in older patients, a uniform fall of 20-30% is observed with aging in maximum voluntary ventilation, maximal expiratory flow rate, maximum mid-expiratory flow rate, and forced expiratory volume at 1 second (Klocke, 1977). A number of investigators have described the progressive increase in alveolar-arterial oxygen difference with age. Shunting, diffusion impairment, and mismatch of alveolar ventilation and pulmonary blood flow are possible explanations for this phenomenon (Klocke, 1977).

Renal System

Decreases in creatinine clearance and renal blood flow occur with increasing age: it has been established that a decline of 46% occurs in these parameters between the ages of 20 and 90 years (Davies and Shock, 1950). Declining renal parameters are relevant to these patients when they are being considered for methotrexate or cisplatin chemotherapy. Another area of geriatric cancer care that requires attention to declining renal function is with the administration of psychotropic medication or antiemetic therapy. Impairment of renal function is reflected in only slight elevation of the blood urea nitrogen in elderly

patients. Raised levels of serum creatinine occur only when clearance levels
are very low because of the reduced creatinine production from a reduced
muscle mass (Sourander, 1980).

Nervous System

Any discussion of aging and cancer treatment must include mention of the
effects of declining mental capacity and the increasing prevalence of
Alzheimer's disease with advancing age. As will be discussed later, patient
compliance, patient decision making, and ethical dilemmas involving the care
of these cancer patients present crucial decisions for clinicians and members
of the extended family.

Within the central nervous system the brain itself atrophies, most markedly
in the frontal halves of the cerebral hemispheres, with coincidental shrinkage
of gyri and widening of sulci. This is commonly seen in patients more than
60-70 years of age with less effect on the brain stem, the cerebellum, or
posterior halves of the cerebral hemispheres (Dayan, 1980). These changes
are found in the brains of "normal," healthy, old people; there is much
debate in gerontological circles about causes, severity, and distribution. Internal CNS changes that correlate with functional changes in a variable way
include basal ganglia and ventricular abnormalities as well as vascular ac-
cumulations of amyloid and fibrosis with hyalinization of the media of intracerebral arteries and arterioles (Baker, 1937). Neurofibrillary tangles, senile
plaques, and granulovacuolar degeneration are recognized as correlates of
presenile and senile dementia of the Alzheimer's type, providing pathologists
with some cellular basis for the changes in cognitive function. The unique
protein within these pathological changes has been likened to the monomers
found in amyloid disease (Prusiner, 1984) but true amyloid is not found in
neurofibrillary tangles (Dayan, 1980). Peripheral and autonomic nerves
demonstrate some degenerative features with increasing age and certainly are
unrelated to other specific causes of neuropathy (Ochoa and Mair, 1969). These
degenerative changes may be important to recognize when treatment includes
cisplatin or vincristine therapy or when radiation therapy is administered to
areas containing large peripheral nerves. These therapeutic interventions
and their effects will be discussed later in the chapter.

Gastrointestinal System

Clinicians who care for elderly patients are well aware of the importance of
many aspects of bowel function including diverticular disease of the colon,
constipation, medication effects on defecation and nutritional deficiencies.
Radiation therapy, control of pain and nausea/vomiting, and nutritional support for postoperative patients require the consideration of aging effects within

this organ system. "Presbyesophagus" is the term used to describe the changes in peristaltic function, increased presence of tertiary contractions, delay in gastric emptying, and dilatation of the esophagus with increasing age (Zboralske, Amberg, and Soergel, 1964). Achlorhydria and decreases in response to stimulation by histamine characterize gastric changes with increasing age (Leeming and Dymock, 1980). It has been conclusively shown that normal elderly patients demonstrate diminished nutrient absorption (Bhanthumnavin and Schuster, 1977). Reduced intake and poor preparation of food may play significant roles in elderly patients who have decreased nutritional status and failure to thrive. However, there have been reports of occult malabsorption occurring in selected groups of frail elderly people, based on bacterial overgrowth in the small intestine (Roberts, 1977; McEvoy, 1983). Broad spectrum oral antibiotic therapy has been helpful in promoting weight gain in some of these patients.

Disturbances in colonic function are quite common in the elderly due to decreased muscle tone and motor function, decreased fluid intake, decreased bulk in the diet, blunting of the defecation reflex, and medications (Manousos, Truelove, and Lumsden, 1967). Conflicting reports exist in the literature concerning changes in liver weight and histology with increasing age. Inducible microsomal enzymes concerned with oxidation and reduction mechanisms (especially the cytochrome P-450 system) are diminished in function with advancing age.

Hematological System

Limited information is available regarding the effects of aging on bone marrow function. Although it has been recognized that anemia increases with age, especially in men, normal features of aging do not seem to include anemia (Lipschitz et al., 1984). Since many variables may affect hematopoiesis including diet, environment, and co-morbid disease, carefully selected groups of aged subjects can now be studied effectively with regard to selected components of their hematopoietic system using long-term bone marrow culture techniques (Lipschitz, McGinnis, and Udupa, 1983).

The dosage of chemotherapy is clearly limited by bone marrow reserve. Healthy, aging patients, when subject to combination chemotherapy may demonstrate a variety of bone marrow responses based on individual susceptibility and physiological reserve. As will be discussed, the assessment of reserve potentials rather than chronological age is more important in the pretreatment evaluation of these patients: however, it is difficult to quantitate this determination.

The proliferative capacity of aged bone marrow cells seems to be limited in a finite manner when studied in bone marrow culture (Mauch et al., 1982).

This finite replication capacity behaves in a manner that is similar to Hayflick's model of limited population doublings in human fibroblast cultures in vitro. However, the hematopoietic stem cell that is selected for repopulation during aging may be recruited from a hierarchy of heterogeneous stem cells based on their previous proliferative history (Botnick et al., 1982).

Mild unexplained anemia was studied in a select group of otherwise healthy elderly patients in an attempt to define the effect of aging on hematopoiesis (Lipschitz et al., 1984). These patients demonstrated fewer bone marrow erythroid precursors than young or elderly controls. An overall reduction in hematopoiesis also was present. This was exhibited by lower peripheral leukocyte, neutrophil, and platelet counts, and a lowered number of myeloid precursors. These elderly patients with mild, unexplained anemia may be demonstrating defects in progenitor cell proliferation or basic cellular abnormalities (Lipschitz et al., 1984). This mild anemia could be a marker to identify at risk hematopoietic systems with limited reserve potentials.

Immune System

Normal immune function declines with age with selective falls in T-cell function, humoral immune responses, and the gradual emergence of disorders involving autoimmune dysfunction, immune complex disease, and cancer. Elderly patients may be more susceptible to bacterial and viral infection after receiving cancer therapy. Mycobacterial infections clearly reactivate in aged, frail, nursing home patients without the added stress of chemotherapy. These declining immune responses can be related to the evolution of the thymus and the shift in balance between idiotypic and autoantiidiotypic antibody production. This is suggested by the observation that levels of natural antibody and antibody to foreign determinants following immunization are reduced in old animals, whereas total immunoglobulin concentration are little affected by age (Weksler, 1982). The contribution of autoantibodies and circulating immune complexes to the pathological changes in aging tissues and organs is less certain.

Thymus-dependent lymphocyte (T cell) function is altered with aging. There is also evidence of increased suppressor cell activity in the peripheral blood lymphocyte pool of aged individuals (Phair, 1983). A number of thymic "hormones" and thymic factors are being investigated to determine the effect of these factors on thymus involution. Other hormone-like substances that modulate immune responsiveness include the interleukins and other lymphokines. Macrophage-derived interleukin-1 promotes the production of interleukin-2 by T cells. This lymphokine (interleukin-2), which augments lymphocyte responses to antigens and promotes T-cell proliferation, seems to be produced in lower amounts in cell cultures of aged lymphocytes compared to those of younger individuals (Thoman and Weigle, 1982). Supplementation of aging animal spleen cells with this lymphokine, interleukin-2, in fact restores the normal high levels of responsiveness of these cells to antigenic stimulation (Thoman and Weigle, 1983).

There is no indication that aging is associated with significant granulo-cytopenia. The milieu of humoral factors within which the polymorphonuclear leukocyte functions can enhance or inhibit this cell's ability to respond to infection. Some of these humoral factors include antiglobulins that inhibit phagocytosis in vitro, and complement and various inhibitors of chemotaxis found in patients with neoplastic and hepatic disease (Till and Ward, 1975). The activity of lymphocytes and polymorphonuclear leukocytes in elderly, healthy patients may differ significantly when the host has developed infection or neoplasia. Therefore, some appraisal of the reserve capacity of these components of the immune system needs to be defined.

II. DIAGNOSTIC AND THERAPEUTIC MANEUVERS AND THEIR IMPLICATIONS IN THE TREATMENT OF ELDERLY CANCER PATIENTS

The scientific model has already been developed which provides the framework upon which this discussion will be built (Engel, 1980). This biopsychosocial model, through its system's hierarchy and levels of organization (see Figure 1), adds on the psychosocial dimension to a traditional biomedical view. The complex, special needs of the elderly cancer patient may be more easily conceptualized when clinicians utilize this comprehensive geriatric model (CGM). Using this framework, the interventions that are external to the organized hierarchy of the elderly cancer patient will be discussed in light of their impact on organ systems, patient host, family, and community.

A. Surgery: Diagnostic and Therapeutic Considerations

When a diagnosis of cancer is considered in the differential diagnosis or has been established by definitive testing, surgical therapy often is a modality used to corroborate the diagnosis, establish the extent of disease, and treat the cancer if appropriate. "Cancer" is a word that may connote an operation, disfigurement, an ostomy bag, a period of dependency, disability, or death. Fears and misconceptions may affect the patient and the support network in terms of the consent to surgery for diagnosis and treatment. These issues are certainly of critical importance to all cancer patients, regardless of age.

The prospect of a surgical procedure in an elderly cancer patient, however, creates new fears and anxieties for middle-aged children who are assisting their parents through the crisis at hand. These children often appear at the bedside to offer consultative advice to elderly parents regarding the decision to undergo surgery. Ethical dilemmas often arise when decision making attempts to coalesce the patient's value system, the family's grief (and often guilt), as well as the physician's best advice. Thoughts of death may be heightened in the patient's mind and may be manifested by anxiety, anger, depression, regression, or inability to cope with uncertainty, pain, or medication side effects. The physician, with the help of other members of the oncology team, can assist the patient and his/her family in an appropriate decision-making process based on the patient's value system or value history (McCullough, 1984). If conflicts are evident within the context of a decision to undergo surgery or not, the physician can use a structured framework to aid the patient and the family in discussing alternative choices. The teleological or utilitarian approach to moral reasoning is especially helpful to physicians who require some formal guidelines in ethical decision making (Candee and Puka, 1984).

As a biomedical intervention, surgery is not contraindicated based on chronological age alone. However, surgical mortality increases in patients over age 70 (Turnbull, 1978; Shein, 1979), with even greater increases in patients over age 80 (Santos and Gelperin, 1975). The physiological condition of the patient and the amount of functional reserve is crucial to determining suitability for major surgery. Selective, preoperative appraisal will assist the surgeon and oncologist in making sound decisions. Goldman et al. (1977) identified nine independent variables that correlate with life-threatening or fatal cardiac complications in noncardiac surgical procedures. These include (1) preoperative third heart sound or jugular venous distention; (2) myocardial infarction in the previous 6 months; (3) more than 5 PVCs per minute; (4) rhythm other than sinus or presence of PACs on a preoperative electrocardiogram; (5) age over 70; (6) intraperitoneal, intrathoracic, or aortic surgery; (7) emergency surgery; (8) important valvular stenosis; and (9) poor general medical condition (Goldman, 1977).

Surgery is recognized as a stress to the host, especially to an elderly host, but this stress can be anticipated as an elective procedure with the added benefit of preoperative, multisystem assessment, maximum physiological preparation, and maximization of physiological reserve. The stress to the host may be more temporally limited with surgery, compared to the chronic stress of longer term modes of therapy.

Invasive preoperative monitoring has been suggested by some authors. One study demonstrated that 23% of the elderly group "cleared" for surgery have unacceptable risks from major surgery involving general anesthesia (Del Guercio, 1980). Risk from major surgery was determined by a staging profile utilizing catheterization and arterial sampling of all patients over 65 for whom major surgery was planned. The subgroup that had unacceptable risks was found to qualify for stage IV status: moderate to severe functional deficits that could not be corrected. A critique of that study which challenges this conclusion and points to a lack of a control population and failure to use age-adjusted physiological variables (Johnson, 1983). Risks could be lowered by better preoperative attention to pulmonary care, management of infectious complications, low-dose heparin therapy, and early mobilization after surgery as demonstrated in one surgical series of 500 patients over age 80 with a hospital mortality of 6.2% within 1 month of surgery (Djokovic and Hedley-Whyte, 1979). In another series of elderly patients undergoing colon resection, it was reported that mortality rates were 5% in the 70-80 age group and 17% for patients over age 80, with a morbidity rate of between 30-35% for all patients over age 50 (Boyd, Bradford, and Watne, 1980). These rates were achieved after thorough evaluation of operative risk factors. Operative mortality was 16% in patients over 70 with 2 or more complicating medical conditions, whereas no patient without a preexisting medical condition died regardless of age. This study supports the feasibility of surgery as a modality in elderly colon cancer patients, especially in those patients without previous co-morbid disease and in those patients with a significant physiological reserve. The functional reserve is even more important in elderly patients undergoing thoracotomies because of a direct age-related compromise in the cardiopulmonary system—a compromise that is separate from specific disease processes (Libow and Sherman, 1981).

Undertreatment of elderly women with breast cancer has been a problem in the past. Since survival rates for women under and over age 70 who have undergone primary surgical treatment are similar, it seems inappropriate to deny mastectomy and axillary lymph node dissection on the basis of age alone (Herbsman et al., 1981).

Besides preoperative evaluation and the risk of perioperative mortality, postoperative care in the recovery room and intensive care units can be troublesome to elderly patients. Disorientation may occur because of round-the-clock activity, absence of daylight, and radical alteration of diurnal patterns (Bowles, 1983). Alterations in pain perception can be manifested by silent, painless myocardial infarctions or pulmonary embolization manifested only by confusion, hypoxemia, and altered mental status. Nursing care to prevent pressure ulcers becomes a crucial issue because of immobility, decreased pain perception, and changes in neurosensory function.

Psychosocial preventive care should be attempted by obtaining some life history details from the patient or family which will assist the oncologist or other members of the oncology team in learning previous coping styles utilized during periods of stress. For example, if belligerence, anger, and regression have been demonstrated during previous illnesses, one can instruct nursing personnel to anticipate such reactions to pain, disorientation, prolonged bed rest, or a lengthy rehabilitation program.

In summary, it is well recognized that surgery for elderly cancer patients is complex and stressful for the patient, the family, and all members of the oncology team. Attention to physiological details and adequate preparation are the cornerstones to minimal pre- and postoperative complications. The oncology physician maintains an essential position in the restoration of biomedical and psychosocial functional status utilizing selective, supportive, medical care, and technology as well as the skills of the oncology nurse and the social worker (Schnaper et al., 1983). Chronological age does not preclude surgery but requires the appraisal of preexistent co-morbid disease and the assessment of functional reserve.

B. Radiation Therapy

Similarities exist between radiation therapy and surgery for elderly cancer patients in terms of the complexity of decision making and informed consent. Physiologically, differences are evident when one compares the temporal relationship between the treatment with radiation therapy, its side effects, and the impact on the host and the hierarchy of systems. It has been learned from irradiation studies of mammalian cell lines that cells from species with the longest life span show the greatest ability to repair ultraviolet-induced DNA damage (Smith, 1978). In aged cancer patients, no evidence exists that a given cancer varies in its radiosensitivity as a function of the age of the patient. As far as normal host tissue is concerned, the radiation effect is said to be enhanced by 10-15% (Gunn, 1980). Radiation of certain aging organ systems does effect the overall well-being of the aging cancer patient. Radiation therapy that involves the oropharynx and oral cavity may produce loss of gustatory function, involution of the salivary glands, and resultant dryness of the mucous membranes. The quality of life for the host is certainly affected with loss of taste and oral gratification as well as the resultant nutritional impact on other aging organ systems. These issues will be complicated by watery diarrhea, abdominal cramps, nausea, fluid-electrolyte imbalance, and malabsorption (Gunn, 1980). Additive systemic effects from simultaneous chemotherapy, radiation therapy, and from the cancer cell mass itself provide the aging host with nutritional stresses that require supplementation, as well as assisted feedings by staff or family.

Since a single large dose or a few massive doses of radiation are less effective than protracted courses of treatment, factors that influence compliance for chronic therapy of any kind exert cumulative effects on elderly cancer patients. Elderly people may have fears and misconceptions about cancer that shape their health beliefs. Concepts such as these are created by culture and age-cohort effects (Kane, 1983). By and large, they are concerned about quality versus quantity of life. Socioeconomic factors that are taken for granted in younger patients such as mobility, transportation, or availability of supportive next of kin are generally more applicable to aged cancer patients.

C. Chemotherapy

Chemotherapy is the treatment modality that may be associated with the greatest negative reaction in elderly cancer patients. There are a number of reasons to explain this association. Drug toxicity effects a number of aging organ systems including bone marrow, lung, kidney, the cardiovascular system, and the nervous system. The aging host contains a heterogeneous group of aging organ systems which have a variety of functional reserve capacities due to co-morbid disease and aging effects. Individualization of chemotherapy based on these variables has not been used effectively in the selection of older patients for treatment protocols. Elderly patients have generally been excluded from these protocols, thus limiting a standard source of information on drug toxicity (Begg, Cohen, and Ellerton, 1980).

Patient compliance for a selected drug regimen is essential to the management of elderly cancer patients. As mentioned above, health beliefs form the basis for much of the observed behavior in any treatment protocol. Although there is little quantitative information available regarding the magnitude of the compliance problem in cancer patients undergoing treatment at any age (Lewis, Linet, and Abeloff, 1983), even less is known about the psychosocial and emotional effects of cancer on older people (Rimer et al., 1983). Other factors such as physician behavior, the patient-physician relationship, and the patient support system need to be investigated in terms of their effect on compliance (Lewis, Linet, and Abeloff, 1983). This is especially important in the management of elderly cancer patients. Practitioners must consider the qualities of the contract "negotiated" between physician and elderly patient to insure compliance. The degree of commitment and the amount of attention devoted to support systems through the efforts of physician extenders and other members of the oncology team greatly effect the willingness of the patient to follow a prescribed therapeutic regimen. These efforts fortify the physician-patient relationship and result in mutual trust and respect. Attention to seemingly small details within the support system reap larger rewards in compliance especially for elderly patients. A small example may be the availability of fresh citrus fruits in the office when patients are receiving intravenous chemotherapy. This taste sensation can do much to alleviate the metallic taste from the administration of these drugs and block other gustatory stimulations of nausea and vomiting pathways. Color coordination and interior decorating, control of extraneous smells and noises in the office setting, and soothing, comforting nursing personnel can all influence the elderly cancer patient in minimizing the side effects of chemotherapy.

Although the body of knowledge continues to expand in geriatric pharma-cology (Ouslander, 1981), little data are available to describe the effects of chemotherapeutic agents in these patients. In effect, because of the variability in the clinical course of cancers in the elderly, few conclusions are available regarding the chemotherapeutic responsiveness of specific tumors as a function of age (Cohen and Crawford, 1984). More information is available on the toxicity of these drugs in geriatric patients.

Most drugs used in chemotherapy are limited by bone marrow toxicity. Reserves in granulocytes or bone marrow precursor cells are decreased in aged patients with anemia (¾ipschitz and Thompson, 1980). In animal studies, long-term cultures of aged mouse bone marrow cells demonstrate a reduced proliferative capacity of normal stem cells (Reincke et al., 1982). In a retro-spective review of elderly patients enrolled in the Eastern Cooperative Oncology Group (ECOG) protocols, excessive toxicity was recognized with the use of only two drugs, methyl CCNU and methotrexate, in the elderly compared to younger patients (Carbone and Begg, 1982). The methotrexate toxicity may have been related to the failure to reduce the dosage to appropriate levels based on age-related physiological changes in renal function. Although the methyl CCNU in the ECOG protocols may have more severely suppressed normal bone marrow stem cells, another nitrosourea, bischlorethyl nitro-sourea (BCNU), was used in combination with cyclophosphamide and pred-nisone and in patients with myeloma there was no increase in toxicity for elderly patients (Cohen et al., 1983). It seems evident that more studies are needed to determine bone marrow toxicity for given drug dosage guidelines in elderly cancer patients based on physiological reserve parameters rather than chronological age.

The lung appears to be at increased risk for toxic fibrosis from bleomycin especially in patients over 70 (Ginsberg and Comis, 1982). Adriamycin has been implicated as having increasing cardiac toxicity for the elderly. One study implicated age as a risk factor for cardiac toxicity in the use of Adriamycin (Bristow et al., 1978), while another suggested co-morbid cardiac disease as the major predisposing factor (Praga et al., 1979). Vincristine often produces peripheral neuropathy as a side effect. However, the age-related changes in peripheral nerves in combination with toxic drug effects create a common situational dilemma for the physician caring for the elderly host. Homeostatic reserves may be so depleted that further impairments are mani-fested as changes in activities of daily living and a changing quality of life. Small losses in neurosensory functioning often produce large changes in the way elderly patients view themselves. In order to maintain a basic level of function which will allow an individual to conduct many of the basic, physical, and instrumental activities of daily living, chemotherapy protocols should be adjusted according to the physiological reserve or tolerance inherent in the organ systems that are more susceptible. Deficits in function that are the direct result of chemotherapy may require supplemental assistance from family, community, or institutional resources in order to maintain a certain "level of functioning and quality of life."

In other clinical situations, such as adjuvant chemotherapy for breast cancer, early trials included provisions for making dose reductions for women over the age of 60. An important early conclusion from these trials was that postmenopausal women did not receive the same benefit from chemotherapy as premenopausal women. Retrospective analysis of these data reveals that a subgroup of postmenopausal women who received the full dose of chemotherapy, similar to premenopausal women, appeared to obtain the same benefit from therapy (Bonadonna and Valagussa, 1980). Full dose chemotherapy may be tolerable to aging organ systems and an aging host, but biological differences in the cancer cell population may require alteration in the therapeutic approach in order to achieve the desired outcome. One example comes from the study of advanced Hodgkin's disease in patients over 60 years of age who were treated with combination chemotherapy. Those elderly patients who received greater than 90% of their projected drug dosages were analyzed and found to have remission rates, median time of recurrence, and duration of survival to be much shorter than younger patients (Peterson et al., 1982a).

In general, there exists an age-related increase in incidence for hematological malignancies. These cancers currently require palliative treatment for many elderly patients. The best approach to management of elderly patients with acute leukemia is very controversial (Peterson, 1982). Although the patient may demonstrate the adverse effects of aggressive chemotherapy, including infection and bleeding from bone marrow aplasia, remission can be achieved with patients under or over age 60 (Foon et al., 1981).

Should the elderly patient receive chemotherapy? Although the answer to this question must be individualized, retrospective reviews have shown instances in which aged cancer patients have demonstrated equivalent responses to younger patients entered into protocols (Begg, Cohen, and Ellerton, 1980; Cohen et al., 1983). In order to prevent the inappropriate exclusion of elderly cancer patients from chemotherapy protocols, *assumptions* about organ function or tolerance based on chronological age alone should not be the sole criterion used for exclusion from such protocols. Future prospective studies must consider the heterogeneity of the elderly population, the changing biology of the cancer cell mass itself, and the need for individualized decision making. The decision to include or exclude elderly patients from specific protocols should be based on sound information from a thorough appraisal of the elderly patient's physiological status and functional reserve.

D. Hormonal Therapy

The oncologist may be assisted in the treatment and management of certain
cancers in elderly patients because of the altered susceptibility of certain
neoplasias to hormonal chemotherapy. Breast and prostate cancers that are
responsive to hormonal therapy may be treated with fewer adverse effects on
aging organ systems than are customary with some chemotherapeutic drugs.
Response rates to hormone treatment in estrogen receptor positive breast
cancer patients can be as high as 50-60% compared to rates of 5% in estrogen
negative patients (Holland and Frei, 1982). Tamoxifen is one example of such
a hormonal intervention with low cardiovascular morbidity and less side effects
than other types of chemotherapy. A separate problem is that the high cost of
this drug may further compromise an already strained fixed budget for many
elderly patients, however.

   In prostate cancer, endocrine ablation can be the most effective treatment
for the patient with metastatic disease. However, the apparent benefit of oral
diethylstilbestrol therapy in palliating the disease is offset by increased cardiovascular mortality (Torti and Carter, 1980). Adjustment of the dosage of
diethylstilbestrol is the key to appropriate management of prostate cancer with
hormonal therapy. Cardiovascular mortality was not observed to be elevated
when 1 mg/day was used. This dose apparently suppressed testosterone as well
as 5 mg/day (Torti and Carter, 1980). Although the mortality associated with
diethylstilbestrol therapy is higher than the mortality with orchiectomy, to
suggest castration for an elderly man carries no less a sense of loss than in a
younger male. Illnesses which affect "physically" significant sites, such as the
reproductive organs, may produce profound disruptions of body image. This
body image is the conceptualization of one's body structure and function; it
includes one's perception, one's ideas or feelings in response to one's own
body. The behavioral reactions that may result include grief, depression,
shame and embarrassment, disturbances in sexual identity, or maladaptive
responses. The net impact of this reaction to one's prostatic cancer may be
the denial of cancer's existence (Verwoerdt, 1981).

III. SELECTED NEEDS AND PROBLEMS OF ELDERLY
CANCER PATIENTS

The theme developed with the use of the comprehensive geriatric model indicates a complex interrelationship between the patient's system organization
and any intervention that is selected as cancer therapy. For the purpose of
organization, these special needs will be addressed in three sections: (1)
biomedical; (2) psychological; and (3) social. Management for each area of
concern may require support and intervention from the other two areas to

maintain homeostasis and functional status. When these special needs are described, we should keep in mind a 15th century description of the role of a physician: "To cure sometimes, to relieve often, and to comfort always," (anonymous; an inscription on the statue of Dr. E. Livingstone Trudeau at Saranac Lake, N.Y.).

A. Control of Nausea and Vomiting

Nausea and vomiting are symptoms that frequently accompany the development of cancer (see also Chapter 5), but these symptoms and their management are especially crucial to the elderly cancer patient for a number of interrelated reasons. It was recorded several years ago that over half of the cancer patients at Duke miss appointments or delay aggressive chemotherapy because of nausea and vomiting (Laszlo and Lucas, 1981). Younger patients with soft tissue sarcoma demonstrated nearly a 90% nonparticipation rate at the point of randomization where significant side effects of therapy were possible (Lewis, Linet, and Abeloff, 1983). The maintenance of adequate enteral nutrition is clearly dependent on the control of these symptoms. The maintenance of adequate nutrition as reflected by a normal serum albumin should be a basic goal for all patients being managed by the oncology team. Elderly patients require the same nutritional support as younger cancer patients but they require more careful monitoring and special encouragement (Ching et al., 1979).

Management of nausea and vomiting in the elderly includes the investigation of other causes of these symptoms (electrolyte imbalance, bowel obstruction) and the use of selected behavioral, pharmacotherapeutic, and supportive methodologies. Environmental changes in room decor and gustatory sensations, small frequent meals, the use of dry crackers or toast after periods of sleep or rest, and avoidance of strongly aromatic foods may all assist in the control of nausea and vomiting (Kaplan, 1984). Cannabinoids (THC) offer effectiveness comparable to prochlorperazine, however, when one uses doses that are antiemetic, this drug (THC) produces sedation and sometimes dysphoria rather than euphoria. These side effects can be especially troublesome in the elderly becuase of additive effects with other analgesics and mood-altering medications. Metoclopramide and glucocorticoids are two other drug therapies that may offer valuable alternatives in elderly cancer patients. A recent report has described the effective control of cisplatin-induced emesis using metoclopramide intravenously to achieve an optimum serum level of 850 mg/ml (Meyer et al., 1984). In fact, despite similar blood levels for patients less than or over age 65, the elderly group (over age 65) demonstrated significantly fewer episdoes of emesis compared to the younger group.

Choices for drug therapy for nausea and vomiting by virtue of the complexity of the symptoms and the character of the population at risk are individualized and discussed elsewhere. A few points relevant to the elderly population will be addressed for completeness. Antidopaminergic drugs, which include many of the phenothiazines, appear to exert their effect centrally on the chemoreceptor trigger zone and can demonstrate a variety of autonomic, anticholinergic effects and extrapyramidal reactions. Since drug levels of phenothiazines may be higher in elderly patients than comparable dosages administered to younger patients, it has been recommended to use lower dosages for elderly patients in addition to closer observation to detect tardive dyskinesia (Ouslander, 1981). Mood-altering drugs of any kind, including phenothiazines and antihistamines, not only provide an increased risk of sedation with declining clearance and metabolism, but also may produce agitation and a heightened confusion in patients with presenile or senile dementia of the Alzheimer's type or other forms of primary degenerative dementia.

Cannabinoids are of limited use in elderly patients because of dysphoric reactions, differences in social acceptability and treatment expectations, and variability in absorption, distribution, metabolism, and excretion of these compounds (Jacknowitz, 1984). Dexamethasone intravenously or orally can be very useful in providing antiemetic effects up to 24 hours. Specific attention should be paid to the elderly cancer patient when using combinations of drugs, sequencing of drugs, or drugs with uncertain mechanisms of action.

The social support of a spouse, adult child, friend, or comforting oncology physician or nurse should not be underestimated in the adjunctive role these people play in the overall management of nausea and vomiting (Lucas and Brown, 1982). Because of the cerebral interconnections of the afferent and efferent pathways for these autonomic responses within the central nervous system, only future investigations can provide the explanations for what is observed at the behavioral level.

B. Pain Control

Neoplastic processes can cause a number of uncomfortable symptoms in elderly cancer patients, not the least of which are syndromes. As described in Chapter 7, pain is the result of a complex interaction of many biomedical and psychologic sensations and defenses. These perceptions of pain are modified by fear, anxiety, despair, or helplessness. Pain responses and the pain threshold seem to be dependent on three sets of factors or dimensions: (1) sensory/discrimination processes; (2) motivational/affective processes; and (3) cognitive/evaluative processes (Harkins and Warner, 1980).

Pain may be secondary to malignancies, but also may be due to treatment-related causes. Interruption of nerves because of surgical procedures can produce pain in post-thoracotomy or post-mastectomy patients. Radiation fibrosis within or surrounding the brachial or lumbar plexus can produce constant, diffuse burning pain that can mimic tumor invasion of these plexi (Klein, 1983). Chemotherapy, especially treatment with vinca alkaloids, podophyllotoxin analogs, and cisplatin, may cause significant, symmetrical neuropathy. Post-herpetic neuralgia is a disabling, neuropathic cause of pain in elderly patients that may warrant special attention. Although a few prospective studies have shown a decreased likelihood of post-herpetic neuralgia in elderly cancer patients receiving corticosteroids during the first 2-5 days of the skin eruption (Keczkes and Basheer, 1980), other effects of prednisone at a dosage of 0.5-1 mg/kg for 21-30 days need to be considered. Dissemination of herpes zoster occurs in 20-40% of cancer patients. Steroids as well as many other forms of cancer therapy may facilitate this dissemination (Merscelis, Kaye, and Hook, 1964).

While painful complaints seem to rise with increasing age, the sensitivity to pain seems to decline with aging. A number of age groups were compared in a pain study using morphine intramuscularly for cancer patients. It was reported that after the administration of 8 and 16 mg of morphine sulfate for these postoperative cancer patients, approximately 1.5-2.5 times as much relief of pain was experienced by the elderly patients compared to younger postoperative patients (Kaiko 1980). Clearly, aging was associated with enhanced analgesia. Fear of the severity of the next attack of pain, depression, as well as many other factors (Table 1) may alter the perception level of pain despite the decreased general awareness of pain in the elderly. Cancer patients with moderate to severe pain should receive a fixed dosage regimen based on the analgesic's age-adjusted pharmacokinetics rather than an "as needed" dosing schedule (McGivney and Crooks, 1984). Experiences with hospice patients at St. Christopher's Hospice in Britain have found that morphine alone is as effective in relieving the pain of cancer as any mixture of drugs such as the Brompton cocktail. Regular use of an appropriate analgesic either orally or parenterally in proper dosages to achieve pain relief *before* the next pain cycle starts can be of extraordinary help in managing the anxiety, hopelessness, and fear that accompany the pain of cancer (Kark and Wardle, 1980). Careful titration is required and mandatory in patients with aged metabolic organ systems in order that side effects of sedation, confusion, constipation, etc., are minimized. The analgesic side effects of nausea and vomiting can be treated by metoclopramide or phenothiazines (as mentioned above) after consideration of polypharmacy and iatrogenic complications in drug usage.

Other geriatric team members can help in the nonpharmacologic management of pain syndromes. Psychologic and psychiatric methods for pain control

Table 1 Factors That Influence Pain Perception

Threshold lowered	Threshold raised
Discomfort	Relief of symptoms
Insomnia	Sleep
Fatigue	Rest
Anxiety	Sympathy
Fear	Understanding
Anger	Companionship
Sadness	Diversional activity
Depression	Reduction in anxiety
Boredom	Elevation of mood
Introversion	Analgesics
Mental isolation	Anxiolytics
Social abandonment	Antidepressants

Source: Twycross (1984).

include distraction, imagery, relaxation, biofeedback, or hypnosis therapy. These methods are included in the comprehensive management of pain control not because of their selective effectiveness in elderly cancer patients, but because these patients should not be denied the benefit of nonpharmacological methods of analgesia based on age alone, provided that cognitive function, mood and thought content are adequate to support the use of these modalities. Heat, massage, pressure treatment, and transcutaneous electric nerve stimulation complete these adjunctive methods of analgesia (Twycross, 1984). A supportive atmosphere of sympathic warmth, intellectual stimulation, and diversion created at home with hospice volunteers or within an institution such as St. Christopher's Hospice of London vastly minimizes loneliness and improves the quality of life for elderly cancer patients and their families.

C. Nutritional Needs and Support

Elderly patients experience a number of physiological, psychological, and sociological changes with respect to nutritional requirements and support. Major variables include personality changes, increased passivity, social isolation, depression, and altered attitudes towards food (Ordy, Harman, and Alfin-Slater, 1984). Changes in taste and smell affect food preferences especially with regard to meats and dairy products. Loss of teeth due to periodontal disease produces an effect not only on mastication but also plays a role by permitting fewer preferences for crunchy foods. These foods may include nuts, fruits, and vegetables which could contribute bulk, vitamins, and carbohydrates for these patients. Less food is purchased in general by elderly patients with the exception of a few items such as coffee. Food consumption seems to be higher at breakfast and lower at dinner. When young and elderly shopping habits were appraised, discrepancies between the two groups in food purchases, reported consumption, and preferences were dependent on: (1) smaller family size; (2) decreased caloric intake; (3) economic factors; and (4) portability factors (i.e., capability of being carried).

Tumors affect the elderly host in a multifactorial manner and ultimately contribute to cachexia in many cancer patients. This physical state is the result of the tumor itself and the presence of anorexia. The degree of cachexia, however, is dependent on a number of other interrelated factors including metabolic changes, altered food intake, malabsorption, and anatomical changes (Young, 1983). A set of guidelines has been proposed (Wretlind, 1981) for nutritional maintenance in hospitalized patients and is also applicable to elderly cancer patients: (1) these patients should maintain good nutritional status as a prerequisite to optimal resistance to infection and response to medical treatment; (2) the diet must be carefully monitored in order that nutrients are being supplied in adequate amounts; (3) good nutrition is easier to maintain than is the treatment of malnutrition; (4) the first choice for nutrition is oral or tube feedings (I.V. feedings should be a second choice); and (5) nutritional support can be maintained through a variety of nutrient formulations.

Despite these general guidelines and the potential benefits of improved nutrition, reversal of weight loss, provision of excess energy needs, and reversal of immune deficiencies, considerable controversy exists about the indication for parenteral nutrition support for these patients. A critical issue that needs to be resolved is the paucity of data to support guidelines for interpretation of anthropometric, biochemical, and functional indices of nutritional status in reference to elderly patients. These guidelines would be helpful to clinicians who require some estimate of nutritional requirements for patients over age 60 who exhibit a specific height, weight, and functional status.

The oncologist must integrate the functional capabilities of a number of aging organ systems when nutritional care plans are instituted. Changes in olfaction, food preferences, economic status, and mental capabilities all can effect an aged host's nutritional state. It is necessary to utilize specialists in nutrition to maximize creativity in meal planning and food supplementation. Responsibility for nutritional care may include not only the dietitian but also the social worker, oncology nurse, and other members of the oncology team.

D. Miscellaneous Medical Needs

Constipation is such an important symptom for the geriatric patient that concern over one's bowel habits often takes precedence over many other needs including cancer therapy. Decreased fluid intake, change in eating habits and preferences, habitual use of cathartics and laxatives, and faulty daily hygiene contribute to the behavioral aspects of constipation. Physiologically, these patients have decreased tone in the bowel wall, diminished peristalsis, and decreased strength in abdominal musculature (Sklar, 1983). Management should include instruction in adequate amounts of fluid per day (2-5 glasses), residue (bran, bulk agents, for example Metamucil) and the avoidance of irritant laxatives.

Elderly patients receiving cancer therapy may certainly demonstrate a compromised immune status and vulnerability in terms of bacterial and viral infections. Herpes zoster has already been mentioned in regard to steroid therapy and management in these cancer patients. Influenza is an epidemic disease that can devastate a nursing home population and impair elderly cancer patients receiving definitive therapy. Prophylactic immunization practices including vaccines for pneumococcal disease and influenza are major adjunctive practices in patients who can tolerate these antigenic challenges and who are not allergic to egg protein. Current recommendations include yearly flu vaccine administration and 1 dose of the 23 valent pneumococcal vaccine (Schneider, 1983; Jahnigen and Laforce, 1982). Tetanus prophylaxis is becoming increasingly important in a population that is neglected in terms of booster doses of tetanus toxoid every 10 years. Tuberculosis screening is a matter of heightened interest for nursing home medical directors because of silent reactivation of old disease and dissemination of new infections in frail elderly patients (Nagami and Yoshikawa, 1983).

Skin changes with aging are important to note in comprehensive cancer care because of the changes with chemotherapy, radiation effects and subcutaneous reactions secondary to extravasation of chemotherapy. Aging of the skin includes dryness (xerosis), wrinkling, laxity, uneven pigmentation, and a variety of proliferative lesions (Gilchrest, 1984). Within the dermis, loss of up to 20% of the dermal volume provides an explanation for the paper thin, transparent qualities of aging skin. Fewer fibroblasts, mast cells, and blood vessels accompany shortened capillary loops and abnormal nerve endings. Changes in support tissue and ground substance rather than changes in blood vessels themselves may be responsible for fragility and so-called "senile purpura" (Tonnesen and Weston, 1982). Since sun-induced damage to the skin is much different from chronological aging, much care must be taken in utilizing peripheral veins in sun-exposed areas for chemotherapy because of dysfunctional, quantitative, and qualitative alterations in collagen and elastin (Gilchrest, 1984).

General rehabilitation of an elderly cancer patient after surgery, radiation therapy, chemotherapy, or combinations of these modalities requires adherence to basic principles of rehabilitation. A definitive diagnosis must accompany prevention of secondary disability while the development of functional abilities and the preservation of the dignity of the individual are pursued (Wolcott, 1983).

IV. PSYCHOLOGICAL NEEDS

Integration of behavioral aspects of the Comprehensive Geriatric Model (CGM) into comprehensive cancer care prevents an oversight of these salient issues. Loneliness, depression, guilt, ethical dilemmas, and effective communication are of critical importance, especially within the context of the care of elderly patients.

A. Cognition–Depression–Grief

In the elderly, disorders accompanied by changes in the brain that lead to profound alterations in memory, decision making, and cognition are more frequent. In many cases of senile or presenile dementia, no specific etiology can be identified (Kane, Ouslander, and Abrass, 1984). The marked increase in media attention for Alzheimer's disease has provided public awareness for a problem that was formerly not recognized. Primary dementing disorders are mentioned in the context of cancer care because of their increasing incidence with age and the coincident usefulness of tools to identify these changes in cognition. A validated series of 10 standard questions (The Short Portable Mental Status Examination) or similar tool can be invaluable to clinicians who care for elderly patients (Pfeiffer, 1975). Changes that are apparent on these mental questionnaires can be noted sequentially over time and may provide economical, efficient ways to gather information on mental performance.

Cognitive changes can be recognized by these measurements and provide very important information in the continual assessment of elderly patients. It is very common to observe clinically subtle changes in cognitive status (often coincident with changes in functional status) when serious infection, pain, drug effects, or postoperative complications occur.

Depression, anxiety, fear, denial, and grief are common problems faced by cancer patients of all ages. Special importance needs to be paid to aged patients in consideration of these behavioral patterns because typical symptomatology is often masked. Depression in the elderly can present with somatic complaints of anorexia, weight loss, constipation, memory disturbance, sleep disturbance, or fatigue, as well as apathy and withdrawal (Kane, Ouslander, and Abrass, 1984). Feelings of guilt are less common in aged patients but may play a large role in the behavior of middle-aged children. Objective data obtained from the history, physical examination, and laboratory assist the clinician in accurately evaluating these complex, often confusing clinical settings.

A course of antidepressant medication is often necessary if severity and duration of these symptoms create functional disability or interference with recovery from cancer management. Grief reactions can be acute or chronic or can be appropriate or pathological. A number of characteristics can be noted in survivors which can predispose these patients to pathological grief reactions: an early traumatic loss in childhood, obsessive personality style, history of previous depression and multiple life crises, a death following an unexpected, short terminal illness, and preexisting relationships characterized by excessive dependency, hostility, ambivalence, or other neurotic conflicts (Brown and Stoudemire 1983). Although these risk factors for pathological grief reactions are not necessarily limited to elderly patients, their occurrence in this age group may indicate a more vulnerable situation because of cumulative losses, isolation, and limited flexibility.

Clinicians caring for elderly cancer patients need to recognize the variety of potential defense mechanisms used by these patients in the adjustment to a number of real losses. These responses may include a retreat from the threat (low energy defenses) which is manifested by regression or giving up. One may exclude oneself from the awareness of the loss by regressing, denying, or projecting the reaction upon someone else. A "high energy" defense may be a mastery or control of the reaction through intellectualization, reaction formation, or isolation of feelings from one's thoughts (Verwoerdt, 1981). The inability to exert any real influence over the aging effects of organ systems and the functional disabilities that follow is a tremendous blow to one's independence and self-sufficiency. Compulsive, rigid personalities who age without disability until a cancer is diagnosed are particularly at risk for despondent reactions, withdrawal, regression, and depression.

B. Death and Dying

While much has been written about the stages of grieving in dying patients (Kübler-Ross, 1969), attention should be focused on the needs of dying elderly patients as well as of the needs of their physicians (see also Chapter 2). These patients need their doctors. Caring as well as curing are the functions of the physician and his oncology team. Health providers who care for elderly cancer patients must come to terms with their feelings about death because death often is not a reflection of medical failure in elderly patients. At other times, the prospect of death raises ethical dilemmas for the patient physician and family. These dilemmas are notably complex by their nature and are often difficult to solve. Distant family members who are geographically removed from the elderly patient often acknowledge these dilemmas and offer their assistance to the decision-making process. The setting tends to become complex and time consuming for the physician. Often it is helpful to assign one person the task of disseminating clinical information to the rest of the family to insure the involvement of appropriate individuals. The entire setting tends to require large amounts of physician time but remains as a major, final role for the oncologist in the care of the elderly patients with cancer.

C. Ethical Decision Making and Informed Consent

When elderly cancer patients refuse medical-surgical therapy, or enteral-parenteral nutrition, and acknowledge the wish to be left alone to die, physicians and other members of the oncology team wrestle with dilemmas that characterize ethical decision making. These problems often contain issues of paternalism, truth-telling, autonomy, and mental competency (McCullough, 1984), especially when an elderly person expresses a desire not to pursue a recommended therapy. These decisions are often opposed by family members or "extended" family members. In order to assist the patient, the family, and the oncology team in resolving these ethical dilemmas, the physician-oncologist needs to follow an orderly, logical series of steps. One such approach is the teleological or utilitarian approach to ethical decision making (Candee and Puka, 1984) (Table 2).

This method is based on sound medical diagnosis and clinical probabilities plus some insight into the value system or value history of the involved patient (McCullough, 1984). This value history describes the moral process used by the patient during previous life experiences. These data tell the family and the oncology team what the patient would have wanted if he/she were able to describe his/her value system. However, it must be recognized that all members of the oncology team carry into a discussion of this type their own biases and perceptions of the patient's needs.

Discussions about the mental competency of the patient are only resolved definitively by a court of law after evidence is presented and testimony is solicited (Smith, 1983). Short of legal proceedings, an opinion from a consulting psychiatrist will assist in determining competence to participate in the decisions that are pending.

Although moral dilemmas are difficult to solve and are prevalent in cases involving elderly cancer patients, a step-by-step approach is available to oncology physicians and other team members. Inherent in this approach is the assumption that personal biases can be acknowledged and can be separated from the biases of the patient and his/her family.

D. Support Systems for the Patient and the Family

In order to effectively provide maximal psychosocial supports for the elderly cancer patient, a variety of approaches is required. Support can be supplied by personally providing information to the patient regarding his/her physical state

Table 2 Teleological Approach to Ethical Decision Making

Gather general claims
List feasible alternatives
Predict consequences (outcomes of each action)
Determine probability of each outcome occurring
Assign a value to each outcome (determine basis of valuing)
Determine utilities (probability multiplied by the ascribed
    value of the various outcomes)

Source: Candee and Puka (1984).

that is timely, accurate, understandable, and reassuring. Other sources can be utilized through sustaining relationships and emotional ties that furnish tangible help for these patients (Kane, 1983). Before a specific approach can be utilized, an appraisal of the entire organizational hierarchy is required from a psychosocial point of view. This comprehensive cancer care should be perceived as a family matter with supports extended to stressed family members, including bereavement when necessary.

Of major concern for the oncology team is the issue of appropriateness and acceptance of available psychosocial services for frail, elderly cancer patients. It is well recognized that patients who are more involved in their medical care are more hopeful, thus freeing themselves from fear and anxiety. A study of cancer patients (ages 20-60+) determined that older patients tended to prefer the nonparticipatory, passive roles in cancer care (Cassileth et al., 1980). The generational differences that were observed in these cancer patients could be the result of more open discussions of cancer and health care that have been recognized as trends in recent decades. Alternative explanations include advancing age per se, with increasingly passive posture, solitude, and isolation.

Direct interviews of patients and families would provide richer pictures of premorbid personality traits, and strengths and weaknesses of the family support system and community resources. These are performed in order to assess risk factors for future care or institutionalization. Interviews such as these would contain the added value of relevancy if the appraisal were held in the patient's home. Although this is not always possible, supportive services within the context of the visiting nurse association and home-based hospice organizations can provide the oncology team with much of this information (Berkman et al., 1983).

Support networks for elderly patients tend to be attenuated and vulnerable (Kane, 1983). Because of economic stresses, bereavement, and social isolation, elderly cancer patients become increasingly dependent on family members. Institutional care often is the only alternative for patients who have no surviving children. Patients differ widely in their needs, depending on whether the cancer is a new diagnosis or whether there is a recurrence of cancer in old age. Cancer can develop in individuals with serious co-morbid disease or it can occur in elderly patients who later develop serious co-morbid disease. Just as treatment needs to be individualized because of the heterogeneity of the population at risk, so also do the psychosocial needs require individualization based on appraisal of the comprehensive geriatric model. Clinicians must keep the complete model in perspective in order to coordinate and orchestrate comprehensive geriatric care.

V. SOCIAL NEEDS

In order to guide the oncologist and oncology team in comprehensive management of the elderly cancer patient, a few basic social support items of great impact will be addressed. This discussion will complete the CGM for the care of the elderly with cancer. Because of the paucity of sociologically oriented information regarding these elderly cancer patients, answers may need to be sought in the literature for elderly patients who have other chronic diseases. Since social supports for the elderly can be variable and lack depth, these support networks must be selectively designed to supplement the elderly individual who has cancer (Kane, Ouslander, and Abrass, 1984). The social functioning and beliefs of the individual are integral parts of the complex series of interrelationships that encompass comprehensive cancer care. The social needs of these patients and their support systems are complex and multileveled, requiring attention to detail and ingenuity.

Debilitated elderly patients receiving cancer therapy often require support from family and community in order to reach therapeutic goals. Assistance with physical activities of daily living (bathing, toileting, dressing, eating, etc.) can be provided by family members home care services, or private fee-for-service contracts. When social networks begin to attenuate because of caregiver stress (usually involving a middle-aged child) or increasing need for higher levels of support, more institutional forms of assistance are required.

The institutional options available to elderly patients range from Life Care (total care) retirement facilities, to traditional nursing home settings, to less dependent styles of residence (rest homes, public or congregate housing). Obviously, financial resources play a major role in determining the number of available options. Fixed, limited incomes and a paucity of financial assets may limit the options to federally supported intermediate or skilled nursing care facilities (Medicaid or Medicare financing). However, decisions to give up one's home, one's possessions, and one's independence are not to be taken lightly, especially for the elderly patient who has experienced a number of physical disabilities in association with the new diagnosis of cancer.

Care at home can be maintained informally through a network of family, friends, and neighbors, or formally with home health services, chore workers, or homemakers. Funding for intermediate or skilled home care can be obtained through Medicare coverage, although criteria for eligibility restrict the use of these services. Interpretation by the physician of the need for *skilled* (not custodial) services for elderly patients is the key to reimbursement (Kane, Ouslander, and Abrass, 1984).

Other alternatives available for rehabilitation of ADLs and social skills in these patients include adult day care centers, which can provide a combination of recreational and restorative activities. Some of these facilities offer more medical components with physical therapy and occupational therapy available on an ambulatory basis.

A clinician is not expected to know about all these services available to elderly cancer patients, but an acknowledgment of the importance of social supports and the CGM will foster delegation of responsibility and accountability for other members of the oncology team. Planning of appropriate measures in advance is the key to successful management of these complicated patients after comprehensive appraisal has been accomplished. These issues are discussed further in Chapter 2.

VI. CLOSING STATEMENTS

Though much remains to be learned about the specific attributes, needs, and problems of the elderly cancer patient, viewing the individual patient in the context of his/her functional status and the state of his/her total hierarchical system can promote more rational decision making. Hopefully, in the future more data specifically pertinent to the elderly cancer patient will become available to lend further strength to this approach.

REFERENCES

American Association of Retired Persons. (1984). Aging America: Trends and projections, Report to U.S. Senate Special Committee on Aging in Conjunction with the American Association of Retired Persons, PL 3377 (584), Washington, D.C., pp. 1-101.

Baker, A. B. (1937). Structure of the small cerebral arteries and their changes with age, *Am. J. Pathol., 13*:453-461.

Becker, P. M., and Cohen, H. J. (1984). The functional approach to the care of the elderly—a conceptual framework, *J. Am. Geriat. Soc., 32(12)*:923-929.

Begg, C. B., Cohen, J. L., and Ellerton, J. (1980). Are the elderly predisposed to toxicity from cancer chemotherapy?, *Cancer Clin. Trials, 3*:369-374.

Berkman, B., Stolberg, C., Calhoun, J., Parker, E., and Stearns, N. (1983). Elderly cancer patients: Factors predictive of risk for institutionalization, *J. Psychosoc. Oncol., 1*:85-100.

Bhanthumnavin, K., and Schuster, M. M. (1977). Aging and gastrointestinal function, *Handbook of the Biology of Aging* (C. E. Finch, and L. Hayflick, eds.), Van Nostrand Reinhold, New York, pp. 709-723.

Bonadonna, G., and Valagussa, P. (1980). Dose-response effect of adjuvant chemotherapy in breast cancer, *New Engl. J. Med., 304*:10-15.

Boren, H. G., Kory, R. C., and Syner, J. C. (1966). The Veterans Administration-Army Cooperative Study of pulmonary function. II. The lung volume and its subdivision in normal men, *Am. J. Med., 41*:96-114.

Botnick, L. E., Hannon, E. C., Obbagy, J., and Hellman, S. (1982). The variation of hematopoietic stem cell self-renewal capacity as a function of age: Further evidence of heterogenicity of the stem cell compartment, *Blood, 60*:268-271.

Bowles, L. T. (1983). Surgical essentials in the care of the elderly cancer patient, *Perspectives in Prevention and Treatment of Cancer in the Elderly* (R. Yancik, ed.), Raven Press, New York, pp. 57-61.

Boyd, J. B., Bradford, B., Jr., and Watne, A. L. (1980). Operative risk factors of colon resection in the elderly, *Ann. Surg., 192*:743-746.

Bristow, M. R., Mason, J. W., Billingham, M. E., and Daniels, J. R. (1978). Doxorubicin cardiomyopathy: Evaluation by phonocardiography, endomyocardial biopsy, and cardiac catherization, *Ann. Intern. Med., 88*:168-175.

Brocklehurst, J. C. (1980). *Textbook of Geriatric Medicine and Gerontology,* 2nd Edition, Churchill Livingstone, Edinburgh.

Brown, J. T., and Stoudemire, G. A. (1983). Normal and pathological grief, *JAMA, 250*:378-382.

Butler, R. N. (1979). Aging and cancer management. III. Research perspectives, *CA, 29*: 333-340.

Caird, F. I., and Dall, J. L. C. (1980). *Textbook of Geriatric Medicine and Gerontology* (J. C. Brocklehurst, ed.), 2nd Edition, Churchill Livingstone, Edinburgh, pp. 125-153.

Candee, D., and Puka, A. B. (1984). An analytic approach to resolving problems in medical ethics, *J. Med. Ethics, 10*:61-70.

Carbone, P. P., and Begg, C. (1982). The elderly cancer patient and cancer therapy—The Eastern Cooperative Group experience, *The Gerontologist, 22*:76 (#29, abstract).

Cassileth, B. R., Zupkis, R. V., Sutton-Smith, K., and March, V. (1980). Information and participation preferences among cancer patients, *Ann. Intern. Med., 92*:832-836.

Ching, N., Grossi, C., Zurawinsky, H., Jham, G., Angers, J., Mills, C., and Nealon, J. F. (1979). Nutritional deficiencies and nutrition support therapy in geriatric cancer patients, *J. Am. Geriat. Soc., 27*:491-494.

Cohen, H. J., Silberman, H. R., Forman, W., Bartolucci, A., and Liu, C. (1983). Effects of age on responses to treatment and survival of patients with multiple myeloma, *J. Am. Geriat. Soc., 31*:272-277.

Davies, D. F., and Shock, N. W. (1950). Age changes in glomerular filtration rate, effective renal plasma flow and tubular excretory capacity in adult males, *J. Clin. Invest.*, *29*:496-507.

Dayan, A. D. (1980). Central nervous system, *Textbook of Geriatric Medicine and Gerontology*, 2nd Edition, Churchill Livingstone, Edinburgh, pp. 158-180.

Del Guercio, L. R. M., and Cohn, J. D. (1980). Monitoring operative risk in the elderly, *JAMA 243*:1350-1355.

Djokovic, J., and Hedley-Whyte, J. (1979). Prediction of outcome of surgery and anesthesia in patients over 80, *JAMA, 242*:2301-2306.

Engel, G. L. (1980). The clinical application of the biopsychosocial model, *Am. J. Psych., 137*:535-544.

Foon, K. A., Zighelboim, J., Yale, C., and Gale, R. P. (1981). Intensive chemotherapy is the treatment of choice for the elderly patients with acute myelogenous leukemia, *Blood, 58*:467-470.

Gilchrest, B. A. (1984). Age-associated changes in normal skin, *Skin and Aging Processes*, CRC Press, Boca Raton, Fla., pp. 17-35.

Ginsberg, S. J., and Comis, R. L. (1982). The pulmonary toxicity of anti-neoplastic agents, *Semin. Oncol., 9*:34-51.

Goldman, R. (1977). Aging of the excretory system, *Handbook of the Biology of Aging* (C. E. Finch, and L. Hayflick, eds.), Van Nostrand Reinhold, New York, pp. 409-431.

Goldman, L., Caldera, D. L., Nussbaum, S. R., Southwick, F. S., Krogstad, D., Murray, B., Burke, D. S., O'Malley, T. A., Goroli, A. H., Caplan, R. H., Nolan, J., Carabello, B., and Slater, E. E. (1977). Multifactorial index of cardiac risk in noncardiac surgical procedures, *New Engl.J. Med., 297*: 845-850.

Goldman, L. (1983). Cardiac risks and complications of noncardiac surgery, *Ann. Intern. Med., 98*:504-513.

Greenblatt, R. B. (1978). *Geriatric Endocrinology*, Raven Press, New York.

Gunn, W. G. (1980). Radiation therapy for the aging patient, *CA, 30*:337-347.

Gutheil, T. G., and Applebaum, P. S. (1982). *Clinical Handbook of Psychiatry and the Law*, McGraw-Hill, New York, pp. 210-252.

Harkins, S. W., and Warner, M. H. (1980). Age and pain, *Ann. Rev. Gerontol. Geriat., 1*:121-131.

Hayflick, L. (1977). The cellular basis for biological aging, *Handbook of the Biology of Aging* (C. E. Finch, and L. Hayflick, eds.), Van Nostrand Reinhold, New York, pp. 159-168.

Hayflick, L., and Moorhead, P. S. (1961). The serial cultivation of human diploid cell strains, *Exp. Cell Res., 25*:585-621.

Herbsman, H., Feldman, J., Seldera, J., Gardner, B., and Alfonso, A. E. (1981). Survival following breast cancer surgery in the elderly, *Cancer, 47*:2358-2363.

Holland, J. F., and Frei, E. (1982). *Cancer Medicine*, Lea & Febiger, Philadelphia.

Holland, J. F. (1981). Cancer in the aged, *Mt. Sinai J. Med., 48*:496-499.

Holmes, F. (1983). *Recent Results in Cancer Research, Aging and Cancer,* Vol. 87, Springer-Verlag, New York.

Holmes, F. F., and Hearne, I. E. (1981). Cancer stage-to-age relationship: Implications for cancer screening in the elderly, *J. Am. Geriat. Soc., 29*: 55-57.

Jacknowitz, A. I. (1984). Gastrointestinal disorders, *Current Geriatric Therapy* (T. R. Covington and J. I. Walker eds.), W. B. Saunders, Philadelphia, pp. 178-238.

Jahnigen, D. W., and Laforce, F. M. (1982). Little things, *Clinical Internal Medicine in the Aged* (R. W. Schrier, ed.), W. B. Saunders, Philadelphia, pp. 305-316.

Johnson, J. C. (1983). The medical evaluation and management of the elderly surgical patient, *J. Am. Geriat. Soc., 31*:611-625.

Kaiko, R. F. (1980). Age and morphine analgesia in cancer patients with postoperative pain, *Clin. Pharmacol. Ther., 28*:823-826.

Kane, R. A. (1983). Coordination of cancer treatment and social support for the elderly, *Perspectives on Prevention and Treatment of Cancer in the Elderly* (R. Yancik, ed.), Raven Press, New York, pp. 227-237.

Kane, R. L., Ouslander, J. G., and Abrass, I. B. (1984). *Essentials of Clinical Geriatrics,* McGraw-Hill, New York.

Kaplan, H. G. (1984). Use of cancer chemotherapy in the elderly, *Drug Treatment in the Elderly* (R. E. Vestal, ed.), ADIS Health Science Press, Sydney, pp. 338-349.

Kark, A. E., and Wardle, D. F. G. (1980). Management of malignant disease in old age, *The Treatment of Medical Problems in the Elderly* (M. J. Denham, ed.), University Park Press, Baltimore.

Keczkes, K., and Basheer, A. M. (1980). Do corticosteroids prevent post-herpetic neuralgia?, *Brit. J. Dermatol., 102*:551-555.

Klein, N. E. (1983). Pain in the concept, *Supportive Care of the Cancer Patient* (P. H. Wiernik, ed.), Futura Publishing Co., Mt. Kisco, N.Y., pp. 173-208.

Klocke, R. A. (1977). Influence of aging on the lung, *Handbook of the Biology of Aging* (C. E. Finch, and L. Hayflick, eds.), Van Nostrand Reinhold, New York, pp. 432-444.

Kohn, R. R. (1977). Heart and cardiovascular system, *Handbook of the Biology of Aging* (C. E. Finch, and L. Hayflick, eds.), Van Nostrand Reinhold, New York, pp. 281-317.

Kübler-Ross, E. (1969). *Death and Dying,* Macmillan, New York.

Lancet, E. (1976). Aging and cancer (editorial), *Lancet, 1*:131.

Laszlo, J., and Lucas, V. S. (1981). Emesis as a critical problem in chemotherapy, *New Engl. J. Med., 305*:948-949.

Leeming, J. T., and Dymock, I. W. (1980). Investigation of the elderly patient with suspected upper gastrointestinal disease, *Textbook of Geriatric Medicine and Gerontology* (J. C. Brocklehurst, ed.), 2nd Edition, Churchill Livingstone, Edinburgh, pp. 344-357.

Lewis, C., Linet, M. S., and Abeloff, M. D. (1983). Compliance with cancer therapy by patients and physicians, *Am. J. Med., 74*:673-678.

Libow, L. S., and Sherman, F. T. (1981). *The Core of Geriatric Medicine,* C. V. Mosby, St. Louis.

Lipschitz, D. A., and Thompson, C. (1980). Leukocyte reserve in anemia elderly, *Clin. Res., 28*:218A.

Lipschitz, D. A., McGinnis, S. K., and Udupa, K. B. (1983). The use of long-term bone marrow culture as a model of the aging process, *Age, 6*: 122-127.

Lipschitz, D. A., Udupa, K. B., Milton, K. Y., and Thompson, C. O. (1984). Effect of age on hematopoiesis in man, *Blood, 63*:502-509.

Lucas, R., and Brown, C. (1982). Assessment of cancer patients, *Assessment Strategies in Behavioral Medicine* (F. J. Keefe and J. A. Blumenthal, eds.), Grune & Stratton, New York, pp. 351-369.

Makinodan, T. (1977). Immunity and aging, *Handbook of the Biology of Aging* (C. E. Finch, and L. Hayflick, eds.), Van Nostrand Reinhold, New York, pp. 379-408.

Manousos, O. N., Truelove, S. C., and Lumsden, K. (1967). Prevalence of colonic diverticulosis in general population of Oxford area, *Brit. Med. J., 3*:762-763.

Marlin, D. H. (1983). Protective service: Legal aspects, *Clinical Aspects of Aging* (W. Reichel, ed.), Williams & Wilkins, Baltimore, pp. 540-542.

Mauch, P., Botnick, L. E., Hannon, E. C., Obbagy, J., and Hellman, S. (1982). Decline in bone marrow proliferation capacity as a function of age, *Blood, 60*:245-252.

McCullough, L. B. (1984). Medical care for elderly patients with diminished competence on ethical analysis, *J. Am. Geriat. Soc., 32*:150-153.

McEvoy, A. (1983). Bacterial contamination of the small intestine is an important cause of occult malabsorption in the elderly, *Brit. Med. J., 287*: 789-793.

McGivney, W. T., and Crooks, G. M. (1984). The care of patients with severe chronic pain in terminal illness, *JAMA, 751*:1182-1188.

Merselis, J. G., Jr., Kaye, D., and Hook, E. W. (1964). Disseminated herpes zoster, *Arch. Intern. Med., 113*:679-686.

Meyer, B. R., Lewin, M., Drayer, D. E., Pasmantier, M., Lonski, L., and Reidenberg, M. M. (1984). Optimizing metoclopramide control of cisplatin-induced emesis, *Ann. Intern. Med., 100*:393-395.

Mor, V., Laliberte, L., Morris, J. N., and Wiemann, M. (1984). The Karnofsky Performance Status Scale: An examination of its reliability and validity in a research setting, *Cancer, 53*:2002-2007.

Nagami, P. H., and Yoshikawa, T. T. (1983). Tuberculosis in the geriatric patient, *J. Am. Geriat. Soc., 31*:356-363.

Ochoa, J., and Mair, W. C. P. (1969). The normal sural nerve in man. II. Changes in the axons and Schwann cells due to aging, *Acta Neuropath. Berlin, 13*:217-239.

Ordy, J. M., Harman, D., and Alfin-Slater, R. B. (1984). *Nutrition in Gerontology*, Raven Press, New York, pp. 4-13.

Ouslander, J. G. (1981). Drug therapy in the elderly, *Ann. Intern. Med.*, 95:711-722.

Perry, M. C. (1982). Toxicity of chemotherapy, *Semin. Oncol.*, 9:1-149.

Peterson, B. A. (1982). Acute nonlymphocytic leukemia in the elderly: Biology and treatment, *Acute Leukemia I* (C. P. Bloomfield, ed.), Martinus Nijhoff Publishers, Boston.

Peterson, B. A., Pajak, T. F., Cooper, M. R., Nissen, N. I., Glidewell, D. J., Holland, J. F., Bloomfield, C. D., and Gottlieb, A. J. (1982a). Effect of age on therapeutic response and survival in advanced Hodgkin's disease, *Cancer Treat. Rep.*, 66:889-898.

Pfeiffer, E. (1975). A short portable mental status questionnaire for the assessment of organic brain deficit in elderly patients, *J. Am. Geriat. Soc.*, 23:433-441.

Phair, J. P. (1983). Host defenses in the aged in infections in the elderly, *Infections in the Elderly* (R. A. Gleckman, and N. M. Gantz, eds.), Little, Brown, Boston, pp. 1-12.

Pitot, H. C. (1977). Carcinogenesis and aging: Two-related phenomena?, *Am. J. Path.*, 87:444-472.

Praga, C., Beretta, G., Vigo, P. L., Lenaz, G. R., Pollini, C., Bonadonna, G., Canetta, R., Castellani, R., Villa, E., Gallagher, C. G., von Melehner, H., Hayat, M., Riband, P., De Wasch, G., Mattsson, W., Heinz, R., Waldner, R., Kolaric, K., Buehner, R., Ten Bokkel-Huyninck, W., Pererodehikova, N. I., Manziuk, L. A., Senn, H. J., and Mayr, A. C. (1979). Adriamycin cardiotoxicity: A survey of 1273 patients, *Cancer Treat. Rep.*, 63:827-834.

Prusiner, S. B. (1984). Some speculation about prions, amyloid and Alzheimer's disease, *New Engl. J. Med.*, 310:661-662.

Reincke, U., Hannon, E. C., Rosenblatt, M., and Hellman, S. (1982). Proliferative capacity of murine hematopoietic stem cells in vitro, *Science*, 215:1619-1622.

Rimer, B., Jones, W., Wilson, C., Bennett, D., and Engstrom, P. (1983). Planning a cancer control program for older citizens, *The Gerontologist, 23*: 384-389.

Roberts, S. H. (1977). Bacterial overgrowth syndrome without blind loop: A cause of malnutrition in the elderly, *Lancet, 1*:1193-1195.

Rockstein, M., Chesky, J. A., and Sussman, M. L. (1977). *Handbook of the Biology of Aging* (C. E. Finch, and L. Hayflick, eds.), Van Nostrand Reinhold, New York, pp. 3-28.

Rodstein, M. (1981). Heart disease in the elderly, *Cardiovascular Aspects of Geriatric Medicine* (L. Libow, ed.), Hoffman-LaRoche, Inc., Nutley, N.J. pp. 7-41.

Rutquist, L. E., Wallgren, A., and Nilsson, B. (1984). Is breast cancer a curable disease: A study of 14,731 women with breast cancer from the cancer registry of Norway, *Cancer, 53*:1793-1800.

Santos, A. L., and Gelperin, A. (1975). Surgical mortality in the elderly, *J. Am. Geriat. Soc., 23*:42-46.

Schag, C., Heinrich, R. L., and Ganz, P. (1984). Karnofsky Performance Status revisited: Reliability, validity and guidelines, *J. Clin. Oncol., 2*:187-193.

Shein, C. J. (1979). A selective approach to surgical problems in the aged, *Clinical Geriatrics* (I. Rossman, ed.), J. P. Lippincott, Philadelphia.

Schnaper, N., Legg-McNamara, C., Dutcher, J., and Kellner, T. K. (1983). Emotional support of the patient and his survivors, *Supportive Care of the Cancer Patient* (P. H. Wiernik, ed.), Futura Publishing Company, Mt. Kisco, N.Y., pp. 1-16.

Schneider, E. L. (1983). Infectious disease in the elderly, *Ann. Intern. Med., 98*:395-400.

Sklar, M. (1983). Gastrointestinal disease in the aged, *Clinical Aspects of Aging* (W. Reichel, ed.), Williams & Wilkins, Baltimore, pp. 205-217.

Smith, I. M. (1983). Infectious disease problems in the elderly, *Clinical Aspects of Aging* (W. Reichel, ed.), Williams & Wilkins, Baltimore, pp. 218-233.

Smith, K. C. (1978). Aging, carcinogenesis and radiation biology, *Prog. Biochem. Pharmacol., 14*:70-75.

Smith, S. M. (1983). Competency, *Psychiat. Clin. North Am., 6*:625-650.

Sourander, L. B. (1980). The genito-urinary system, *Textbook of Geriatric Medicine and Gerontology,* 2nd Edition, Churchill Livingstone, Edinburgh, pp. 291-306.

Thoman, M. L., and Weigle, W. O. (1982). Cell mediated immunity in aged mice: An underlying lesion in IL-2 synthesis, *J. Immunol., 128*:2358-2361.

Thoman, M. L., and Weigle, W. O. (1983). Deficiency in suppressor T-cell activity in aged animals, reconstitution of this activity by Interleukin-II, *J. Exper. Med., 157*:2184-2189.

Till, G., and Ward, P. (1975). Two distinct chemostatic factors in human serum, *J. Immunol., 114*:843-847.

Torti, F. M., and Carter, S. K. (1980). The chemotherapy of prostatic adenocarcinoma, *Ann. Intern. Med., 92*:681-689.

Tonnesen, M. G., and Weston, W. L. (1982). Aging of skin, *Clinical Internal Medicine in the Aged* (R. W. Schrier, ed.), W. B. Saunders, Philadelphia, pp. 296-303.

Turnbull, A. D., Gundy, E., Howland, W. S., and Beattie, E. J., Jr. (1978). Surgical mortality among the elderly. An analysis of 4,050 operations (1970-1974), *Clin. Bull., 8*:139-142.

Twycross, R. G. (1984). Control of pain, *J. Royal Coll. Phys. London, 18*: 32-39.

Verwoerdt, A. (1981). *Clinical Geropsychiatry,* 2nd Edition, Williams & Wilkins, Baltimore, pp. 130-141.

Weisfeldt, M. L. (1980). *The Aging Heart,* Raven Press, New York.

Weksler, M. E. (1981). The senescence of the immune system, *Hosp. Pract., 16(10)*:53-64.

Weksler, M. E. (1982). Age-associated changes in the immune response, *J. Am. Geriat. Soc., 30*:718-723.

Williams, M. E. (1984). Clinical implications of aging physiology, *Am. J. Med.*, 76:1049-1054.

Wolcott, L. E. (1983). Rehabilitation in the aged, *Clinical Aspects of Aging* (W. Reichel, ed.), Williams & Wilkins, Baltimore, pp. 182-204.

Wretlind, A. (1981). Parenteral nutrition, *Nutr. Rev.*, 39:257-265.

Young, V. R. (1983). Some nutritional considerations with reference to treatment prevention of cancer in the elderly, *Perspectives on Prevention and Treatment of Cancer in the Elderly* (R. Yancik, ed.), Raven Press, New York, pp. 189-201.

Zboralske, F. F., Amberg, J. R., and Soergel, K. H. (1964). Presbyesophagus, cineradiographic manifestations, *Radiology, 82*:463-467.

11

Support Services for Hospitalized Patients

Beverly K. Rosen, Louise Bost, and Paul W. Aitken
Duke University Medical Center, Durham, North Carolina

I. FAMILY SUPPORT: A HIDDEN ALLY (OR ANTAGONIST?) IN CANCER CARE*

A. Introduction

It is frequently written that cancer is a family disease, and like other serious and prolonged illnesses, it is a source of severe stress that demands major adjustments, not only by the patient but by family members. Concerns about family complications in cancer care have increased in the last decade as major research studies have attempted to document the "impact, costs, and consequences," and multiple problems that cancer imposes on family functioning (Cancer Care, Inc., 1973; Gordon et al., 1980; Greenleigh, 1979). These studies indicate that cancer disrupts personal functioning; work; marital and family relationships; educational plans; career advancements; financial stability; social and sexual relationships; and can lead to multiple health and emotional adjustment problems for family members.

While clinical concerns about the harmful and stressful effects of cancer treatment on the family have increased, so has the recognition that although stressed and distressed themselves, the family is becoming more and more an integral participant in the comprehensive care of the cancer patient. While some authors feel that evaluation of the cancer patient cannot be considered complete unless family members are included, most caregivers agree that cancer management requires major participation by the family. Rosenbaum

---

*This section was written by Beverly K. Rosen.

and Rosenbaum (1980) claim that traditionally the patient's family was over-looked as a resource in the planned treatment process. They were asked to "wait outside;" the patient was expected to keep the family informed. This concept is now as archaic as the passive patient.

First of all, family support is now recognized as a critical factor in predict-ing how patients will cope with the treatment process (Weisman, Worden, and Sobel, 1980). Virtually all studies that examine predictors of good coping and adjustment to cancer have found that individuals who are able to maintain close interpersonal relationships with family and friends despite their illness are more likely to cope effectively with their disease (Wortman and Dunkel-Schetter, 1979; Weisman, 1974). Second, how a cancer patient adjusts to and manages his/her treatment course is dependent, in part, on the behavior of the individuals closest to him/her (Cohen, 1982; Kaplan, 1982). A woman's re-action to breast cancer and surgery, e.g., may affect the response of her family and the response of her family may in turn affect her ability to cope (Spiegel, Bloom, and Gottheil, 1983). Third, the nuclear family continues to remain the most important social support source for the patient and has the most powerful effect on mediating and buffering the multiple stresses of cancer treatment. A life-threatening illness is an event that forces the patient to rely even more on family resources, and studies show that family members have the most sustained contact with the patient (Aitken-Swan, 1959; Binger et al., 1969; Klein, Dean, and Bogdonoff, 1967; Dyk and Sutherland, 1956).

Finally, health professionals need the family's support as a necessary ally in cancer care. Family members pressure the patient to seek out initial medical examinations for cancer treatment; they participate in the therapeutic decisions made by the patient; they provide the practical and financial assistance for patients to receive cancer therapy; and they can provide care-givers the best information about the patient as an individual. If health pro-fessionals do not utilize this potential ally well, they will waste a valuable resource that can facilitate the patient's recovery.

Family support, however, is not the same as family availability, and the mere presence of a large and hovering group of individuals in a waiting room does not necessarily mean access to helpful social resources on whom the patient and professional can rely in the treatment process. A family can either facilitate or obstruct the cancer patient's efforts to master the task of coping with cancer. Therefore, knowing how to mobilize and strengthen the family's support potential is an effective preventative tool in cancer care. This section will examine the function of the cancer family as the patient's source of social support, discuss common complications in this process, and review how caregivers can use preventative interventions with families to enhance the patient's adjustment, compliance, and response to his/her care.

B. Social Support and Cancer

There has been increasing evidence that points to social support playing a central role not only in preventing disease and maintaining health but also in alleviating the impact of illness on both the stricken individual and those close to him/her (Bloom, 1982). Research by Cobb (1976); Kaplan, Cassel, and Gore (1977); and Dean and Lin (1977) has emphasized the stress buffering role of an individual's social support system with health problems. They define this concept in terms of the protective psychological process that social supports provide in the presence of stressful situations.

Since cancer precipitates a highly stressful situation, it is no surprise that during the last decade, investigations of social support have begun to appear in the cancer literature and social support systems have been increasingly identified as critical elements in determining how a patient will cope (Revenson, Wollman, and Felton, 1983). Wortman and Dunkel-Schetter (1979) comprehensively reviewed all available literature on interpersonal relationships and cancer, and found that there is apparently a positive relationship between the quality of the patient's interpersonal relationships and his/her ability to cope with the illness. However, at the same time, they found that cancer patients have considerable difficulty in their interpersonal relationships because of their disease. Weisman and Worden (1976) observed 120 cancer patients for a 3-4 month period immediately after diagnosis and found that the presence of interpersonal support was viewed as a psychological asset that contributed to successful coping.

Woods and Earp (1978) made similar findings for post-mastectomy patients. Their study of women 4 years after breast surgery showed that social support mediated the effect of surgical complications and the mental outlook of the mastectomy patients. Clark (1983), in a study of 171 cancer patients examining the importance of one's social environment in the adaptation to specific problems related to cancer, concluded that a "strong interpersonal support system is a psychosocial asset for cancer patients." Furthermore, the evaluation of the social environment is important in identifying high risk patients whose potential for adaptation may be impaired. Cohen and Wellisch (1978) observed that the more that family members were able to share information and communicate with one another, the greater the likelihood families could adjust effectively after the death of the cancer patient.

There may be many sources of social support for the cancer patient such as his treatment team, spouse, family, friends, neighbors, community groups, and institutions. Whether certain behaviors are perceived to be supportive by the cancer patient may depend on who is offering the support (Wortman, 1984). In a study of perceived support among patients with breast or colorectal malignancies, Dunkel-Schetter (1981) found that advice was perceived as very helpful when provided by the physician but was regarded as not helpful when offered by relatives.

Not only does every patient's need for support vary over time, but different types of support are needed for reducing different areas of cancer-related stress. Distinct types of social support include maintenance of social identity, emotional support, tangible and environmental support, and informational support. A cancer patient who is very ill or is experiencing physical changes may find emotional support quite necessary. Alternatively, for a patient who has been hospitalized a long time and is distressed about role requirements he/she cannot meet, tangible help may be more comforting than reassurance (Cohen and Wills, 1983).

While the relevance, magnitude, source, and type of social support wanted and needed will vary with the individual, the uncertainties and fears experienced by a cancer patient result in an enhanced need for overall social support for many disease-related reasons. First, as the cancer patient contends with anxieties about pain, physical changes, treatments, or recurrence, the need for emotional support increases. Second, perhaps with no other disease, the societal attitudes toward cancer and its etiology form the interpersonal experience of the cancer patient and his/her family. The intense stigma still associated with a cancer diagnosis and the lingering myth of contagion make cancer patients fear rejection and isolation. In fact, this is one of the greatest fears patients have during the early stages of cancer (Sutherland and Orbach, 1953). Hence this creates a greater need to maintain one's social identity through social support. Third, given the multiple demands of cancer treatment regimens and the potentially incapacitating side effects of the treatment there is increased need for tangible support. Fourth, there are many new decisions to be made concerning cancer treatment choices, physician and treatment center selection, equipment purchases, job decisions, financial applications, etc., which all require social activities due to illness and treatment may lead inevitably to reduced social support from friends. For all of these reasons, family support can become a critical factor for the cancer patient.

C. The Family: The Hidden Ally in Social Support

The cancer caregiver needs the family to be their ally for there are many ways that the family can prevent complications in the patient's medical management. The family may be crucial in getting the patient to seek medical treatment for cancer once it is recommended. In a study by Michielutti (1976) of 242 cancer patients who delayed seeking care, he found the three most important variables were education, frequency of visits from relatives, and whether someone encouraged him/her to see the doctor. The last two variables suggest family interaction may be the key factor in encouraging people to follow through with medical recommendations to seek cancer care. Once the diagnosis has occurred, family support can influence how the event can be appraised. Integrating the reality of having cancer can be quite anxiety provoking, particularly when the patient is socially isolated or lacks emotional support from the family (Noble and Hamilton, 1983). Family members can influence how threatening the diagnosis is viewed by the patient by providing information about the disease or the resources available to cope with stress, such as where to obtain a wig for hair loss. If the treatment plan is interpreted to both the patient and the family, frequently it will be the family member who will hear and remember it better and can help correct the patient's distortions or encourage him/her to ask necessary and clarifying questions.

The family can help encourage treatment compliance in several ways. As Cobb (1976) states, feelings of obligation to family members can encourage patients to keep going when the going gets rough, to maintain chemotherapy regimens, exercise, nutrition, or other different treatments. If a patient's family understands the ramifications of compliance and encourages it, the patient's chances of following medical treatment are increased. Alternatively, family members can also interfere with treatment compliance if not provided with knowledge. If they do not understand medical procedures, they may not be able to offer encouragement or support, such as interpreting the tiredness that normally accompanies chemotherapy as laziness (Wortman and Dunkel-Schetter, 1979). Family issues are often the key to understanding refusal of treatment. The patient may be fearful of burdening his/her family. Family myths about illness may be a powerful determinant of a patient's behavior, or a patient's refusal may be a displacement of anger for some family problem (Goldberg, 1983). Therefore, difficulties in noncompliance are more likely to occur where there is family disharmony, instability, or lack of family support (Gillum and Barsky, 1974).

Finally, family support can help resist the tendency to a marked lowering of self-esteem, a precursor of depression in cancer care (Caplan, 1976). When family members appear relatively calm and reassuring, it may moderate the cancer patient's emotional arousal, and keep it within manageable limits during treatment.

D. Complications in Family Support: Three Case Examples

The "Overcompensating Smotherers"

There is strong clinical evidence that interpersonal relationships for the cancer patient may often act as a source of stress as well as a source of support. Social interactions between family members and cancer patients are often colored with ambivalence and family members may have vast discrepancies between their outward behavior and inner feelings (Wortman and Dunkel-Schetter, 1979). Social support by families may create a process whereby cancer patients are victimized by ineffective efforts to help, such as the "overcompensating smotherers."

During the first day of a course of inpatient chemotherapy for Mr. S, a newly diagnosed 62-year-old man with Hodgkin's disease, the staff was greeted at the door by his wife, Mrs. S, a hostile, protective, obese woman, and her nervous 34-year-old daughter. At home, the daughter lived with her parents and was their sole provider. She worked as a discharge planner in the local hospital. At the treatment center, the daughter's role was to stop, screen, and interrogate each staff member as to their function and purpose. The wife had moved the patient's bed away from the window to prevent pneumonia, although this made it farther for the patient to walk to the bathroom. The patient, at first, acquiesced to the family's blocking his communications with his physicians. When asked about his understanding of the therapy plan, he said, "Mama will tell me what needs to be done," referring to his wife. The daughter made unreasonable requests on the staff, insisting that only one nurse knew how to insert an I.V. without hurting her father. Mr. S, over time, became increasingly demanding on his family, making his daughter feel responsible for hospital delays and demanding special foods that he then refused to eat. As he became more angry and dissatisfied with his family's efforts, they became more confused and hurt by him. Meantime, his daughter's daily presence was jeopardizing her job at home. The staff felt they needed to understand more about this complex family's background to know how to assist them with their problems in family support. A family history revealed a life-long pattern of a passive, dependent alcoholic patient with weakened marital ties. The daughter revealed that she felt extremely helpless and hence threatened outside her own hospital system, and felt enormously burdened by the responsibilities she thought she had to perform. Understanding the vulnerability of this family for providing effective social support, the staff set up a brief weekly conference time for Mrs. S to talk with a nurse about the patient's needs. The trust that ensued from this increased contact with the nursing staff allowed the wife to participate in the weekly cancer ward support group. This provided her with some structured time away from the patient and the opportunity to gain a better understanding of normal reactions to cancer as well as peer support from the other families. Through further individual counseling sessions, Mrs. S began to express directly her negative feelings about the patient and began to modify her covert hostile behavior. While the daughter did decide to return home to her job, separation from her parents was very traumatic. She was given a copy of the treatment protocol in order for her to be able to understand and follow her father's treatments and she was sent home with instructions to plan for the patient's home care needs. This task allowed her to feel she was doing something competently to hasten his recovery.

When families react to the cancer diagnosis, some of the behaviors can include both covert and overt hostility, depression, panic, guilt, and the inability to resume normal activities. The S family exhibited many of these reactions. They tended to be too close, to pamper the patient, overwhelming him in an effort to ward off guilt feelings about their past relationship. This behavior tended to increase the patient's depression as well as deplete the family. The staff mitigated these problems by limiting their own expectations of change for this family based on the family assessment; helped them understand the patient's real needs for help through education; and reduced their anxiety with increased contact with the staff, structured activities, and peer support.

The "Denying Helpers"

There is a tendency for families to operate according to a set of rules designed to minimize discomfort, and the discussion of true emotions between the cancer patient and his/her family is often very difficult. Families have a natural need to protect the patient from the realities of cancer and to feel it is essential to remain cheerful and optimistic. Yet while the negative feelings of anger, sadness, and depression may be too difficult to express, this may result in family support problems by the "denying helper."

Mrs. R was a 50-year-old woman undergoing therapy for recurrent breast cancer. Mr. and Mrs. R had the utmost confidence in their physician. They felt he had "cured" Mrs. R after her mastectomy 5 years ago. The Rs were quite wealthy and were active in local cancer fund-raising events. It was a tremendous shock to both of them when, during a routine checkup, positive lung metastases were found on the chest x-ray. During daily radiation therapy visits, Mr. R voiced extreme optimism, cutting off any teariness from his wife with assurances about recent advances in cancer treatment. Mrs. R, who was worried about her husband's heart condition, tended to keep her distress from him and her physician, fearing that they would both regard her as a nuisance. As Mrs. R's disease progressed and did not respond to therapy, Mr. R continued to minimize her physical problems, fearing she would terminate all treatment. He would tell the physician what a good "trooper" she was and that he felt she would never give up fighting. He did focus on her refusal to eat and went through elaborate efforts to prepare uneaten gourmet meals. The clinic nurse and social worker provided supportive counseling to

Mrs. R and her son and daughter-in-law, but were unable to involve Mr. R. It was obvious that in this family the provider and recipient of support differed in the perception of what was supportive, and the well-intended efforts of Mr. R to keep up his wife's spirits were resulting in reduced self-esteem and isolation. Given the potential for continued problems in honest communication, the physician called the family together for a family interview. The physician, who was a powerful figure for Mr. R, was able to serve as a catalyst in helping the family discuss the realities of the patient's disease and side effects of her therapy. During the interview, Mr. R was shocked to learn that his wife and children had been discussing plans for future terminal care. After several family sessions with the physician, Mrs. R was able to be more direct with her husband about her needs and felt she could express her true feelings without fear of rejection. Mr. R was better able to work with the public health nurse and dietitian to provide realistic and supportive home care.

Bringing a family together for such a discussion can be of great value in mitigating communication problems within a family and the importance of the medical physician in facilitating this process is often overlooked or minimized (Worby and Babineau, 1974). As the chief health care provider, the physician can evoke special responses from a family based on what he/she says, and his/her suggestions will have a great impact in a supportive climate. Families frequently believe that any discussion about death will be intolerable and they worry that they will break down and betray their feelings (Parkes, 1972). Studies find that discussion about illness in general is frequently guarded and confused in late stage disease (Krant and Johnston, 1978). When there is progression or recurrence of disease, family members should have a renewed opportunity to meet and discuss their fears with the physician and be taught how to minimize disruptive effects on the marital relationship and the patient him/herself.

The "Rejecting Avoiders"

While most families initially mobilize around the cancer patient to obtain services and treatment, some are temporarily immobilized and flounder and others may reject the patient and abandon him. There are families who are emotionally unsupportive and tend to evade, shun, or neglect the patient either because they were never close, they fear catching cancer, or they want to protect themselves from hurt by giving the patient up at an early stage. The treatment team can become the patient's surrogate family, but only after they have evaluated their own motivations and interventions and assessed what might be workable for the patient and family.

Miss K was a 16-year-old newly diagnosed young woman with acute myelogenous leukemia. She was the oldest of five children from a low-income family where both parents worked alternating plant shifts. She was admitted for inpatient chemotherapy and ended up staying in the hospital for 5 months before obtaining a partial remission. During that time, her parents claimed they could only afford the time and money to see her once or twice a month. She was a very quiet, somewhat passive young woman, who apparently caused her family much embarrassment by becoming pregnant in high school. She frequently spent her time watching the soap operas on a portable television given to her by her boyfriend. He attempted to see her as much as possible, but worked two jobs and did not own a car. The patient had little money to spend on long-distance calls. She became increasingly detached, depressed, and nonverbal as time wore on. All attempts by the nursing staff and intern to increase her parent's involvement or visitation failed, and after enough pressure, they became openly hostile and defensive. They claimed they had no money and had to attend to the needs of the other children. The staff was becoming increasingly frustrated and tended to project their anger by overwhelming the patient with their concern and pressuring her to talk about her feelings towards her parents. A ward meeting was held to discuss what problems the staff, patient, and family might be getting into and to assess their motivations and behaviors with the patient. Plans were made to provide a more relaxed atmosphere for the patient, for the staff realized they needed to reduce the emotional charge of the family situation for the patient. Miss K was additionally referred to the cancer recreation therapy program where peer volunteers could provide diversion and company. The social worker was designated the main liaison contact with the family as she could provide the tangible assistance that the family and boyfriend needed and wanted for gas and lodging. This resulted in increased weekend visits.

Not every family can be open and loving to every cancer patient, and it is difficult for staff to work with families when they have their own ideal preference for family support. It was impossible to penetrate the Ks' family system where offers of help were interpreted as intrusion by others and parental failure. For families with preexistent intergenerational problems, providing concrete services may develop a sense of trust and decrease family stress. Creative interventions for alternate forms of support may need to be the goal.

E. Preventative Interventions for Maximizing Family Support

Family Assessment

Caregivers need to understand the cancer family's interactions if its members
are to be assisted with the cancer experience. Too often when we attempt
to inquire about the patient's family background, network, styles of communication, and past and present level of functioning, we do so without explaining why we are asking these questions, or by "interviewing" them. The staff
then takes their information and makes an intervention plan based on their own
beliefs about what help the family may need without allying the family in this
process. Since studies (Weisman, Worden, and Sobel, 1980) have shown that
family assessment of social support is a good predictor of future emotional
stress, the best way to do a family assessment is to explain this rationale and
allow the family to participate with open and clear objectives.

Many offices, clinics, and hospital centers do not have the ideal situation
where well-trained personnel have the time to meet with each family to do a
"participatory self-assessment" soon after diagnosis, or administer a validated
instrument such as the family environment scale (Moos and Moos, 1981).
Alternative strategies can include training office or ward personnel to administer a simple family support screening questionnaire which can include the
following question areas: (1) Who does the patient define as his family?
(2) Who are some significant others? (3) Who does the family/patient perceive
to be the major decision makers and stabilizers? (4) How does information get
communicated and problems resolved in the family? (5) What are the family's
proximity and availability? (6) What are the family's beliefs and past history
with cancer treatment? Other factors that can be assessed include marital
structure, religious beliefs, ethnic and cultural orientation, description of
residence and home community, financial resources, insurance coverage, premorbid family problems, and potential extrafamilial support and assistance.
Utilizing public health nurses to further evaluate potentially vulnerable
families through home visits and observation has been a useful tool (Wellisch,
1984). In any case, every cancer treatment team needs to have systematic
and routine methods for screening families at risk for complications in social
support.

Family Counseling

Early detection of potential problems and high risk families should be followed
by psychological services that are made available immediately and provided
routinely. In one needs survey (Greenleigh, 1979), many families stated that
they would have liked to talk with a mental health professional about their
concerns but were fearful of being stigmatized. Patients frequently complain
of a lack of understanding and support from their spouses and decreased ability

to communicate with them (Lee and Maguire, 1975; Meyerowitz, 1980; Silberfarb, Maurer, and Crouthamel, 1980). It is important that families are routinely offered these services with the sanction and authority of their physician and that they know these services are regularly needed and used by many families coping with cancer. Whether it is several family interviews using a short-term crisis intervention model, or in-depth, long-term family therapy, both can help make cancer patients and families aware of complications that may exist in their social environment, and encourage resolution. Unfortunately, while the physician is central to providing the cancer treatment, he/she is not always trained in the psychosocial aspects of medicine, yet third-party health coverage for nonphysical services are not conducive to the resolution of social problems. Despite this, timely intervention with families can relieve their burdens of guilt and anxiety, foster better communication, and help prevent future support complications.

Family Education

Caregivers need to know how to mobilize existing family resources by making them active and educated members of the treatment team. Education needs to be offered on three levels. First, the modern cancer treatment system is complex and families need to learn the role and function of the team members with a translation of their services. This can be done by orientation and written materials or via orientation support groups such as those held prior to admission at Memorial Sloan-Kettering Cancer Center in New York.

Second, families need to be provided with hands-on information about the course of illness, the cancer diagnosis, the treatment sequence, the potential side effects, and the ways in which they can be involved and active in the physical care of the patient where appropriate. Whereas some caregivers may be reluctant to discuss undesirable side affects or negative emotions unless requested, Mitchell and Glicksman (1977) found that many family members felt it was inappropriate to express their own concerns to doctors for fear they were too busy or would react negatively. Information can do much to alleviate family members' anxiety and correct misconceptions and is especially good for those who handle crises intellectually. While many caregivers present the initial diagnosis and treatment information to the patient and family in an initial meeting, it is imperative to plan for follow-up meetings in order to give the family as much information as possible which they can hear and remember. This legitimizes the family as part of the treatment team and helps them support the patient.

Third, families need to understand not only the nature of the disease and the medical procedures, but also the common emotional reactions to cancer in order to offer encouragement and support. If they attribute the patient's negative feelings and fears to their own inadequacy, they may become unwilling or unable to help. With regard to primary prevention, families need to be both psychologically prepared and medically educated in a sensitive manner for the stresses they may encounter.

Supporting the Supporters

Helping family members to support each other and to effectively use other sources of support is essential to preventing family burnout. Families of cancer patients may be strained, anxious, and fearful about the patient but too guilt ridden and burdened to attend to their own needs. Research on long-term problems of social support documents the deleterious consequences on providers' mental and physical health and the frequent cycling of the cancer process can cause extreme fatigue. Dimatteo and Hayes (1981) found that the extent to which family members may support a patient may depend on the degree of support they receive in turn. This can be provided in several ways.

Families need to receive a consistent message from the treatment team that illness should not deprive the family of all pleasurable activities or totally disrupt the household. There needs to be some balance between the efforts devoted to cancer and the treatment and the continuation of normal living. During remission, there needs to be some relief from the illness and a period of replenishment, instead of totally focusing on the possibility of recurrence.

In the hospital, all efforts should be directed towards maintaining family solidarity even though the treatment of the patient may necessitate long stays away from home. Patients should be encouraged and assisted in making long-distance calls and hanging family pictures on the wall. Caregivers should avoid segregating and isolating family members who may be remaining with the patient for in- or outpatient treatment by encouraging frequent visits from other family members.

While social agencies do not assume the responsibility for the family, family members do need information about outside groups wich can be available to augment their support. It is important to correct faulty assumptions that government programs are available to totally cover patients' physical, emotional, and financial needs (Cassileth and Hamilton, 1979). However, care-givers need to guide families to use appropriate community resources. This involves a thorough assessment of the individual family situation so that families are not misdirected to programs for which they are ineligible. This also involves strategy in teaching families how to understand, approach, and work alongside multiple community systems.

Finally, increasing family access to others who have experienced cancer is frequently quite helpful. Peer support through one-on-one cancer counseling and educational programs, and visitation services such as the American Cancer Society's I Can Cope and Can Surmount programs, may be available. Family support groups affiliated with treatment centers can bring similarly affected families together and break through the isolating effects of cancer, and foster the delivery of common concerns and the development of mutual aid (Galinsky, 1984). Talking with others in similar circumstances can help families get through rough times as they are faced with increased responsibilities, financial difficulties, and changes of lifestyle. New coping skills required to manage the demands of the disease such as "what to tell the children," how to apply for Social Security Disability," and "how to talk to employers," can be acquired from groups.

F. Conclusion

For the individual who has cancer, the family appears to be an integral part of his/her treatment process and many families rally and rise to this challenge. Where family support exists, it can result in patient compliance with regimens and progress toward recovery. Lack of family support or unrealistic expectations can slow and even undermine caregivers' efforts. But just as families influence the course of illness for the patient, cancer has a direct impact on the entire family. The family is then an interacting and transacting organization, and the relationship between cancer, the patient, and family support is reciprocal and complicated, and deserves the attention of all caring cancer caregivers.

II. THE ONCOLOGY PATIENT: USING RECREATION THERAPY TO ALLEVIATE SOCIAL ISOLATION AND DEPERSONALIZATION*

Much can be done to mitigate the isolating and depersonalizing effects of cancer and cancer treatment by providing an environment in which the uniqueness of the patient is recognized and opportunities for social involvement and creative use of leisure time are offered.

Cancer patients cite fear of isolation, abandonment, dependency, and loss of individuality and status among their greatest worries. The recreation therapist, working with other health professionals, can alleviate these fears and bolster flagging morale by means of providing leisure education, companionship, and opportunities for pleasant and stimulating choices. Comprehensive recreation therapy programs recognize the strengths and abilities of the individual patient and provide activities such as arts and crafts, games, music, out-trips, and group diversions. These help to relieve tension and boredom, provide constructive outlets for emotions, and afford opportunities for learning and for developing social relationships. Encouraging the patient and family to focus on abilities rather than disabilities and helping them have positive experiences within the hospital contributes greatly to the patient's general well-being,

---

*This section was written by Louise Bost.

adaptation to illness, and rehabilitation (Bost and Brown, 1982; Willetts and Sperling, 1983).

A cancer patient's social and personal relations are often subjected to severe pressure by the confinement, dependence, and loss of productive individuality brought about by the disease and its treatment. The patient can experience a devastating sense of isolation. Friends usually rally around the sick bed for a short while and then drift away (Weisman, 1979). Many people are uncomfortable in the presence of ill people and are unsure of what is needed or expected. Also, the bonds built by previous work and recreational activities may grow weak as opportunities for shared experiences diminish. The "enforced" free time that often accompanies chronic illness may be an additional burden for both patient and family.

The feeling of being cut off from the world during hospitalization is expressed by patients repeatedly and in many ways.

> "You've never been in prison? Well, this is the way it is. It's like you know the street is out there, but you can't get on it."

> "It's like being on a spaceship—and it's o.k. for a few days, but then you want to touch the earth again."

> "It's like a zoo—a real zoo. The cage is clean and the food comes on time. The attendants are kind. But it is not a natural habitat."

There is no way to completely overcome such feelings of displacement and confinement, but at least the recreation therapist can bring a little of the nonmedical world into the hospital and can get those who are physically able out of the institutional environment to "touch the earth," enjoy "real food" and entertainment, and gain relief from the sights, sounds, and smells of the institution. Opportunities for some measure of control and options for pleasant choices are offered in a setting in which patient control is usually minimal (Figure 1). Such positive intervention can make a difference:

> "My father was claustrophobic—he needed space and nature—and being confined to one room for so long was extremely hard for him. Jane (the recreation therapist) brought so much into his days. I am convinced that his will to fight would not have been so strong had it not been for people like her. Her crafts and teas and bingo and many things helped to brighten a long, scary day."

> "I had only known about the cancer 5 days. A week before that I was up doing all types of activities. Imagine finding yourself with lung cancer, plus possible other cancers over your body in a hospital bed in less than a week. Suddenly you have someone walk in your room and say, 'Come on up and make baskets with us.' The person asking having such a pleasant smile, also mentioning baskets. Soon you are with a group of seemingly happy, pleasant

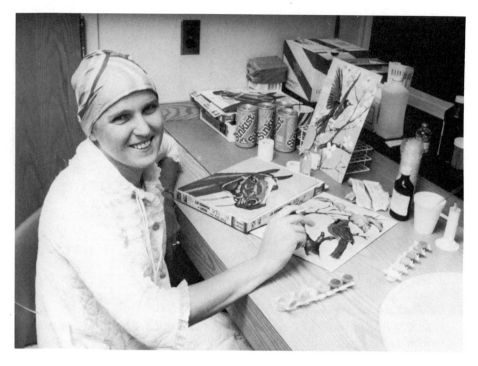

Figure 1 Offering patients a choice of leisure activities facilitates coping mechanisms and allows them to feel in control in a hospital setting.

people. You don't forget your problems, but soon they do seem so much lighter. Only after going through this can others understand."

Social isolation is a significant factor in increased anxiety. Anxiety, in turn, is a barrier to communication and can be an impediment to treatment. "It causes distortion, unwarranted shifts of emphasis and inability to comprehend, remember, and even to hear" (Bard, 1966). Anxiety-ridden patients cannot comply with instructions because they cannot understand them. In addition, anxiety is one of many factors influencing the experiencing of pain. It is usually reflected in skeletal muscles, and tense muscles make pain worse (Schafer, 1984).

Although existential questions are an ongoing, underlying cause of worry, more immediate and pragmatic problems can also cause great anxiety. We once found a timid patient extremely agitated because he did not know how to convert a check into cash for bus fare. Social interaction with a caring person, staff, family, or other patient can easily solve such straightforward problems

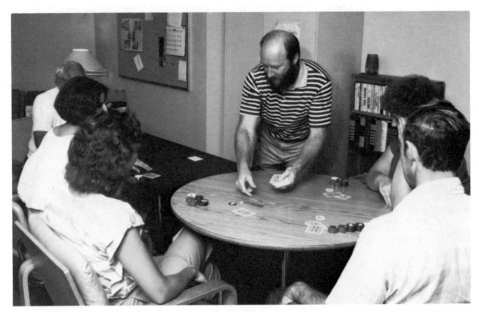

Figure 2 Patients and families retreat from the medical atmosphere and relieve tension during group activities in lounges and game rooms.

and alleviate the general level of anxiety caused by the accumulation of smaller problems.

The hospital has an obligation to expend every effort to create an environment of trust and mutual support within the institution. Patients and family members chatting over coffee or enjoying a game or puzzle share mutual concerns and information. Questions believed to be not important enough to ask physicians or nurses may safely be asked of other patients or the recreation staff. The recreation therapist in the role of a nonthreatening friend is often able to alleviate anxiety by encouraging the patient to ask medical questions of appropriate medical personnel, by referring the patient to social workers or chaplains, and by alerting the nursing staff to fears and questions expressed by patients and families.

Activities that provide temporary relief from anxiety and tension are renewing for the family as well as the patients. Baking cookies, playing cards, making popcorn, or singing on the patient unit can be catalysts for the growth of a caring community of patients, families, and staff who gain strength from one another as they laugh and cry (Figure 2). Self-help skills are shared as family members learn from other patients' families how to communicate with the withdrawn or angry patient. Staff members see this happening.

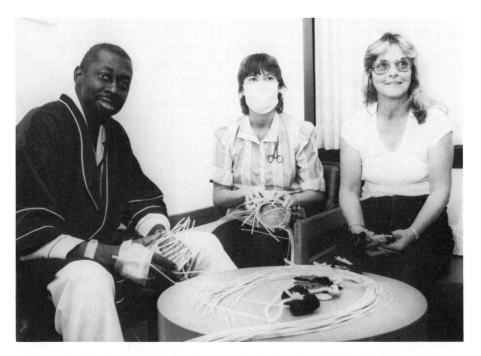

Figure 3   The sharing of experiences and the forming of friendships between patients, family members, and staff are by-products of busy hands.

The oncology patient's family also receives much benefit from recreation service. It gives them a time away from caring and worrying over a loved one. It also allows them to meet and share with each other in fun activities. This often opens the door for much deeper support for, after being out of a stressful situation for a period of time, the family members are able to cope much better with their loved one.

Activity is also valuable in opening the channels of communication for expression of concerns and fears. Busy hands in a nonthreatening environment make it easier to communicate (Figure 3).

A young man expressed his fears for his wife only while at the pool table. As he sighted the ball he talked, almost as if to himself, "They say she may not live through another treatment. She has to decide what to do. How can I help her, I only have a third grade education. I just want her to live . . . ."

A 60-year-old patient meticulously painted Christmas ornaments, carefully including her initials and the date. She acknowledged that she would

probably not see another December. The therapist sat quietly working on
a project of her own and provided a sounding board for the patient as she
reviewed her life—the joys, the time of great sorrow, and the dreams of the
young girl carried forward through the years, now never to be fulfilled.

Laughter is one aspect of social and personal relations that often disappears
under the intense pressures and pains of severe disease. Common sense, however, has long told us that it has beneficial effects on the patient. Mark Twain
expressed this idea in *Tom Sawyer*: "The old man laughed loud and joyously,
shook up the details of his anatomy from head to foot, and ended by saying
that such a laugh was money in a man's pocket, because it cut down the
doctor's bills like everything." There is a growing body of knowledge to
document this belief. We now know that "hearty laughter can clear the
respiratory system, exercise vital organs, reduce tension, and provide a
positive emotional release" (Bresler and Trubo, 1979, p. 312). Norman Cousins,
a pioneer in the field of personal control of pain, made the oft-quoted statement
that 10 minutes of laughter would give him 2 hours of pain-free sleep (Cousins,
1976).

Humor should be a planned part of the therapeutic environment. A staff
with a sense of the ridiculous can lighten the atmosphere and help patients
cope with the inevitable assaults on dignity and control that beset them. A
liquid-diet meal tray delivered with a flourish and "Here's your gourmet
special for the day" provides a bond of understanding that hospital life is not
ideal. As Ellis writes, "Humor is curative. A joke can be more effective than
a pill and certainly makes a pill more efficacious" (Ellis, 1978). Laughter is
not only therapeutic, it is also contagious. That is why canned laughter is inserted into radio and television programs. Light comedy movies are funnier when
viewed with others; ridiculous songs bring more laughter when sung with a
group; and patients may rise above some of their problems by exaggerating them
and recounting them to the laughter of others.

In *Megatrends,* John Naisbitt states that there is a need to balance the
powerful forces of technology with the spiritual needs of human nature
(Naisbitt, 1982). The "high-tech/high-touch" correlation described seems particularly applicable when the technology is concerned with life itself as is the
sophisticated technology of cancer diagnosis and treatment (Paulen, 1984).
Personal and social relations—sharing a laugh, lending a hand, "smelling the
roses" with others—become increasingly important in the world of the cancer
patient.

The disruption of social and personal relations combines with several other
factors to produce in the cancer patient a "loss of self." This loss is identified
by Charmaz (1983) as a fundamental form of suffering in the chronically ill. A
loss of self-esteem is experienced as former self-images crumble away and are not
replaced by equally valued new images. Experiences upon which former positive

self-images were based may become unavailable. Patients may perceive their role in the family, at work, and in the community as diminished, and they may no longer be able to pursue valued leisure-time activities. In addition, the cancer patient may find humiliating and depersonalizing the necessity to depend on the judgment of others for treatment of a disease he/she does not understand (Rosenbaum, 1975). The required hospital routines and procedures and the need to rely on the judgment of others contribute to a climate of dependence in which the patient's sense of individuality may diminish (Purtilo, 1973; Mauksch, 1975). The universal need to be valued as a unique person is expressed in words spoken by Hubert Humphrey to his children: "Until they open me up, the doctors won't know how far the cancer has spread. But whatever it is, I want you to know that I'm not a statistic, I'm your Dad, I'm Hubert Humphrey, and I'm not a statistic" (Thomas, 1977).

Helping patients to maintain a positive self-image is an essential component of good cancer care. Weisman (1979) includes in 10 directives for good coping with cancer, "self-concept is as important as symptom relief" and "hope is self-pride, not self-deception." Letting patients know that we appreciate the knowledge and skills they have acquired in the past and that we value them as special and unique individuals helps to bridge the gap between life before cancer and the present. This transition can be facilitated by talking with them about areas of interest or expertise, by asking for their advice, by acknowledging their interests in communal life in the hospital, and by leisure education to explore the meaning of leisure-time activities in their precancer lives and in the present. Recreation therapists can help patients to understand that recreation is essential for mental, emotional, and physical well-being of all persons, and that the need for recreation—for refreshing experiences—is often intensified by illness. Patients and therapists can consider together new avenues for self-expression and for achieving a sense of mastery and a feeling of accomplishment. These are basic human needs (Frye and Peters, 1972).

It is to be expected that the patient will mourn the loss of the premorbid self and its potential. This mourning is in fact a necessary step toward structuring a future-oriented existence with new and realistic goals (Feldman, 1980). Recreation therapy can provide a supportive and protective microcosm in which cancer patients can begin to forge more realistic goals and initiate activities appropriate to their present state of health. Noncompulsive, unhurried, and nonrestrictive leisure activities can create an atmosphere in which patients dare to look at their present selves and eventually grow to accept and even like what they see (Frye and Peters, 1972). The case histories that follow illustrate the process of adaptation and growth fostered by recreation therapy through appropriate activities and social interaction.

A. A.K.

A.K., a lively, 75-year-old patient with colon cancer, presented a challenge to the recreation therapy staff. She wanted to learn a new craft of or skill that could be continued at home during each of her many periods of hospitalization. She liked to pass the skills on to friends and organized groups and to make holiday and birthday gifts for her large family and her friends. A.K. was accustomed to being a leader in her community and wanted to continue to contribute, to be a "doer" and not just "done unto." This attitude was evident during hospitalization also, as she looked for persons with whom she could share the skills she learned, and often made small gifts for other patients. Even when terribly ill, A.K.'s eyes would light up when we visited, and she would take our hands and tell us that the crafts had "brought so much joy" into her life.

B. W.L.

W.L., a 49-year-old man with leukemia, appeared rather quiet and shy when Jane, the recreation therapist, first met him. He stayed in his room much of the time. Jane encouraged him to come to a coffeebreak. He came and sat very still, responding only to direct questions. Late that week Jane visited with W.L., learning about his family and his illness. Then they walked and talked in the halls.

The following week W.L. came to a craft workshop but was very quiet and chose only to observe activity. He soon returned to his room. This behavior continued for much of the 4 weeks that he was hospitalized.

When W.L. returned to the hospital for consolidation chemotherapy, he was friendlier and more talkative. He came independently to activities and asked for things to do in his room. He seemed to feel rather free and happy with the recreation therapy staff, nurses, and doctors.

After some weeks at home, W.L. was hospitalized with fever. During this admission he spoke freely with Jane about his medical problems and talked with her about his worries and fears. He began to encourage other patients on the floor to come to group activities. He helped to lead craft workshops and showed other patients how to do projects in their rooms. He visited patients whom he had met during previous admissions.

W.L. slowly assumed control where possible. He began to call home and tell others exactly what to do. He became very much in control of the home front and his teenage daughter. His family seldom visited during the first few admissions. During later admissions they visited more frequently, and he planned things for them to do (go to the chapel, the cafeteria, the gift shop, group activities, and so on).

W.L. became very much at home in the hospital. He welcomed newcomers to the unit, led activities, and encouraged patients and families to attend. The highlight of his many weeks of hospitalization came when Jane arranged for him to meet visiting celebrity Dinah Shore, his longtime "dream girl." He enjoyed the notoriety that he received on the unit and was very proud of a picture made with the star.

C. J.T.

A nursing referral to recreation therapy for 32-year-old J.T. stated that the patient was exceedingly apathetic during recent admissions for chemotherapy, even though she tolerated treatments well by objective measurements. The nurse suggested that J.T. might be interested in using an electric keyboard as she was known to have an interest in music.

The therapist who performed the recreation therapy evaluation learned that J.T. aspired to a career as a gospel singer. J.T. responded with enthusiasm to the idea of using the keyboard and began to play and sing as soon as the instrument was put in her room. Subsequently, during many months of treatment, she sang on the unit for the pleasure of patients, families, and staff. Group calendars were planned to accommodate to her schedule so that she could perform before treatments started, or, if that was not possible, at the next best time for her. J.T. also attended other group activities and enjoyed simple craft activities in her room.

J.T. became a regional celebrity. She was filmed singing in the hospital by a local television station, was featured on a television talk show, and was helped to make recordings of her songs. She was also featured in television promotions of cancer awareness.

D. S.R.

We had known S.R., a young woman with aplastic anemia, for more than 5 years prior to her hospitalization for a bone marrow transplant. Over the years we had taught her many arts and crafts skills, accompanied her on trips out of the hospital, and provided companionship when she was confined to her room. S.R. was heavily dependent upon her immediate family for her social support. Our staff was concerned that she would not tolerate lengthy confinement and separation from her family, and none of her family could afford to spend extended periods at the hospital.

S.R. surprised us by coping remarkably well through the period of protective isolation. Although there were days when the treatment consumed all of her energies, there were other days when she made gifts for her family, listened to gospel music, and played cards. She seemed to accept the staff as a surrogate

family. There was some regression and unreasonable insistence on specific
activity supplies, but her morale was generally good throughout confinement.
She helped with plans and made decorations for a Halloween party on the
unit. The party coincided with her first venture out of her room (complete
with a Halloween protective mask) and the party became a celebration of her
newly regained freedom and well-being.

A few days after the party the nursing staff noticed that S.R. seemed
depressed. She was talking less and staying in bed more than seemed appropriate. The nurses believed that facial discoloration and other physical changes
were demoralizing and that something needed to be done to improve her self-image. A plan was made to encourage S.R. to teach crafts skills to new volunteers in the security of her room. She responded to the challenge to become
the teacher instead of the pupil. As she taught small groups, she gradually
began to rejoin communal life on the unit.

E. T.M.

T.M., a 55-year-old patient with colon cancer, was an outdoor person. His
favorite leisure-time activities were hunting and fishing. He spend as little time
as possible in his room during his many 5-day admissions for chemotherapy and
could often be found on the porch or in a patient lounge where there were floor-to-ceiling windows. He attended most of the group activities on the unit, and
his lively sense of humor added life to the occasions. T.M. liked popcorn,
freshly baked cookies, bingo, cards, slide shows, leather crafts, and basket
making; and the recreation staff made efforts to have a "menu" of the activities
he enjoyed each time he was admitted.

T.M. was an avid observer of the world about him. He expressed particular
appreciation for slide shows of foreign countries shown by volunteers who had
traveled abroad, saying, "This is the only way I will ever see these countries."
His lively curiosity about the slides stimulated the interest of other patients, and
his questions delighted the volunteers who shared their travel experiences.

F. R.B.

R.B. was a 22-year-old college junior when he was diagnosed as having acute
myelogenous leukemia. He was the leader of a skydiving club in his home community and said that "skydiving is an obsession, my great love."

During early treatments, volunteers and students on the recreation therapy
staff visited him frequently, often discussing sports or comparing notes on
college life. R.B. spent much of his free time on his college studies and occasionally asked for assistance in obtaining information from libraries near the
hospital. He also received assistance in contacting local skydivers.

R.B.'s mother was with him during most of his many days of hospitalization and enjoyed working on craft projects while in his room. R.B. was proud of his mother's work and was particularly pleased in a needlework sampler of his school's motto and a decoupage picture of his school's mascot.

Following months of remission, R.B. returned to the hospital for a bone marrow transplant. The rapport built with the recreation therapy staff during earlier admissions helped to make confinement and isolation more tolerable during the long and difficult treatment. Companionship, music cassettes, and games were provided when appropriate.

R.B.'s younger brother, also a skydiver, brought a videocassette featuring their skydiving club to the hospital and the recreation program provided viewing equipment. R.B. enjoyed showing the film in his room to friends and hospital staff and was pleased to be the star of "Skydiving with R.B." when the film was used at several group activities. His brother helped coordinate activities and answered questions at the group showings. He appeared to enjoy the recognition of his own feats and took particular pride in R.B.'s leadership role.

G. Summary

An environment that provides opportunities for social interaction and personal growth is a humanistic and necessary adjunct to optimum cancer treatment. Treatment team recreation therapists who are comfortable in the presence of cancer with all of its ramifications can be strong allies for patients as they struggle to be valued, and to value themselves, as unique, evergrowing and changing individuals. Adaptation to illness and hospitalization is enhanced by alleviating the social isolation and depersonalization that is so often a part of the cancer experience. A basic premise of a social support system to facilitate this adaptation can be expressed in the words of Sir William Osler: "It is more important to know what kind of a person has a disease than what kind of a disease a person has" (Bresler and Trubo, 1979, p. 4).

III. RELIGIOUS BELIEFS: A HELP OR A HINDRANCE?*

A young divorced mother of two children, in her middle thirties, had melanoma. Believing herself to be fatally ill, she returned to the community where several of her family members lived. She wanted to be close to her family in order that they might assist her with the care of her children while she devoted as much time as necessary to her own health care. The family were all members of a conservative religious community. The patient, Mrs. A, attended the church with her family, not because she believed all that was taught in the church but

---

*This section was written by Paul W. Aitken.

because she wanted to participate with her family in activities that were important to them. Mrs. A also wanted to feel the security of having a good relationship with God. She felt that a good way to begin such an effort was to attend church with her children. She did not have the courage to attend a different church or religious community whose beliefs might have been more compatible with hers. She attended the church of her parents and that religious community had a "healing service" for Mrs. A. She attempted to participate as conscientiously as possible in the service. Following the service, she truly tried to believe that she was healed as the religious community had declared. There was much celebration and thanksgiving by all. Problems started when Mrs. A gave evidence of relapse and recurrence of her disease. Mrs. A was certain that she needed to get back to her doctors at Duke Hospital. Her family and the church challenged her "lack of faith" and insisted that she was healed and that she should not yield to her sinful doubts. Mrs. A dared to return to the hospital, with no support from her family or from her small children who believed that she did not need to return to the hospital. Mrs. A's fears about her disease were confirmed and new treatment plans were proposed by her physician. She consented to the new treatment program and also began discussing her religious troubles with the hospital chaplain. She felt very comforted and sustained by the medical team, the social worker, the chaplain, and all other members of the allied health team. She felt isolated from her family and was in great distress because it was her family who was taking care of her children. They would continue to care for her children after her death if the treatment was not successful. Mrs. A was greatly troubled by her dilemma.

Mrs. A returned to her family home for a few days before coming back to the hospital for bone marrow transplant. She dreaded the tension that she anticipated between herself and the family. One of her physicians, with her permission and with the approval and support of the entire health care team, called the family who lived several hundred miles away. He spoke with them in clear and specific terms about the circumstances Mrs. A faced regarding her relapse with her melanoma. He spoke candidly and firmly. The family, impressed by the courage of this physician, were able to admit to themselves that Mrs. A had not been healed and that she was desperately in need of further treatment. They enthusiastically rallied around Mrs. A and provided family support and assistance that Mrs. A needed. It is doubtful that the whole church community reversed its position on the claim of healing Mrs. A. However, the unanimous stand of the health care team at Duke, including the hospital chaplain, and voiced by the physician, gave the family sufficient support to let go of their desperate desire for a magical transformation.

It is not surprising that some patients and family members revert to denial as a method of coping when they have to face the harsh reality that there has been a relapse and a recurrence of the disease. They may continue to cling to the unrealistic hope that some magic will relieve them of their dreadful reality. Most will move beyond this denial rather quickly and begin to cope more effectively, especially if they receive proper support from all of the health professionals. Talking and thinking aloud about these matters can be facilitated by any of the health care team. The more formal struggle with religious beliefs and issues can best be facilitated by a clinically trained clergyperson. Most patients and family members will gradually let go of their desperate wish and hope for a magical "cure." The physician and the health care team should be sensitive to the religious struggles of the patient and family members and by so doing, avoid complications. One of the most common complications that occurs is the misuse of religion as a magical formula when patients and families need so desperately to deny the reality which they face.

Patients and family members often review their religious belief early in the course of their experience with cancer. They tend to do this at the onset rather than in the terminal phase of the illness. Every human being has a need to explain to him/herself what is happening in life and why. Such a serious review of one's beliefs is seldom undertaken unless life itself is threatened. There are more casual reviews at other times in life, but nothing compares with the search to know and to understand when life is threatened. The patient must attempt to answer such questions as: "If I cannot control or correct my health problem and physicians cannot control or correct my health problem, who is either causing or letting this happen to me? Why is this happening to me? Can I influence or effect in any way whoever or whatever is causing or letting this happen to me? What will happen to me when I die?" The major examination of these beliefs comes rather early in the illness.

In the great majority of cases, religious beliefs do help people answer the questions mentioned above. Patients and family members alike are able to draw conclusions that will enable them to cope effectively with their cancer. Reviewing their religious beliefs, practicing their rites and rituals should enable them to have faith and courage as they launch into the treatment program. Effective use of religious beliefs should enhance their sense of security and safety even while taking a variety of treatments that may have severe side effects. Effective religious beliefs should help patients and family members have the courage to participate actively in their treatment and make wise decisions when needed. Effective religious beliefs should help patients and family members celebrate remissions, and withstand the suspense of waiting, perhaps for years, to see if they have accomplished a cure. All religions advocate that people should live life to its fullest each day whether or not there is a tomorrow. Such religious beliefs will be a source of comfort and courage to patients and family members and should enhance good health care. The result will be increased faith, with a renewed sense of security and safety that is an all-encompassing feeling. It will help the patient and family cope with even the most difficult and painful of experiences. It will also contribute to the quality of those good and worthwhile times, as seldom as they might occur, during the later stages and the terminal phase.

Mr. B came into the hospital one morning to visit his wife who was critically ill with cancer. He announced that God had appeared during the night and informed him that his wife was going to be healed. Mr. B was very excited and enthusiastic. I accepted his announcement and suggested that he be certain to tell his wife's physician. We could all observe his wife over the next few days to see whether this was a real experience or whether he had had a dream (desperation and denial). Mrs. B did not begin to improve; in fact, her condition steadily worsened. It appeared more and more obvious that she was moving into the terminal phase of her life. She lamented over the fact that her husband was so enthusiastically proclaiming that she was being healed that she had no opportunity to talk with him about her fears of death and separation. She said, "B is so convinced that I am being healed that I can't even tell him goodbye." The home minister reinforced all that Mr. B was saying by having a special service of thanksgiving at the church when Mr. B first announced the "good news" about the healing.

When Mr. B could no longer deny the fact that his wife was losing ground rapidly, he became angry with the staff (especially with the chaplain) and said that if the staff had as much faith as he had, his wife would be getting well and would be healed. Even though we did not hold the same beliefs as Mr. B and discussed the difference with him quite frankly, we never did belittle his position. We just kept pointing out the discrepancy between his belief and the daily condition of his wife.

Mrs. B never was able to talk to her husband about her impending death, nor was she able to gain any support from him. The staff, on the other hand, was able to maintain open communication with her and assist her with much gentle care until the time of her death.

Mr. B gradually let go of his denial and his anger toward the staff. He rationalized his position by stating that the death of his wife was evidence that God had fulfilled his promise. "God had taken Mrs. B to be with him."

The physician and the health care team should be sensitive to the religious struggles of the patient and family members. In the majority of cases, the patient and the family will not need special assistance with these struggles. They will rely on the relationship they maintain with their family and friends, their home clergy, and the general staff who are treating them at the hospital. If special assistance is needed, the hospital chaplain should be qualified to provide it. If the patient or family prefers a representative from their own religious community or faith group, every effort should be made to locate that person. Most community clergy want to be an ally of the physician and the health care team. However, not all community clergy have had clinical training, nor have they acquired any clinical experience. If a community clergyperson is invited to participate, it is usually helpful to include him/her in conferences regarding treatment goals.

Physicians who treat patients with cancer are confronted with two dilemmas. One is telling the whole truth or not telling the whole truth to patient and family. The other dilemma is deciding whether to continue or terminate the physician-patient relationship when the physician decides to discontinue treatment in the terminal phase. Both of these problems are complex and have the potential for causing complications even when they are handled well. First, the issue of truthfulness.

All of the great religions of the world stress the importance of truthfulness among people. At the same time, the great religions of the world also stress the importance of the value and worth of the human being and the importance of respectfulness and kindness toward one another. Being kind and considerate toward a person and being utterly honest with that same person are not always compatible. For example, the person's emotional state may be so fragile that stark truth may shatter the psychological defenses and coping mechanisms of the person rather than assist that person. The physician is always faced with the challenge to temper the truth because of his/her awareness of the state of mind of the patient and family.

Not too many years ago, physicians had to make independent decisions about what they would tell or not tell their patients about their illness. Patients had a greater need to hide from the truth and physicians felt that it was more respectful to accommodate the wishes of the patient. This has changed considerably in the practice of modern medicine, especially as it pertains to medical treatment that is still considered to be experimental. Informed consent statements require that complete, explicit, and detailed information be given the patient about his/her condition and the treatment proposed. Since a good portion of the treatments available to patients with cancer is still considered research, much has been learned about the resilience of patients when they are told the truth about their condition. They handle it quite well. Thre is very little, if any, opportunity to hide from the truth about one's health problem when reading the informed consent prior to participating in a treatment procedure. Of course, the denial mechanism of severe grief becomes operative rather quickly as a means of protecting the patient from the fearfulness of life-threatening truth. In other words, what the patient has been told is frequently quite different from what the patient remembers having been told. As one patient stated, "I cannot retain my sanity or maintain any hope if I live with the probability of death in my conscious mind all of the time. I must set it aside and live as if I am going to live forever in order to remain sane and hopeful."

In spite of the risk of shocking or upsetting the patient or the family, the dilemma for the physician certainly seems to be weighted on the side of telling the truth. In the Christian religion, Jesus on one occasion tells some of his followers that if they know the truth, the truth will make them free. This teaching or principle has become the axiom upon which informed consent statements have been built. It is the conviction of Institutional Review Boards that the more clearly, completely, and understandably the truth is told, the more free the patient is to make a decision. Even so, the burden of the responsibility for deciding what to tell in many cases rests with the attending physician. Reality still must always be tempered with compassion.

Now let us consider the dilemma of deciding whether to continue a physician-patient relationship when no more treatment to extend life or rescue the patient from the disease is indicated. The patient is in the terminal phase of his/her life and the question is "What is left for the physician to do?" Some physicians terminate the relationship and refer the patient to a home care service or to Hospice. The rationale for this frequently is that it is unethical for the physician to continue to charge the patient for consultations when there is essentially no treatment that the physician can be administering. In other incidents, the physician remains available to the patient if the patient or family call for such consultation. In both cases, there is always the question about what the physician should do and why.

Permit me to share some of my experiences with a patient in order to illustrate what I would like to suggest to physicians and to other health care professionals. Mrs. K was a lady who battled with cancer for approximately 2 years and was in and out of our hospital on a variety of occasions. I met her first when she was struggling with cognitive issues and was actively wrestling with her religious beliefs and attempting to integrate her experience with those beliefs. Throughout those early visits, I frequently held her hand when she was feeling emotional pain or distress. It was a comfortable and mutual act and it became an integral part of our conversational relationship. She would talk at length with me but would reach out and take my hand the moment she began to feel some emotional pain triggered by the content of our conversation. As she became sicker and began to lose her battle with cancer, there was less reason for us to talk but increased reason for us to be together for emotional and spiritual support. We would talk less and hold hands more. My visits became briefer, perhaps 3-5 minutes in length on many occasions, but she would reach for my hand when I walked to her bedside and I would hold her hand throughout those brief minutes. It was as if all that had transpired between her and me was reduced to the ritual of holding hands. The importance of the relationship was not lost, it just took a different form and the ritualistic form maintained its importance for the remainder of her life. In fact, the last physical manifestation of her consciousness was evident when I spoke her name at her bedside shortly before her death. There was feeble movement of her hand, obviously a ritualistic effort to take hold of my hand. I responded by holding her hand and no words were spoken. Hours later she died.

I would suggest that there are many physician-patient activities that can be ritualized in a way that will allow the relationship to be maintained in some significant form.

Bobby was a 15-year-old cancer victim who was in the terminal phase of his illness and moments before his death had suffered hemorrhages in his eyes so that he could no longer see clearly. He asked for his favorite physician and when the physician and his team entered the room, the young patient stated, "Would the real Dr. Barnes (not his name) please stand up!" Bobby could not distinguish Dr. Barnes from the other members of the staff and was asking him to step apart from them so he could identify him properly. The doctor immediately came over to Bobby's side and began to examine him and he went through several physician-patient rituals that were not medically indicated or essential. It was obvious that the substance of the significant relationship between Dr. Barnes and Bobby was being acted out in the ritual between them. There was obvious warmth, tenderness, and sensitivity on the part of both. Within 30 minutes Bobby was dead.

When there are no words left to be said, it may seem senseless to examine the body of the dying patient. On the other hand, if there was any substance to the relationship between the patient and the physician then there needs to be ways other than conversation for acting out and celebrating that substance. Dying is anticipated by so many people as being a lonely and frightening experience. It is extremely important for people to feel safe even in the midst of a frightening and lonely experience. A 3-5 minute ritual may be all that is left of a relationship but on a given occasion that ritual can be as important as a 45-minute physician-patient conversation. All of the acts that a physician performs in giving a patient a physical examination are potential rituals for the terminal phase of life. It is for the physician and the patient to determine what is most meaningful and satisfying for the two of them. If the physician has a significant relationship with a patient before the terminal phase of the patient's life, hopefully that relationship will not be terminated. The compassionate "treatment" of rituals may hold much potential for maintaining the relationship until the very moment of death.

REFERENCES

Aitken-Swan, J. (1959). Nursing the late cancer patient at home, *Practitioner*, *183*:64-69.

Bard, M. (1966). Psychological adaptation to the stress of cancer and its treatment, *The Swedish Cancer Society Yearbook 4* (H. Bergstrand, ed.), Almquist & Wiksells, Uptsala, Sweden, p. 462.

Binger, C. M., Ablin, A. R., Kushner, J. H., Feurerstein, R. C., Zoger, S., and Mikkelson, C. (1969). Childhood leukemia: Emotional impact on patient and family, *New Eng. J. Med., 280*:414-418.

Bloom, J. R. (1982). Social support systems and cancer: A conceptual view, *Psychosocial Aspects of Cancer* (J. Cohen, J. Cullen, and L. Martin, eds.), Raven Press, New York, pp. 129-149.

Bost, L., and Brown, E. (1982). Recreation therapy: A humanistic adjunct to oncology treatment, *Oncol. Nursing Forum, 9*:45-49.

Bresler, D. E., and Trubo, R. (1979). *Free Yourself from Pain*, Simon & Schuster, New York, p. 312.

Cancer Care. (1973). *Impact, Costs and Consequences of Catastrophic Illness in Patients and Families*, Cancer Care, Inc., New York.

Caplan, G. (1976). The family as a support system. *Support Systems and Mutual Help* (G. Caplan and M. Killilea, eds.), Grune & Stratton, New York, pp. 19-36.

Cassileth, B. R., and Hamilton, J. (1979). The family with cancer, *The Cancer Patient—Social and Medical Aspects of Care* (B. R. Cassileth, ed.), Lea & Febiger, Philadelphia.

Charmaz, K. (1983). Loss of self: A fundamental form of suffering in the chronically ill, *Sociol. Health Ill., 5*:168-194.

Clark, E. (1983). The role of the social environment in adaptation to cancer, *Social Work Res. Abstr., 19*:32-33.

Cobb, S. (1979). Social support for the cancer patient, *Forum Med., 1*: 24-30.

Cohen, M. (1982). Psychosocial morbidity in cancer: A clinical perspective, *Psychosocial Aspects of Cancer* (J. Cohen, J. Cullen, and L. Martin, eds.), Raven Press, New York, pp. 117-122.

Cohen, M., and Wellisch, D. (1978). Living in limbo: Psychosocial intervention in families with a cancer patient, *Am. J. Psychother., 32*:561-571.

Cohen, S., and Wills, T. (1983). *Social Support, Stress, and the Buffering Hypothesis: An Empirical Review*, Carnegie Mellon University, Pittsburgh, Pa.

Cousins, N. (1976). Anatomy of an illness, *New Engl. J. Med., 295*:1457-1462.

Dean, A., and Lin, N. (1977). The stress-buffering role of social support, *J. Nervous Mental Dis., 165*: 403-416.

DiMatteo, M. R., and Hayes, R. (1981). Social support and serious illness, *Social Networks and Social Support* (B. Gottlieb, ed.), Sage Publications, Beverly Hills, Calif.

Dunkel-Schetter, C. (1981). *Social Support and Coping with Cancer*, unpublished doctoral dissertation, Northwestern University, Chicago.

Dyk, R. B., and Sutherland, A. M. (1956). Adaptation of spouse and other family members to colostomy patient, *Cancer, 9*:123-128.

Ellis, S. (1978). Humour the wonder drug, *Nursing Times, 2*:1792-1793.

Feldman, D. J. (1980). Chronic disabling illness: A holistic view, *Role of the Family in the Rehabilitation of the Physically Disabled* (P. W. Power and A. E. Dell Orto, eds.), University Park Press, Baltimore, pp. 14-20.

Frye, V., and Peters, M. (1972). *Therapeutic Recreation: Its Theory, Philosophy, and Practice,* Stackpole Books, Harrisburg, Pa., pp. 99-110.

Galinsky, M. J. (1984). Groups for cancer patients and their families: Purposes and group conditions, *Individual Change Through Small Groups,* (P. H. Glasser and M. Sundal, eds.), 2nd Edition, The Free Press, New York.

Gillum, R. F., and Barsky, A. J. (1974). Diagnosis and management of patient noncompliance, *JAMA, 228*:1563-1567.

Goldberg, R. J. (1983). Systematic understanding of cancer patients who refuse treatment, *Psychother. Psychosomat., 39*:180-189.

Gordon, W., Fridenbergs, I., Diller, L., Hibbard, M., Wolf, C., Levine, L., Lipkins, R., Ezrachi, O., and Lucido, R. (1980). Efficacy of psychosocial intervention with cancer patients, *J. Consult. Clin. Psychol., 48*:743-759.

Greenleigh, Inc. (1979). *Report on the Social, Economic and Psychological Needs of Cancer Patients in California,* American Cancer Society, San Francisco.

Kaplan, B., Cassel, J., and Gore, S. (1977). Social support and health, *Medical Care, 15*:47-58.

Kaplan, D. M. (1982). Predicting the impact of severe illness in families, *Health and Social Work, 1*:72-82.

Klein, R. F., Dean, A., and Bogdonoff, M. D. (1967). The impact of illness upon the spouse, *J. Chron. Dis., 20*:241-248.

Krant, M. J., and Johnston, L. (1978). Family members perceptions of communications in late stage cancer, *J. Psychiat. Med., 8*:203-216.

Lee, E. G., and Maguire, G. (1975). Emotional distress in patients attending a breast clinic, *Brit. J. Surg., 62*:162.

Mauksch, H. (1975). The organizational context of dying, *Death the Final Stage of Growth* (E. Kübler-Ross, ed.), Prentice-Hall, Englewood Cliffs, N.J., pp. 16-22.

Meyerowitz, B. E. (1980). Psychosocial correlates of breast cancer and its treatments, *Psychiatry Bulletin, 87*:108-131.

Michielutti, R. (1976). *Factors Associated with Delays in Decision to Seek Medical Treatment for Cancer,* Research Report, Bowman-Gray School of Medicine, Winston-Salem, N.C.

Mitchell, G. W., and Glicksman, A. S. (1977). Cancer patients: Knowledge and attitudes, *Cancer, 40*:61-69.

Moos, R., and Moos, B. (1981). *Family Environment Scale Manual,* Consulting Psychologists Press, Palo Alto, Calif.

Naisbitt, J. (1982). *Megatrends,* Warner Books, New York.

Noble, D. N., and Hamilton, A. (1983). Coping and complying: A challenge to health care, *Social Work, 28*:462-466.

Parkes, C. M. (1972). The emotional impact of cancer on patients and their families, *J. Laryngol. Cytol., 89*:1271-1279.

Paulen, A. (1984). High touch in a high tech environment, *Cancer Nursing*, *June*:201.

Purtillo, R. (1973). *The Allied Health Professional and the Patient*, W. B. Saunders, Philadelphia, pp. 44-45.

Revenson, T., Wollman, C., and Felton, B. (1983). Social supports as stress buffers for adult cancer patients, *Psychosomat. Med.*, *45*:321-331.

Rosenbaum, E. H. (1975). *Living with Cancer*, Praeger Publishers, New York, p. 53.

Rosenbaum, E., and Rosenbaum, I. (1980). *A Comprehensive Guide for Cancer Patients and Their Families*, Bull Publishing, Palo Alto, Calif.

Schafer, D. W. (1984). Pain, emotions and the cancer patient, *Surgery Annual* (L. M. Nyhus, ed.), Appleton-Century-Crofts, Norwalk, Conn., pp. 57-67.

Silberfarb, P. M., Maurer, L. H., and Crouthamel, C. S. (1980). Psychosocial aspects of neoplastic disease. I. Functional status of breast cancer patients during different treatment regimens, *Am. J. Psychiat.*, *137*:450-455.

Spiegel, D., Bloom, J. R., and Gottheil, E. (1983). Family environment as predictor of adjustment to metastatic breast cancer, *J. Psychosoc. Oncol.*, *1*:33-44.

Sutherland, A. M., and Orbach, C. E. (1953). Psychological impact of cancer and cancer surgery. II. Depressive reactions associated with surgery for cancer, *Cancer*, *6*:958-962.

Thomas, H. (1977). A talk with Senator Hubert Humphrey, *Family Circle*, *Sept. 20*:60.

Weisman, A. D. (1974). Coping with cancer, *This Question of Coping, No. 5*, Roche Laboratory Series, Nutley, N.J.

Weisman, A. D. (1979). *Coping with Cancer*, McGraw-Hill, New York, pp. 42, 43, 79.

Weisman, A. D., and Worden, J. (1976). The existential plight in cancer: Significance of the first 100 days, *Int. J. Psychiat. Med.*, *7*:1-15.

Weisman, A. D., Worden, J., and Sobel, H. J. (1980). *Psychosocial Screening and Intervention with Cancer Patients*, Research Report, Project Omega, Boston.

Wellisch, D. (1984). Work, social, recreation, family and physical status, *Cancer, 53(10)*:2290-2302.

Willetts, H. C., and Sperling, A. (1983). The role of the therapeutic recreationist in assisting the oncology patient to cope, *Supportive Care of the Cancer Patient* (P. H. Wiernik, ed.), Futura Publishing Co., Mt. Kisco, N.Y., pp. 35-55.

Woods, N., and Earp, J. (1978). Women with cured breast cancer, *Nursing Res.*, *27*:270-285.

Worby, C. M., and Babineau, R. (1974). The family interview: Helping patient and family cope with metastatic disease, *Geriatrics, 29*:83-94.

Wortman, C. B. (1984). Social support and the cancer patient: Conceptual and methodologic issues, *Cancer, 53(10)*:2339-2360.

Wortman, C. B., and Dunkel-Schetter, C. (1979). Interpersonal relationships and cancer: A theoretical analysis, *J. Social Issues, 35*:120-155.

12

Care of the Dying Patient

Paula Balber
Triangle Hospice, Durham, North Carolina

I. INTRODUCTION

There comes a time in treating many cancer patients when the physician realizes that no matter how expertly managed the therapy, the patient will die in weeks or months. The time also comes for those under treatment and for their families when they too realize no matter how much they have acted to comply and to enhance the chances of a successful outcome, death is inevitable. Even for those who have thoughtfully reflected on this possibility before, the shift to the terminal phase in the illness provokes renewed fear and anxiety. There are many ways in which physicians and the health care team can intervene to lessen those responses. Concomitantly, staff can act to provide well-considered palliative treatment that will enhance the remainder of the life of patient and family and prevent needless complications.

This chapter focuses on care of the dying patient and family. The first section explores some of the factors to be considered when telling patients and families that there is a short prognosis; a second section examines the effect of that information on patients and families and describes some ways to enhance good coping skills throughout the remainder of the patient's life. The rest of the chapter discusses Hospice as one alternative for the care of those with a short life span.

II. DISCUSSING PROGNOSIS

At some point, perhaps after a relapse or with the recognition that the disease is progressing despite treatment, it becomes evident that prolongation of life beyond weeks or months is no longer likely. This awesome possibility may be suspected or clearly understood by the dying person or family before they are told. The patient or family may be the first to mention concerns about prognosis and they may do so in overt or covert form. Sometimes there are pleas for honesty and support which are cloaked in a long list of requests for factual information. The covert communication may come merely through an indication by the patient or family that the pain is not getting better, the tumors are not shrinking, or the weakness is increasing. They might ask questions that indicate an understanding that the patient's condition is deteriorating: "Will you be able to give me something for the pain later on?" "What happens when the tumor in the liver gets bigger?" If the physician or staff hear such questions, they should realize that time needs to be set aside for a conference to discuss prognosis and care options as quickly as possible.

Generally, it is the physician who controls the dissemination of the "official" information. When the physician first becomes aware of the limited life expectancy, he/she must decide how and when to talk to the patient and family. Rarely these days do physicians in the United States not tell their patients at least some of the crucial information. However, this specific task and other dealings with the family are still so discomfiting to many doctors that the interactions are often handled unskillfully.

In a study by Gold (1983) of 40 terminally ill patients and families, only about half the doctors were perceived as being honest and thoughtful. Similar perceptions and results have been noted by other authors and researchers as well (Kincade 1982; Dickinson and Pearson, 1980; Neimeyer, Behnke, and Reiss, 1983; Wanzer et al., 1984; Redding, 1980). In many cases, important information is obscured by medical language or conveyed in a blunt or patronizing manner. At times patients or families have described being told over the phone that "nothing more can be done to help you." One ex-fighter pilot described the experience of being told his prognosis as similar to the time his plane was shot down over Vietnam and exploded in flames killing the navigator, his best friend.

An effective way to tell a patient and family about a short life expectancy is to schedule one or more conferences. In preparation for such a conference it will help if the physician and staff understand the social, emotional, and spiritual impact of the disease on the family constellation. Knowing how the family has dealt with earlier crises will help predict their reactions to this crisis. The physician, who often takes responsibility for the discussion, may not have all the necessary information and will need to gather it from nurses, social workers, and clergy, who often have valuable insights into family reactions and coping skills.

Clearly, such conferences will work better if physician, staff, and patients have already established a climate of open dialog about the course of the disease, options in treatment, and possible outcomes. Hertzberg (1972) points out that for most people uncertainty surrounding the illness is hardest to bear. Open dialog reduces some of the uncertainty.

When meeting to talk about prognosis it is helpful to provide a supportive environment where there is complete and gentle honesty, as well as clear statements reflecting realistic hope. Questions should be encouraged and answered in a straightforward, understandable manner. Various types of ongoing care should be explored; this will decrease fears of abandonment by the health care team.

Having a second staff member present at the conference who is trusted by patient and family along with the doctor is often useful. The second person can monitor the conversation for misconceptions and correct them, can reiterate information if it is not being heard by the family, patient, or physician, and can return to the family after the conference to reinforce information and generally provide continued support.

Finally, it is important to include both patient and family in these initial conferences, for several reasons. First, this reduces the likelihood of splitting or continuing an already existing split of patient and family into lonely, isolated entities by ensuring that all receive the same information; this often helps increase cohesiveness and mutual support. Second, families and patients may be in different phases of dealing with the illness and impending loss. The family often maintains hope for cure or prolongation of life longer than the patient, and this makes for a painful disparity. It is important to acknowledge to all that a disparity may exist and that this is not unusual. For the denying family or patient, it is helpful to note that concerns voiced by the patient or outcomes outlined by the physician *may* never need to be addressed, that the plans for his/her worsening condition may never need to be put into effect. Merely stating this will lessen the resistance and increase the tolerance for the discussion.

III. REACTIONS OF PATIENTS AND FAMILIES: USEFUL APPROACHES

Either as a result of the conferences or from a worsening in the condition of the patient, knowing that one is dying often precipitates an "existential plight" as Weisman and Worden (1976, p. 3) term these times: "a time of great change in emotional responses and in interpretation of how one relates to the network of people and things that comprise the immediate world." As the patient and family deal with the probability that cure will not occur, fears become intensified. As Pattison (1967, pp. 35-40) points out, the fears of the dying are fears of the unknown, of loneliness, loss of identity, suffering and pain, and fear of regression. These heightened fears and feelings often take on a chronic form that "consists of awareness of progressive erosion of body and mind, depletion of resources, accumulation of regrets, preservation of the past, obtuseness in the present, and blunted appetite for the future (Weisman and Hackett, 1961, p. 249).

These fears are not the only psychological changes. Time no longer passes uniformly, and the acceleration and deceleration lead to further feelings of insecurity, threat, and helplessness (Feigenberg and Schneidman, 1979). "The world suddenly becomes alien, disjointed and runs along without us" (Weisman and Hackett, 1961).

Despite the increased vulnerability and the emotional distress that waxes and wanes, most people manage to live the remainder of their lives with a surprising amount of grace and courage and without extremes of behavior. As has often been pointed out, people die in the style in which they have lived (Schneidman, 1978; Scott, Goode, and Arlin, 1983). For some, chronic depression, high levels of anxiety, hypochondriasis, excessive anger, or regression may occur and these need to be responded to appropriately.

Families also continue as best they can, but stress levels are equally high for them. Fear of the loss of an individual who maintained a certain emotional and social role in the family, fear of loneliness, fear of inability to provide the necessary care, or tolerate the dying process in the best way possible are the most pervasive fears. Family members deal with the reality of a terminally ill relative as they have dealt with other crises, and with other times of accommodation to crises (Freedman, 1982, pp. 120-121).

Given these considerations, a family-centered approach that acknowledges their courage and ability to "carry on" and at the same time responds to their fears is essential. It is important to understand which of the many fears and feelings of loss are most troublesome to the particular patient and family, and focus attention on those concerns first. Different fears may surface as the family continues through the terminal phase. Sometimes by knowing family history, it is possible to anticipate which concerns are most likely to arise and address those to the family as commonly occurring feelings thereby giving them reassurance that they are not "going crazy" or "should be doing better." One way to provide such support and to reduce the fear of loneliness and suffering is to continue to schedule conferences with the patient and family.

During this terminal period staff members must consistently try to determine that information given is correctly perceived and understood by patient and family. To accomplish this, the staff must be willing to reiterate and listen to family's reiterations several times. This enables the emotionally charged, anxiety-producing information to become synthesized into the family system, thereby reducing some of the fear of the unknown.

There is also a large body of research (Suls and Mullen, 1981; Schneidman, 1978; Rebok, 1979) which indicates that having some control, being able to make some determination of care management, is most valued by families and plays a large part in decreasing feelings of helplessness. Considering the family constellation as expert about their own needs and therefore partners with the health care team is one way of achieving shared control. This stance is perfectly consistent with allowing the patient and family to lean heavily on the staff's expertise during times of extra stress or difficult decision making.

Finally, Weisman and Sobel (1979) describe good coping, which increases tolerance for the dying process as an active, problem-solving approach through which one deals with a problem by defining it, creating several possible solutions and imagining how each one might fit, and then choosing the most acceptable at the time.

It is important to help families who are often medically naive frame the problems they are likely to encounter in the coming weeks, explore several care options, and together with staff decide on a course of action with the understanding that as conditions change, this process can be repeated and alternatives reconsidered.

It is beyond the scope of this chapter to examine all the options for care and treatment of the dying patient and family. Instead we will focus on Hospice as one alternative for palliative care.

IV. HOSPICE

In the last several years there has been phenomenal growth in the number of Hospice programs in this country. In 1984 the National Hospice Organization estimated there were over 1000 hospices, whereas 10 years before there had been none (Fact Sheet, 1984). This growth represents a response to the many needs of dying persons and their families for information and support, which are not met by other institutions and cannot be. The needs are too great to be handled by one physician or even by a small health care team. Now throughout the country Hospices work in cooperation with the entire team to extend sensitive and comprehensive care to both patient and family. Hospice reflects a particular philosophy of care. It is defined as a "centrally administered program of palliative and support services which provides physical, psychological, social, and spiritual care for dying persons and their families. Services are provided by a medically supervised, interdisciplinary team of professionals and volunteers. Hospice services are available in both the home and inpatient setting. Home care is provided on a part-time, intermittent, regularly scheduled, and round-the-clock or on-call basis. Bereavement services are available to the family" (Standards of a Hospice program of care, National Hospice Organization, 1979).

Although the definition above is accurate and complete, it does not quite
capture the essence of Hospice care as Peter Mudd does in this description:
"Hospice works best when the family and Hospice team confront the reality
of death together. That is the magic. Hospice workers should help the
family to realize their potential in caring for the dying person (and the dying
person for himself) and for each other and they should try within reason to
do whatever the family (and person) cannot accomplish. In keeping within
this guideline the family assumes the prime responsibility for its own fate,
with Hospice team members as valuable resources to draw on" (Mudd, 1982,
p. 12).

People hear about Hospice in many ways. Friends, family, professionals,
and the media are sources of information for the dying person and family.
They must choose Hospice care together with their physician, and both must
sign a consent form. The form clearly states that care is palliative in nature.

Once the physician and family make the sometimes difficult decision that
symptom control is the major goal, several other factors must be considered
especially when the choice involves home-based Hospice care, the most prevalent form of Hospice in the United States.

First, studies show that most symptoms can be managed at home (Brescia,
Sadof, and Barstow, 1984). Most needed equipment is rentable. Intravenous
feeding, injections, suctioning, and other skills can be taught to families or
managed by professionals.

Professionals need to take into account the care needs of the patient and
the family resources available to meet those needs (Rosenbaum and Rosenbaum,
1980). Small families can become exhausted and unable to continue especially
with a prolonged dying period. Elderly families sometimes do not have the
stamina to provide even minimal care. Finally, if family members need to
work, there must be someone who can be with the patient during the time
the family is away from home. If other family members or friends cannot
cover work time, the family will need to have the financial resources to pay
someone to stay with their relative.

Professionals thinking about Hospice for particular families might also consider that some Hospices have resources for respite and some do not. Some
provide aide service; others provide none. Those Hospices that are Medicare-
certified must provide certain specified services (see "Final Medicare Regulations—Hospice" in the Appendix). Therefore, it is important to know
exactly what is provided by the local Hospice before recommending its use.

There are also admission criteria designed by each Hospice which may keep
out people who probably could use the service. Gold (1983) noted that
although there is flexibility in admission criteria, there are several categories
of people who find it difficult to gain admission to a Hospice program: (1)
the unattached single, widowed, or divorced person; (2) the very old who have

survived their families and support groups; (3) those for whom prognosis is uncertain or whose physicians decline to reveal the prognosis to patients and families; (4) those who do not wish to verbalize their own awareness of dying; (5) those who have been deceived by physicians or families about diagnosis or prognosis; (6) those with little or no insurance coverage; (7) those whose physicians oppose Hospice care or are not accurately or fully informed about Hospice care; (8) those lacking linkages to make referrals; and (9) those living in areas not served by a Hospice program (Gold, 1983, p. 55).

Although Hospice is not for everyone, and there are barriers for some who are appropriate candidates, for the most part Hospice is a viable choice, a life-enhancing choice. Two families cared for by Triangle Hospice, a home-based program, can serve to further illustrate Hospice care more fully.

Triangle Hospice serves two counties in central North Carolina. The care it provides is medically directed by the patient's own physician. An interdisciplinary team of nurses, who function as care coordinators, social workers, clergy, and lay and professional volunteers provide most of the service with financial and legal advisors available as needed. About 50% of the families also employ nursing services provided by a home health agency. The following case presentations illustrate many facets of care at Triangle Hospice.

Mr. R, a 64-year-old retired small business manager, had been diagnosed as having oat cell carcinoma of the lung several months before. Despite chemotherapy, the cancer was rapidly advancing and had metastasized to his liver and elsewhere in the abdomen. It was clear that he had only a few months to live. At his married sons' request, Mr. R was referred to Hospice by the physician.

In an hour-long visit to the Hospice office, the sons expressed their concerns about the ability of both their parents to function in the coming weeks. Both sons, busy executives (one living in a town 10 miles away, 1 from out of state), described their father as a stubborn, autocratic ruler who "refused to face his condition." They spoke of their mother as a "dingbat," an anxious woman who had been given ECT years before for depression and since then had not functioned well socially. They described their parents as having acquaintances but no close friends and their home life as quiet with few visitors allowed in. They also made clear that their own role in the care of their father would be minimal. The younger and geographically closer son—J—planned to take over financial matters and would "advise" both parents in a weekly visit home.

Later that week, in a short interview in the family dining room, Mr. R, a grayish-looking, thin man, made very clear in his terse but polite Southern style that although he had periods of pain and was anorexic, he felt relatively well at present. He also hoped he might "lick this thing," although he was not sure; thus he refused Hospice care. Mrs. R, a neatly dressed 60-year-old who paced constantly in the immaculate room, spoke pleasantly enough but her conversation was circumstantial and sometimes difficult to follow. She had begun to make eye contact and offer brief nods as we described Hospice care, but quickly deferred to her husband's refusal.

The combination of Mr. R's denial of his condition, his need for control, his somewhat common perception that Hospice equals death, and the family's tightly circumscribed boundaries resulted in, "Don't call us; we'll call you."

Mr. R's wavering denial of his condition is typical of many patients: in some it persists until their death. People move in and out of denial and acceptance, sometimes in the same sentence. Mr. R's need for control was greater than most, yet control is an important issue for most people who are dying. As mentioned earlier, the more "in control" people feel, the better they can cope with the myriad of symptoms and changes in life style. Finally, although the R family boundaries were more circumscribed than most, it is common for families to complain of enforced isolation as the illness wears on and friends/neighbors/family resume their own lives and visit less.

Obviously, families always have the choice to accept or reject Hospice care. The role of Hospice personnel is to present information and to help sort out feelings, values, and preferences so that families can make a reasoned decision on any care issue. The actual decision making resides with them in consultation with their physician, no matter how futile or unwise the decision seems to us, except where there is obvious incompetence or lack of safety. The role of Hospice personnel is to attempt to help the family enact care based on their own decision.

Sometimes families who refuse Hospice care at first will later reconsider. This often occurs when the patient's condition deteriorates or a crisis in caregiving ensues, and feelings of being overwhelmed mount. Such was the case with the Rs.

Hospice became actively involved with the Rs 4 days after Mr. R's discharge from the hospital 2 weeks later. He had been admitted for dehydration and poorly controlled pain. The pain was due to an enlarging liver and abdominal metastases and he was treated with Dilaudid q4h with relief. His dehydration, secondary to vomiting and poor fluid intake, had been treated with I.V.s and antiemetics that controlled the nausea and vomiting. It was clear to his physician that one factor contributing to his poor fluid intake was depression and he was placed on a tricyclic antidepressant which also often enhances pain control. A few days after discharge, he was again in pain and dehydrated. At this point he acceded to his sons' request (order?) to accept Hospice care.

When we saw Mr. R this time he was a bed-bound, cachectic man huddled in fetal position. Mrs. R and J deluged us with questions about care. She apparently had been bombarding the physician in twice-daily calls as well. During this visit, Mrs. R sat fairly quietly and made good eye contact as we

answered oft repeated questions. Both she and the care coordinator wrote
down answers to questions, since it was clear that her anxiety level was high
enough to lead to misperceptions and forgetfulness. We also responded
approvingly, if with some surprise, to her good, common-sense approaches to
managing her husband's needs. Revealingly, it was J who consistently mis-
interpreted our responses and then angrily contradicted his mother's correct
understanding. It was also interesting to note that his care planning was much
more rigid than hers; yet she would consistently, if somewhat resentfully, bow
to his command.

From these two encounters and later observations, our mutual and professional goals were delineated. The whole family expressed an urgent need for
better pain control. Physical symptom control is obviously of primary
importance in Hospice care for all families. Mr. R's Dilaudid had been prescribed
on a prn basis, despite extensive literature that indicates that administration of
pain medication on a regular round-the-clock schedule is most effective in the
treatment of chronic pain in the terminally ill. The reasons for the effectiveness
of such a schedule follow:

1. Patients spend less time in pain as a result of obtaining a relatively
    steady plasma level of analgesic.
2. Doses of analgesic can be lower than if pain is allowed to increase or
    become severe; therefore, there are fewer side effects.
3. Decreased anxiety about the return of pain erases the memory of pain
    and its anticipation.
4. Patients experience decreased concern about obtaining relief when
    needed; thus there is a concomitant decrease in craving the drug.
5. Patients can therefore increase their physical activity (McCaffrey, 1984;
    Blumberg, 1983).

With Mr. R we briefly discussed the theory of pain control in simple and
concrete terms, noting to him how effective this had been while he was
hospitalized. We also reassured all family members that his doctor would ap-
prove of the modified schedule (as we knew from discussing the issue with him
before). Mrs. R quickly agreed to try a regular every 4-hour schedule. She
was, however, not at all certain that her husband would accept the medication
and was openly skeptical of her son's "order" to "order him" (father) to
take it.

There are many reasons why patients do not take pain medication on a
regular basis even when prescribed: (1) fear of addiction; (2) fear of side
effects; (3) fear of loss of control and stoic acceptance of pain as an integral
part of the condition; (4) feelings that one must "hold out" until the pain
"really gets bad;" and (5) fear that there will be nothing to take when the
pain "really gets bad" (McCaffrey, 1984).

Mr. R stated that he was, indeed, most afraid of becoming addicted, but did respond to a suggestion that he try the medication on a regular basis for a few days. We also gave him a very brief explanation of supporting research. We made sure to note that he could adjust the schedule of administration as soon as the pain was decreased, thereby addressing the issue of control to some extent.

Clearly, this totally family-centered approach to pain control, a cornerstone of Hospice care, was useful. Mr. R's pain was quickly and well controlled with smaller amounts of medication until a couple of weeks later, when he again would refuse the medication until the pain was excruciating. In reevaluating with him, we found that his new fear was of "not enough medication for later when it gets bad." By this time we had developed an alliance with him and he responded to our reassurance that there would be enough medication available to control his pain. We had told him this early in our work with him; however, then his high anxiety level and lack of trust in us made this information value-less to him.

Mr. R remained largely pain-free until his death; for the last few days, when he was comatose, he received Dilaudid suppositories because he had moaned and seemed restless. Although we can never be certain that pain was the cause of this behavior, at Triangle Hospice we treat it as such. No harm comes from this tactic, and it provides much comfort to bystanding caregivers.

Concomitantly, when Mr. R's pain was controlled he also had good fluid intake, until close to the end of his life. This may have been due in part to the resulting decrease in vegetative signs of depression. It may have also been another sign that he was less in need of control by noncompliance. He and his wife responded well to our concrete suggestions about the amounts of fluid he needed to take in order to remain hydrated and as comfortable as possible.

Gradually, as he neared death, he stopped taking fluids and became lethargic, then comatose. This lack of intake was not distressing to Mr. or Mrs. R per se, although his nearing death obviously was. For many families and doctors the issue of whether "to hydrate, feed or not" is crisis producing. Feeding is perceived as such an important part of caring for someone, yet lack of food or fluid does not seem to engender pain as such. Dehydration can produce some beneficial effects such as reduced nausea and vomiting especially with bowel obstruction, decreased pulmonary secretions, decreased choking from pharyngeal secretions, and decreased peripheral and pulmonary edema. De-hydration can also lead to electrolyte imbalance with increased lethargy, con-fusion, neuromuscular irritability, and cardiac arrhythmias (Zerwekh, 1983). As we noted before, we present the information about the pros and cons of feeding/hydrating to families, then help them come to a decision with which they are comfortable in consultation with their physician.

We continued to teach Mrs. R to care for her husband in three-times-a-week visits and almost daily phone calls. When there was a crisis, such as when he was restless and moaning, the nurse-on-call (who is available 24 hours/day) obtained a prescription for suppositories and taught Mrs. R to use them. Had we planned far enough ahead, as we routinely do now, we would have recommended having some suppositories on hand to prevent that kind of panic call. Our frequent encounters with the Rs demonstrated that intense nursing intervention decreased the need for pain medication and decreased Mrs. R's reliance on the physician.

We also provided a volunteer, Ann, who bathed and cared for Mr. R for several hours, twice a week. This gave Mrs. R respite from the 24-hour/day, 7 days/week grind. Ann was an R.N. who could also assess changing physical status, reinforce symptom control tenets, and troubleshoot the myriad aspects of care involved with a dying person. She also supported Mrs. R in her ongoing, if anxiety-ridden, attempts to encourage Mr. R to take his medication, to turn and position him as his skin started to break down, and to monitor his fluid intake.

Hospice-trained lay and professional volunteers are an essential component of any home care Hospice. Lay volunteers provide relief time and errand running for caregivers. They also provide ongoing support that decreases the isolation that comes with the narrowing of field of the dying and their caregivers. Volunteers accomplish all this by utilizing skills of nonjudgmental listening and hours of friendly concern shown in a variety of ways that demonstrate to all family members that they are valued and of concern just as the patient is.

Mindful of how little energy most family members have to start new relationships at this time, we try to carefully match the volunteer to the family. Because of the constricted R family boundaries, we especially wanted to introduce the least stressful intruder. Fortunately, Ann was a trusted nurse who worked in the hospital in which Mr. R had been treated. She had cared for Mr. R and had provided support for Mrs. R while her husband was hospitalized. We were pleased at how quickly and comfortably she was accepted, indeed relied upon by the Rs.

With Ann's support, Mrs. R also agreed to allow fellow church members to come in. They had volunteered to clean the house and cut Mr. R's hair, mundane tasks, but ones vitally important to Mr. and Mrs. R's emotional well-being. Thus Hospice helped this family tap into informal community resources. Hospice personnel also coordinate care and can help families locate and utilize more formal community resources including legal and financial services when necessary.

One of our goals with the R family was to decrease the clearly apparent emotional distress. We know from a study by Wellisch et al. (1983a) that after somatic side effects, mood disturbance is the most commonly cited distressing symptom of the homebound cancer patient. Many authors discuss issues of emotional distress in the terminally ill and their families; among them are Simonton and Simonton (1975), Schneidman (1978), Weisman (1979), Holland (1982), and Tornberg, McGrath, and Benoliel (1984). Since the issues of cancer and dysphoria are addressed in more depths in Chapter 8, we will simply highlight a few pertinent aspects.

Our observations were that Mr. R became emotionally incapacitated rapidly, and that he was a depressed man for whom antidepressants were effective in relieving the vegetative signs of depression but not as a mood elevator. It was evident that even before he became physically incapacitated, he had collapsed into regression.

One factor that may partly account for this was the rapidity of disease progression which overwhelmed his usual coping skills. Another factor that may have had some role in his massive regression was the rigidity of his defenses. He had always been known as a quiet, very controlled and controlling man who paid meticulous attention to detail. He lived his life in unvarying routine where doing one's duty was paramount. "A sense of powerlessness is particularly threatening to the type of individual who has characteristically denied or minimized dependency need" (Kiely, 1972, p. 113). Finally, one cannot rule out unknown organic factors that may have played some role in his regression.

Our approach to this taciturn man who never did talk about death or dying was to treat him as a man who still needed to be responsible and have some choices in matters affecting him and his well-being. This approach seemed to work well in some areas such as those described before in the example of pain medication. It is an approach supported by Goldberg (among others), in his article "Management of Depression in the Patient with Advanced Cancer," where he discusses the use of joint control as a treatment strategy with depressed patients (Goldberg, 1981).

Our approach also included demonstrating our utmost trustworthiness and meticulous attention to detail and to his wishes in order to decrease his fear of the intruder. We also made sure to let him know, to the extent that we could, what symptoms to anticipate, and how we planned to intervene, while being careful to allow and encourage him to express his preferences. This approach worked well also; the reassurance it gave him combined with his pressing need at that time for knowledgeable caregivers allowed us to enter the system and be perceived as dependable, panic-easing and loneliness-decreasing figures.

It is also clear to us that all members of any family are entwined in an ever narrowing and sensitively balanced system. It is pertinent to this particular case to note a study by Wellisch et al. (1983b) which demonstrates that elderly families and families caring for a male with lung cancer are most overwhelmed, depressed, and frightened. They attribute these findings to the decreasing stamina of older age and the rapid physical decline of lung cancer patients, which necessitates many adaptations in a short time span. Despite all, as mentioned above, at Triangle Hospice we are often impressed by the strength that many patients and families exhibit at this stressful time; Mrs. R, surprisingly, was no exception. She fit all the criteria for a disastrous Hospice-at-home case study; she was a relatively older woman caring for a male with lung cancer, and she had a psychiatric history with still-evident high levels of anxiety, obsessiveness, and dependency.

Despite all this, she was motivated by her strong need to continue to function and to maintain herself for her husband and provide exceptional care for him. This was clear in the meticulous notebook she kept of his daily routine. She was knowledgeable about basic care and practiced her knowledge somewhat obsessively but with concern and sensitivity to his moods.

Since she was so overwhelmed at first, her natural or learned inclination to "keep the intruders out" was only a small factor once we established our trustworthiness and our wish to engage with her to keep her husband comfortable. She quickly transferred some dependence from the physician to us. In response to her many phone calls, we established a schedule of frequent visits and calls. This cut down calls to the doctor to once or twice a week and meant only one panicky nighttime call to us despite many long, lonely hours she spent caring for her husband.

We also told her frequently that she was giving excellent care and reassured her of our genuine admiration. With our help, she was also beginning to make all the role shifts she needed to in order to successfully carry on presently and survive without her husband after his death. It is a commonly used strategy of Hospice personnel to support patient and family strengths and to minimize attention to pathology as much as possible; this works well in a supportive role.

This stance was most tested when mother and son were together. With the help of a family therapist (who meets with us, our medical director, chaplain, representatives from other nursing agencies, and volunteers in a weekly team conference) we devised a strategy of continued support for Mrs. R with as little threat and as much acknowledgment for her son. It was a difficult balancing act at times, but it had become fairly clear that she was, in many ways, the family scapegoat, "the sick one." It was immensely gratifying after Mr. R's death when J told us how important we were in helping him realize how competent his mother was and how special she was to him.

Part of the role of Hospice is to prepare family members for the event of death and its aftermath and provide support at the actual time of death and later, during bereavement. As Worden (1982), Sanders (1982), and Seigal and

Weinstein (1983) point out, too long a time of anticipatory grief can be just as traumatic as sudden death. For Mrs. R there seemed to be enough time for her to grieve in anticipation without the prolonged decline that can result in overwhelming pressure, guilt, detachment, and exhaustion on the part of the caregiver. She was able to plan the funeral, take care of other necessary arrangements, somewhat rehearse her life without him, and begin to mourn his passing. Parkes (1972) discusses how active participation in making arrangements eases immediate adjustments to a death. She was also able to tell him that she loved him and would miss him; from her statements, it sounded as if he had been able to tell her this also.

At the actual time of death, Mrs. R called the Hospice care coordinator who pronounced Mr. R dead, called her doctor and the funeral home, and waited at the house until after the funeral home took the body, and the family had arrived. Mrs. R tolerated the whole process with tears and, beginning acceptance of the reality of the loss, said, "I will miss him; we've been together a long time." She had no obviously pathological distress, despite her son's constant worry that she was not "all right."

Hospice personnel went to the funeral and continued for the next several months to maintain frequent contact; we do so for at least 1 year if we assess this as necessary. Mrs. R is now involved in a volunteer project in the community and is functioning quite well in her usual somewhat socially distant manner. She seems to be moving through at least three of the four tasks of mourning: (1) accepting the reality of the loss; (2) experiencing the pain of grief; (3) adjusting to an environment in which the deceased is missing; and (4) withdrawing emotional energy and reinvesting it in another relationship (Parkes, 1972, pp. 15-18). She is often lonely and sad but is burdened with surprisingly little anger and excess despair. Perhaps as Doka (1984) points out, constant involvement in a relative's care eases acceptance of death.

Perhaps too her relationship with her husband was not a highly ambivalent one, although given Mr. R's personality and her role in the family, one might expect it to have been so. In any case, thus far she does not exhibit any of the clues of complicated grief which Worden (1982, pp. 64-65) enumerates:

1. The person cannot speak of the deceased without experiencing intense and fresh grief.
2. Some minor event triggers off an intense grief reaction.
3. The person is unwilling to move material possessions belonging to the deceased.
4. The person develops physical symptoms like those of the deceased often at anniversary times or when reaching the same age as the deceased.

5. The person makes radical changes in lifestyle or excludes those who were involved with the deceased.
6. The person presents a long history of subclinical depression earmarked by persistent guilt and lowered self-esteem.
7. The person has a compulsion to imitate the dead person.
8. The person may have self-destructive impulses.
9. The person may experience unaccountable sadness at a certain anniversary time each year.
10. The person experiences a phobia about illness or death often related to the specific illness that took the deceased.
11. The person may have avoided death-related rituals or activities.
12. Themes of loss come up in interviews (Worden, 1982, p. 68).

Most patients are not like Mr. R, who was unable or unwilling to talk about his life or his dying. Most patients, if they are not burdened by symptoms such as pain or dyspnea, want to talk about their past life and their dying, even if not named as such by them.

"Encounters with the dying are frequently characterized by some narration of their life story. In terms of family, job, sense of self or religion, these stories are interpretations of how the process of disease and death fit, or fail to fit, into a larger account of things. Only the dying can narrate or tell the story, because only they know how the story goes" (Churchill, 1979).

One of the most valuable services Hospice provides is the people, volunteers or staff, who have the time, desire, and the sensitivity to listen well to patients' and families' life stories. At times the symbolism in the stories is clearer than at other times, but knowing the symbolism is often not important to the process.

Mr. M was a man who talked directly and clearly about his illness, multiple myeloma, once he trusted the Hospice personnel. However, he also spent time talking in great detail about his career in the police department, a career of which he was proud. He was a man who had become a sergeant when few black men were promoted to that post and he had created functional, well-run squads from groups of sometimes hostile men.

With most people, Hospice involvement begins with a focus on symptom control. It was no exception with Mr. M. He had been diagnosed with myeloma 3 years before and had been through many rounds of chemotherapy, with sepsis occurring several times as a result of leukopenia. He had also received radiation therapy to many sites of his body, "chasing" the plasmacytomas as they appeared.

By the time Hospice was involved, he was in mild chronic renal failure, had no use of his left arm due to bony disintegration, and had peripheral neuropathies as a result of vincristine. During the time we worked with him, the beginning of each meeting was spent dealing with new symptoms, reviewing old symptoms, and sorting out symptom management in conjunction with his physician.

It was clear that these discussions of symptoms, as much as they were an end unto themselves, were also a bridge to Mr. M's need to tell his story. As his symptoms increased and his usual ability to maintain a stoic affect and controlled demeanor was tested, his stories about the police force became more detailed and ongoing. He talked a lot about his strategies for shaping the police squads. He related how he evaluated each person's ability, sorted out who could work well together, defused hostile reactions to him, and stroked various commanders and subordinates.

As he became sicker his stories ceased and he, as the usual family care-taker, focused on preparing his family for his approaching death. He planned his funeral with them and instructed his wife as to his wishes in several other practical matters important to him. They spent a lot of time talking and cry-ing together. As with others, in many ways, Mr. M still maintained the surface of "fighting on; I'm not tired." Yet his behavior had obviously changed and he clearly had moved on, for the most part, to the next phase before his death.

During the last stage of his life Mr. M, as do many patients, gradually with-drew from those around him. He spoke little, slept a great deal, and seemed unconcerned with the daily life of his family. This caused some distress in his wife who wanted more time with him in the way he had once been with her. We spent time daily with her at this point telling her that he was prepar-ing for the final phase of his living-dying. Simply being there with her and allowing her to ventilate her feelings was providing some of the support she needed to be able to let go of him.

That Hospice personnel have the time and ability to recognize the value of storytelling and to understand without direct statement that a patient has moved on to a new phase in the living-dying process and to help families come to terms with this process is part of the magic of Hospice.

V. CONCLUSION

For those who are dying and their family members there are many times of crisis and intense need; there are also many times of strength and growth. Physicians and the health care team can intervene to promote the strength and to provide support in times of need. They can deal sensitively with informa-tion giving; they can promise and deliver continued expert care as partners with patients, families, and by extension with Hospice personnel and those not formally associated with a Hospice, but who know how to give Hospice care.

REFERENCES

Blumberg, B. (March 1983). Control of cancer pain, *Fact Sheet,* National Cancer Institute, Bethesda, Md.

Brescia, I., Sadof, M., and Barstow, J. (1984). Retrospective analysis of a home care Hospice program, *Omega, 15*:37-44.

Churchill, L. (1979). The experience of dying, *Sounding,* University of North Carolina Faculty Lecture Series Reprint, Chapel Hill.

Dickinson, G., and Pearson, A. (1980). Death education and physicians attitudes toward dying patients, *Omega, 11*:167-174.

Doka, K. (1984). Expectations of death, participation in funeral arrangements and grief adjustment, *Omega, 15*:119-129.

Feigenberg, L., and Schneidman, E. (1979). Clinical thanatology and psychotherapy: Some reflections on caring for the dying person, *Omega, 10*: 1-8.

Freedman, T. (1982). *The Role of the Family Therapist in Clinical Care of the Terminal Cancer Patient* (B. Cassileth and P. Cassileth, eds.), Lea & Febiger, Philadelphia, pp. 119-127.

Gold, M. (1983). *Life Support: What Families Say About Hospital, Hospice, and Home Care for the Fatally Ill,* Institute for Consumer Policy Research, Consumers Union Foundation, Mt. Vernon, N.Y., pp. 15-28, 55.

Goldberg, A. (1981). Management of depression in the patient with advanced cancer, *JAMA 246*:373-376.

Hertzberg, L. (1972). Cancer and the dying patient, *Am. J. Psychiat., 128*: 808-810.

Holland, J. (1982). Psychosocial aspects of cancer, *Cancer Medicine* (J. Holland and E. Frei, eds.), Lea & Febiger, Philadelphia, pp. 1181-1190.

Kiely, W. F. (1972). Coping with severe illness, *Adv. Psychosomat. Med., 8*: 105-118.

Kincade, J. (1982). Attitudes of physicians, house staff and nurses on care for the terminally ill, *Omega, 13*:333-344.

McCaffrey, M. (1984). Pain: Assessment and intervention in nursing practice, Presentation at Duke University, Durham, N.C., December 6, 1984.

Mudd, P. (1982). High ideals and hard cases: The evolution of a Hospice, *Hastings Center Report, 2*:11-14.

National Hospice Organization. (1979). *Standards of a Hospice Program of Care,* National Hospice Organization, Arlington, Va.

National Hospice Organization. (1984). *Fact Sheet,* National Hospice Organization, Arlington, Va.

Neimeyer, G., Behnke, M., and Reiss, J. (1983). Constructs and coping: Physicians responses to patient death, *Death Education, 7*:245-264.

Parkes, C. M. (1972). *Bereavement: Studies of Grief in Adult Life,* International Universities Press, New York, pp. 15-18, 68.

Pattison, M. (1967). The experience of dying, *Am. J. Psychother., 21*:32-43.

Rebok, G. (1979). Clients nearing death: Behavioral treatment perspectives, *Omega, 10*:191-201.

Redding, R. (1980). Doctors, dyscommunication and death, *Death Education*, *3*:371-385.

Rosenbaum, E. H., and Rosenbaum, J. R. (1980). Principles of home care for patients with advanced cancer, *JAMA*, *244*:1484-1487.

Sanders, C. (1982). Effect of sudden versus chronic illness death on bereavement outcome, *Omega*, *13*:227-241.

Scott, D., Goode, W., and Arlin, Z. (1983). Multiple remissions, *Cancer Nursing*, *6*:202-206.

Schneidman, E. (1978). Some aspects of psychotherapy with dying persons, *Psychosocial Aspects of Terminal Care* (C. Garfield, ed.), McGraw-Hill, New York, pp. 201-218.

Seigal, K., and Weinstein, L. (1983). Anticipatory grief reconsidered, *J. Psychosoc. Oncol.*, *1*:61-73.

Simonton, C., and Simonton, O. (1975). Belief systems and management of the emotional aspects of malignancy, *J. Transpersonal Psychol.*, *7*:1-4.

Suls, J., and Mullen, B. (1981). Life events, perceived control and illness: The role of uncertainty, *J. Human Stress*, *7*:30-34.

Tornberg, M., McGrath, B., and Benoliel, J. (1984). Oncology transition services: Partnerships for nurses and families, *Cancer Nursing*, *7*:131-137.

Wanzer, S., Adelstein, S., Cranford, R., Federman, D., Hook, E., Moertel, C., Safar, P., Stone, A., Taussic, H., and Van Eys, J. (1984). The physicians' responsibility toward hopelessly ill patients, *New Engl. J. Med.*, *310*:955-959.

Weisman, A. (1979). A model for psychosocial phasing in cancer, *Gen. Hosp. Psychiat.*, *1*:187-195.

Weisman, A., and Hackett, T. (1961). Predilection to death, *Psychosomat. Med.*, *23*:232-256.

Weisman, A., and Sobel, H. (1979). Coping with cancer through self instruction: A hypothesis, *J. Human Stress*, *5*:3-8.

Weisman, A., and Worden, J. (1976). The existential plight in cancer: Significance of the first 100 days, *Int. J. Psychiat. Med.*, *7*:1-15.

Wellisch, D., Landsverk, J., Guidera, K., Pasnau, R., and Fawzy, F. (1983a). Evaluation of psychosocial problems of homebound cancer patients, *Psychosomat. Med.*, *45*:11-23.

Wellisch, D., Fawzy, F., Landsverk, J., Pasnau, R., and Wolcott, D. (1983b). Evaluation of psychosocial problems of the homebound cancer patient: The relationship of disease and sociodemographic variables of patients to family problems, *J. Psychosoc. Oncol.*, *1*:1-17.

Worden, J. W. (1982). *Grief Counseling and Grief Therapy: A Handbook for Mental Health Practitioners*, Springer-Verlag, New York, pp. 15-18, 64-65, 87-90.

Zerwekh, J. (January 1983). The dehydration question, *Nursing*, *13*:47-51.

APPENDIX: HOSPICE MEDICARE BENEFITS

On December 16, 1983, the Department of Health and Human Services (HHS) published the final rules providing coverage for Hospice care for terminally ill Medicare beneficiaries who elect to receive care from a participating Hospice. The regulations establish eligibility requirements and reimbursement standards and procedures, define covered services, and delineate the conditions a Hospice must meet to be approved for participation in the Medicare program. Highlights of the rules, which are effective retroactively to November 1, 1983, are set forth below.

1. Eligibility and Conditions of Coverage

A terminally ill Medicare beneficiary may elect to receive Hospice care in lieu of most other traditional Medicare benefits for up to two periods of 90 days each, plus an additional 30 days. An individual must be certified as terminally ill within 2 days of initiating Hospice care by both his attending physician (if the individual has one) and the Hospice medical director or the physician member of the Hospice interdisciplinary team for the first 90-day benefit period. A beneficiary is considered terminally ill if there is a medical prognosis that his life expectancy is 6 months or less.

2. Election of Hospice Care and Revocation

Eligible individuals must file an election statement to receive Hospice care with a particular Hospice. An initial election will remain in effect for the first 90-day coverage period as well as the additional authorized 90- and 30-day periods as long as the individual remains in the care of the Hospice and does not revoke the election to receive Hospice care. The election statement must include acknowledgment that the individual understands that certain Medicare services are waived by the election. An individual could revoke an election to receive Hospice care at any time. The individual would then resume regular Medicare coverage until such time as the individual reelects to receive Hospice care. A revocation of Hospice coverage results in a forfeiture of the remaining days of possible coverage for Hospice care in that election period.

3. Waiver of Other Benefits

During the time the Hospice election is in effect, the beneficiary will be deemed to have waived entitlement to any Medicare services related to the treatment of the individual's terminal illness or services equivalent to or duplicative of Hospice care. Coverage will continue for services provided by the individual's attending physician if the physician is not employed by the Hospice program. While coverage may also continue for certain other benefits in exceptional and un-usual circumstances as HHS may provide, HHS does not yet know the specific types of circumstances that may warrant the use of this exception. Addition-ally, HHS is authorized to establish guidelines to stipulate what services are waived which relate to the treatment of the individual's terminal condition or are the equivalent of Hospice care. While HHS has not issued such guidelines, it has acknowledged that there are many illnesses that may occur when an individual is terminally ill which may be brought on by the underlying weakened condition of the patient (e.g., pneumonia). Treatment of such illness would be considered a Hospice service and payment of other Medicare benefits would be waived by the Hospice election.

4. Covered Services

In order to be covered, Hospice services must be reasonable and necessary for the palliation or management of the terminal illness as well as related conditions. The services must be consistent with a written plan of care to be established for each individual by the individual's attending physician, the Hospice medical director, and the interdisciplinary Hospice team group before care is actually provided.

Covered services are nursing care, medical social services, physician services, counseling services, short-term inpatient care ("respite" care), medical appliances and supplies including drugs and biologicals, home health aide services, physical therapy, occupational therapy, and speech language pathology services. Nursing care, home health aide, and homemaker services may be provided on a 24-hour continuous basis only during periods of crisis and only as necessary to maintain the terminally ill individual at home. Respite care is short-term inpatient care provided only when necessary to relieve family members or other persons caring for the individual. It must be provided only on an occasional basis and cannot be reimbursed for more than 5 consecutive days at a time. Bereavement counseling is a required Hospice service, but is not reimbursable under Medicare.

5. Conditions of Participation

Hospice programs are eligible to participate in Medicare if they are public or private organizations primarily engaged in providing Hospice services. They are required to make these services available on a 24-hour basis, in individual's homes, on an outpatient basis, and on a short-term inpatient basis.

A Hospice must have a governing body that assumes full professional and management responsibility for determining, implementing, and monitoring policies governing the Hospice's total operation. It also must have a doctor of medicine or osteopathy who serves as medical director and who assumes overall responsibility for the medical aspects of the Hospice's program. An interdisciplinary group of Hospice employees must be designated to provide or supervise the care and services offered by the Hospice. A Hospice must assure that substantially all of the following services, referred to as "core" services, are provided directly by Hospice employees: nursing care, medical social services, physicians' services, and counseling services. The remaining "non-core" services may be provided either directly by the Hospice or under arrangements with others.

Other administrative and organizational requirements for Hospices include an ongoing, comprehensive, integrated quality assurance program; appropriate licensure for the Hospice and its employees; compliance with standards for the establishment and maintenance of central clinical records; use of volunteers, in defined roles, under the supervision of designated qualified Hospice staff members; use of appropriate informed consent forms; and provision of an ongoing program for training and education of its employees. A Hospice must also agree not to discontinue or diminish care provided to Medicare beneficiaries because of their inability to pay for care. This means that Hospice services would have to be provided even after the individual exhausts the Medicare Hospice benefit as long as the person wants to receive the services and is terminally ill.

6. Reimbursement

HHS has established payment amounts to reimburse specific categories of covered Hospice care. The Medicare payment for Hospice care per year may not exceed an average of $6500 per beneficiary. This amount is the Hospice "cap." Payment amounts for services are established for the following categories:

Routine home care (per day)	$ 53.17
The first 8 hours of continuous home care	$119.56
(Hourly rate after 8 hours)	$ 14.94
Inpatient respite care (per day)	$ 55.33
General inpatient care (per day)	$271.00

For each day an individual is not an inpatient the Hospice will receive a routine home care day payment (regardless of whether any services are provided). The patient must receive continuous care for a period of at least 8 hours for that care to be paid for at the continuous care rate of $19.56. For each additional hour or portion of an hour of continuous care, the Hospice will be paid on the basis of the hourly rate. The Hospice rates include the general supervisory services of the medical director and the interdisciplinary group physician member. Payment will be made for 100% of the reasonable charge for physician services furnished by Hospice employees or by other physicians under arrangements with the Hospice. Physicians who are neither employed by the Hospice nor providing services under arrangements are paid 80% of reasonable charges. All physician reimbursement is included in determining whether payments exceed the cap.

The Hospice is required to provide assurances that the aggregate number of inpatient (both general and respite) days provided in any 12-month period not exceed 20% of the aggregate number of days of Hospice care provided to Medicare beneficiaries during that period. The Hospice will receive payment at the routine home care rate for those inpatient days in excess of the 20% limit.

Except for a 5% coinsurance payment for drugs, biologicals, and inpatient respite care days, Medicare payment to a Hospice relieves an individual of liability for payment for any Hospice care services. The individual will be responsible for Medicare coinsurance for services received before or after the Hospice election and for physician services if the physician is not working under arrangement with the Hospice.

FINAL MEDICARE REGULATIONS—HOSPICE (ADDENDUM #1)

Final regulations implementing the Hospice benefits were issued by HCFA in the December 15, 1983, Federal Register. The final rules set lower daily Medicare payment rates for routine home care and respite care, while continuous home care rates were increased and the general inpatient care rate was unchanged. A comparison of the final rates is presented below. These rates are subject to adjustment for differences in local area wage rates utilizing the wage indices published in the Prospective Payment System Regulations.

	Final
Routine home care (per diem)	$ 53.17
Continuous home care	
Total continuous care rate	$311.96
8-16 hour interval	$156.96
16-20 hour interval	$233.97
20 through 24 hour interval	$285.96
Inpatient respite care (per diem)	$ 61.65
General inpatient care (per diem)	$271.00

In addition, the aggregate cap on Hospice coverage of $6500 per beneficiary per year, as set by P.L., 98-90 was adopted. The final rule provides for the cap to be adjusted by the Medical Care Component of the Consumer Price Index on November 1 annually.

There were a few changes made to certain provisions, which have been summarized below:

Short-term inpatient care—may only be provided in a hospital, SNF, or free-standing Hospice that meets the strengthened conditions.

Required services—only "critical services" need to be furnished on a 24-hour basis (i.e., nursing, physician, drugs, and biological services) and other services on an as-needed basis.

Election statement—may be signed by a representative when the patient is mentally unable to make the decision.

Medical supplies and drugs—may be administered by family members subject to state and local laws.

Medicare cost reporting—HCFA will require the filing of cost reports by all certified Hospices.

Fiscal intermediary—free-standing Hospices will be serviced by Blue Cross of California in states west of the Mississippi including Minnesota and Louisiana and by Prudential Insurance Company of America in states east of the Mississippi. Other free-standing Hospices will be serviced by the same fiscal intermediary as their parent organization.

Index

Achlorhydria, 54, 247
Activities (*see also* Leisure activities),
    8, 11, 31, 198, 204, 208, 243,
    254, 267-268, 280, 283,
    288-300, 305
ADLs (activities of daily living), 243,
    254, 267-268, 289
Adrenal insufficiency, 53
Adriamycin (*see* Chemotherapy)
Aging, 238-239, 241-249, 252-253, 255-
    256, 259, 261-264, 268-275
  Alzheimer's disease, 246, 258, 263,
    273
  blood urea nitrogen, 245
  bone marrow function, 247
  brain atrophy, 246
  cardiovascular system, 244-245,
    253, 271
  constipation, 122, 189, 211, 213,
    246, 261, 263
  creatinine, 125, 245-246
  diagnostic maneuver, 249
  emotional effects of cancer on, 253
  excessive toxicity in, 254

[Aging]
  immune function, 88, 248
  mortality, 37, 47-48, 54, 58, 93,
    108, 204, 212, 215-216,
    237-238, 245, 250-251, 256
  nutritional deficiencies, 246, 260-
    261, 269
  overtreatment, problem of, 224-
    231
  pain sensitivity, 259
  preoperative appraisal, 250-251
  prophylactic immunization, 262
  pulmonary changes, 245
  resources, financial, 267, 286, 314
  responsiveness of specific tumors,
    254
  skin changes, 262
  smell, changes in, 260
  support networks, 266-267
  taste, 252-253, 260
  therapeutic environment, 249, 294
  treatment protocols, selection of
    elderly for, 253
Alimentary tract sterilization, 91

Alkylating agents, 63, 77, 80, 82-85,
    87, 111, 113, 115, 129, 131,
    191, 228-229
  busulfan (Myleran), 76, 78, 83,
    111, 113-114, 130, 132, 165
  chlorambucil, 78, 83-84, 131-132,
    137, 228
  cyclophosphamide (Cytoxan), 27,
    63, 68, 80, 83-84, 109-110,
    114-116, 124-127, 130-131,
    136-137, 140, 143, 228, 254
  melphalan (Alkeran), 83
  nitrogen mustard, 63, 82-83, 138
Allergic reactions, 114-115
Alopecia, 6, 106-107, 136, 138
Alzheimer's disease (see Aging)
Amenorrhea (see Chemotherapy)
Analgesia, nonpharmacologic means,
    260
Anaphylactic reactions, 114-115
Androgens, hematologic effects, 87
Anemia, 75, 80-84, 87, 174, 247-248,
    254, 272, 297
  microangiopathic hemolytic, 81
Anesthesia, general, 244, 250
Ankylosis, 157, 173
Anorexia, 27, 44, 48, 50, 57, 65-67,
    168, 201, 261, 263
Anthracycline cardiomyopathy (see
    Chemotherapy)
Anticancer drugs, safety in handling,
    134
Anticipatory grief, 321-322, 326
Anticipatory nausea and vomiting,
    64, 67, 142
Antidepressant, 28, 187, 199, 210-212,
    216-217, 260, 264, 320, 361
Antidopaminergic drugs, 258
Antiemetic (see also Nausea, THC,
    Vomiting), 63-65, 68-73, 114,
    137-144, 168, 245, 257-258,
    316

Antihistamines, 53, 69-71, 115, 258
Antimetabolites (see also Chemo-
    therapy), 68, 77, 81, 84-85,
    122
Anxiety, 28, 71, 75, 119, 184, 188,
    202-206, 209, 217, 222, 233,
    250, 258-259, 263, 266, 281,
    283, 287, 291-292, 309, 312,
    317-319, 321
Apomorphine, emesis-inducing effect
    of, 70
Apprehension, 62, 205
Aspermia (see Chemotherapy)
Auditory canal (see Radiation therapy)
Autoimmune dysfunction, 248
Azoospermia (see Chemotherapy)

BCNU (see also Nitrosourea), 85, 116,
    129, 137, 165, 194, 254
Behavioral reactions, 256
Beliefs, 31, 207, 267, 286, 299-305
Bereavement, 204-206, 213, 215-216,
    266, 313, 321, 325-326, 328
Biliary obstruction, 55
Biochemical tumor markers, 181
Biopsy, 21-22, 30, 56, 109, 123, 164,
    171
  endomyocardial, 109, 269
Biopsychosocial profile, 237, 249, 270
Bladder, 9, 127, 169
Bleomycin (see Chemotherapy)
Blindness (see Radiation)
Blood-brain barrier, 225, 234
Blood urea nitrogen (see Aging)
Blood volume alterations, 45
Body image, 9, 96, 106, 207, 256
Body water excess (see Surgery)
Bone marrow protection (see Chemo-
    therapy)
Bone necrosis (see Radiation)
Bowel function (see also Radiation,
    246

Brain atrophy (*see* Aging)
Brain damage, 225
Brain metastases, 180-182, 194, 196
Brompton cocktail, 259

Cachexia, 48-49, 65-66, 261
Caldwell-Luc (*see* Radiation)
Cancer
    breast, 13, 20, 33, 38, 61, 64, 77,
        85, 132, 136, 174, 179, 215,
        251, 255-256, 269-270, 273,
        278-279, 283, 308
    care (curable), 237, 277
    care (incurable), treatment of (*see
        also* Hospice), 15
    estrogen receptor positive, 256
    fears of, 252
    head and neck, 148
    lung
        cost of, 13
        deaths from, 13, 17
    misconceptions about, 252
    prostate, 77, 181, 256,
    psychosocial and emotional
        effects of, 5, 253
    testicular, 10, 61, 64, 72, 125,
        179
    thyroid, radiation-induced, 228
Cannabinoids (*see also* Antiemetic,
        Tetrahydrocannabinoid,
        THC), 72, 257
Carcinoma (*see* Cancer)
Cardiac monitoring (*see* Cancer)
Cardiac monitoring (*see* Chemo-
        therapy)
Cardiomyopathy (*see* Chemotherapy)
Cardiotoxic agents, 245
Cataracts, 130, 132, 149-150
Catheter, 52, 55, 57, 58, 88, 94,
        96-97, 102, 193
    central venous, 96, 102
    Hickman, 96

[Catheter]
    implantable, 96
    sepsis, 52, 96-97
    subclavian, complications of, 51
    subclavian vein, thrombosis of, 52
CEA, 19-20, 23-24
Central nervous system (CNS), 70, 95,
        139, 179-182, 186-187, 191-
        192, 194-196, 207, 224-227,
        246, 270
Central venous access devices, 102
Cerebrospinal fluid (CSF), 180-181,
        186-187, 191-195, 225, 233
Chemoreceptor trigger zone (CTZ),
        70-71, 258
Chemotherapy, 1-2, 4, 9-10, 13-14,
        33-34, 49, 55, 61-146, 148,
        166-167, 172, 224-227,
        234-237, 244-245, 247-248,
        252-257, 259, 262, 268-271,
        273-274, 281-282, 285, 296-
        298, 315, 323
    adjuvant, 13, 24, 33, 61, 64, 132,
        184, 255, 269
    Adriamycin, 245, 254, 273
    alkeran, 83
    amenorrhea, 128
    anthracycline cardiomyopathy,
        107-108
    aspermia, 172
    azoospermia, 128, 229
    BCNU, 85, 165, 254
    bleomycin, 53, 59, 62, 110-112,
        114-116, 120, 127, 130,
        137-138, 165, 245, 254
    busulfan (Myleran), 83, 111,
        113-114, 130, 132, 165
    bone marrow protection, 83, 86
    cardiac monitoring, 107, 109
    cardiomyopathy, 107-109, 269
    cardiotoxicity of, 107-109, 139,
        144, 211, 273

[Chemotherapy]
chlorambucil, 78, 83-84, 131-132,
137, 228
cisplatin, 43, 62-64, 70-73, 114-
115, 125-127, 141, 189-
190, 195-196, 245-246,
257-259, 272
complications of, 62
cyclophosphamide (Cytoxan), 83,
115, 117, 124-127, 130,
228, 254
cystitis, 26-28, 126-127
diphenhydramine, 71, 115, 121,
187
drug extravasation, 62, 96-97
encephalopathy, 130, 185-192
fetus and, 129, 144
gastrointestinal toxicity, 120
haloperidol (see also Nausea),
70, 74
hematologic effects of, 75
hepatotoxicity, 122-123, 142, 145
hormonal, 131, 237, 239, 256
immunosuppression, 88
infections, 37, 87-97, 137, 139-
140, 186-187, 194, 206,
248, 262, 273
fungal, 93-95
GI, 122
prophylaxis program, 91
intrathecal, 95, 114, 190-192,
194, 224-227, 233, 235
late effects, 130, 176, 224-231
malabsorption, 43, 48, 247, 252,
261, 272
marrow aplasia, 76, 130, 255
mastication, 260
methotrexate, 63, 81, 84, 86, 106,
114, 116, 120-125, 130, 132,
144, 165, 191-192, 194, 196,
225, 233-235, 245, 254
methyl CCNU, 254

[Chemotherapy]
metoclopramide, 70-74, 139-140,
144, 187, 257, 259, 272
minimizing side effects of, 253
mitomycin-C, 81-83, 103, 106, 111-
114, 125-126, 130, 140
mucositis, 26, 48, 95-96, 121-122
mutagenesis, 131, 133
Myleran (busulfan), 83, 111, 113-
114, 130, 165
myelodysplastic bone marrow, 131
nausea and vomiting, 39, 44, 48, 57,
63-75, 84, 125, 139-145, 213,
253, 257-259, 316, 318
nephrotoxicity, 125, 127
neurotoxicity, 132, 187-189, 191,
194-196
nitrogen mustard, 63, 82-83, 138
nitrosourea, 76, 80, 85, 110, 122,
127, 254
ocular effects, 132
opportunistic organisms, 95
pigmentation, 116, 118, 262
procarbazine, 129, 131, 189-191, 194,
211, 290
prophylactic antibiotics, 90, 92, 95
retinopathy, 133, 140
risk to personnel, 133-136
scalp hypothermia, 106, 138, 143,
145
scalp tourniquets, 106
secondary malignancies, 129-132
shunts, 95, 186
skin toxicity, 116-119
stomatitis, 120-121
tissue necrosis, 97
vein care, 96-106
ventriculostomy reservoirs, 96
vinca alkaloids, 106, 122, 188-189,
259
vincristine, 68, 106, 122, 125, 133,
188-189, 246, 254

Chlorpromazine, 70
Cholestatic jaundice, 130
Choroid, 149
Chromosomal damage, 175
Ciliary body, 149
Cisplatin (*see* Chemotherapy)
CNS infections, 187
Coagulation defects, 82
Cognitive function, 246, 260, 263
Communication, 5-7, 9, 128, 136,
        213, 263, 282, 284, 286-
        287, 291-293, 302, 307,
        310, 326
Community clergy, 303
Community resources, 288, 319
Compliance, 10-13, 63-64, 246,
        252-253, 272, 278, 281,
        289, 307, 329
Comprehensive geriatric model
        (CGM), 239, 241-242, 249,
        256, 263, 267-268
Computerized cranial tomography
        (CT), 57, 180, 186, 225,
        235
Conduction system (*see* Radiation)
Conjunctivitis (*see* Radiation)
Constipation (*see* Aging)
Control, 8, 12, 201, 205, 290-291,
        294, 296, 301, 313, 316-
        320
Coping skills, 209, 221, 289, 309-310,
        320
Coping strategy, 7, 9
Cordotomy, 185, 193-194
Corneal ulceration (*see* Radiation)
Coronary arteries (*see* Radiation)
Corticosteroids, 72, 87, 94, 112, 115,
        120, 122, 130, 132, 181, 184,
        188, 192-193, 259, 271
Costs
    direct and indirect, 11-12, 15-16
    fees, 11, 15, 18, 31
    psychosocial, 11
    savings, 10, 13, 17, 26, 28, 32

Cranial irradiation, 132, 191, 195, 224-
        228, 234
Creatinine (*see* Aging)
Cure
    cost of, 12
    effect a, 12, 14
Cystitis (*see* Chemotherapy)
Cytomegalovirus, 187

Death, 6-7, 11, 17, 21, 29, 34, 38, 41-
        42, 49-51, 64, 84, 88, 108,
        145, 183, 197, 204-205, 215,
        233, 237, 249-250, 264, 271,
        279, 284, 300, 302-303, 305,
        307, 309, 314, 316, 318,
        320-326
    preparation of family for, 321
Decision making, 234, 246, 255, 265,
        268, 313, 316
Dehydration, 29, 39, 51, 57, 66, 73,
        316, 318
Delirium, 200, 206-208, 211
Dementia, 191, 200, 206-208, 225
Denial, 7, 147, 202, 215, 256, 263,
        300-303, 316
Dental care, 94, 142,
        157
"Denying helpers", 283
Depersonalization, 289, 299
Depression, 10, 44, 184, 188, 197-
        217, 231, 250, 256, 259-260,
        263-264, 281, 283, 312, 315-
        316, 318, 320, 323, 325
    defined, 197-199
    incidence of, 10
    measurement of, 202
    treatment of, 209-210
    "vegetative symptoms" of, 201, 208,
        210
Dexamethasone, 258
Diagnosis, 2, 5, 9, 15, 17, 19-22, 50,
        77, 93, 132, 179-181, 183-
        184, 186, 188, 192, 196-198,
        200-202, 204-206, 208-209,

214, 216, 237, 249, 262,
    265, 267, 279-281, 283,
    286-287, 294, 307, 315
  approaches to, 7, 16-17
  of lung cancer, 13
Diethylstilbestrol, 256
Diphenhydramine (see Chemotherapy)
Disease-Related Groups (DRG), 26, 63
Disorientation, 206, 251
Disseminated intravascular coagulation,
    81
Dopamine receptors, 70
Drug extravasation (see Chemo-
    therapy)
Dying, 9, 205, 212-213, 215, 264,
    271, 305, 307, 309-316,
    319-320, 323-326
Dyskineses, 71, 258
Dysphoria, 72, 198, 244, 257

Ear, middle, 150
Ectropion (see Radiation)
Elderly (see also Aging), 3, 211, 237-239,
    242, 244-275, 314, 320-321
Electroconvulsive therapy, 199, 212
Electroencephalogram (EEG), 42,
    186, 190-191, 225
Electrolyte losses (see Surgery)
Emotional support, 9, 106-107, 274,
    280-281
Encephalopathy (see Chemotherapy)
Endocrine system, 227-228
Enteral nutrition, 257
  complications of, 51
Environment, 68, 91, 134, 136, 201,
    206, 238, 242, 244, 247, 257,
    279-280, 286-287, 292-294,
    299, 306-308, 311, 322
Epidural metastases, 181, 193
Epiphora, 149
Erythropoiesis, 75, 78, 82,
    87
Esophageal tears, 65

Esophagitis, 22, 159
Esophagus, 159, 247
Ethical decision making, 246, 250,
    263-266
Euphoria, 257
Expectations, change in, 3, 12
Experimental therapy, defined, 28
Extravasation, 97, 99-103, 144, 262
Extremities, 97, 172, 188

Family
  assessment, 283, 286
  burnout, 288
  counseling, 286
  education, 287, 293, 295
  environment scale, 286, 307
  interaction, 280
  grief, 250
  solidarity, 288
  support, 277-278, 280-281, 286,
    288-289
Fees (see Costs)
Fetal malformation (see Radiation)
Fetus, chemotherapy and (see
    Chemotherapy)
Fever and antibiotics, 88, 90-91
Fistulas, rectovaginal, vesicovaginal,
    170
Flu vaccine, 262
Foods, 23, 27, 66, 190, 257, 260,
    282
"Foot-drop", 182
Functional reserve status, 239
Functional status, 238, 242-244,
    252, 257, 261, 263, 268
  homeostatic core of, 242-244, 254
Functioning, level of, 255

Gastrointestinal infections, 122
Gastrointestinal system, 246
Gastrointestinal toxicity (see
    Chemotherapy)
Gastrostomy, 159

Glaucoma, 150
Glucocorticoids, 257
Goals
    disparity, 6
    health team, 8
Gonadal
    aspermia, 172
    dysfunction, 128, 228-229
    function, 129
    hypogonadism, 130
    infertility, 128, 130-131, 228-
        229
    oophoropexy, 229
    ovarian function, 128, 138, 228
    ovaries, 172
    pubertal development, 228
    sexual dysfunction, 128
    sperm banking, 128, 130
    sterility, 128, 172
Granulocyte transfusions, 78, 90
Granulocytopenia, 61, 76-79, 83,
        85, 90-93, 143, 249
Grief, 204-205, 209, 215, 250,
        256, 263-264, 303,
        322, 325-326
    anticipatory, 321-322
    complicated, 322-323
    reactions, 264
    risk factors of, 264
Growth hormone deficiency,
        227-228
Guilt, 7, 198, 202, 205, 220,
        233, 250, 263, 283,
        287-288, 322-323

Haloperidol (see Chemotherapy)
Hayflick's model, 239, 248
Healing service, 300
Health beliefs, 252-253
Hearing loss (see Radiation)
Heart, 160
Hematopoiesis, aging, 248, 272

Hematopoietic system, 174, 247-248
Hepatotoxicity (see Chemotherapy)
Herpes simplex, 96, 187
Herpes zoster, 187, 259, 262, 272
Hoarseness (see Radiation)
Hodgkin's disease, 16, 18, 34, 59, 85-
        86, 94, 130-131, 138, 141,
        148, 161, 175-176, 181, 186,
        227, 229, 234-236, 273, 282
Hormonal therapy, 227-228, 237, 256
Hospice, 2, 4, 9, 259-260, 266, 304,
        309, 313-331
    admission criteria, 314
    concept of, 25-26
    programs that provide, 313-324
    standards of care, 313
Humor, 213, 294, 298
Hyperbaric oxygen, 157
Hypercalcemia, 125, 185
Hypermagnesemia, 44
Hypernatremia, 40-41
Hyperphosphatemia, 43, 125
Hyperuricemia, 125
Hypnosis, 73, 145, 260
Hypogonadism (see Gonadal)
Hypokalemia, 42, 65
    potassium depletion, 42
    potassium excess, 41-42
Hyponatremia, 40-41, 43, 48, 185
Hypopharynx, 158
Hypothalamic pituitary axis, 227
Hypothyroidism, 227-228
Hypoxemia, 185, 251

Immune complex disease, 248
Immune system, 248-249
Immunosuppression, 88, 95
Inanition, 66
Inappropriate ADH syndrome, 130
Infections (see Chemotherapy)
Infertility (see also Gonadal), 128,
        227-229

Influenza, 262
Informed consent, 5, 12-13, 38,
    221-238, 265, 303, 329
Infusaid, 21, 25
Institutional Review Board, 304
Institutional options, 267
Insurance, 27-29, 34, 286, 315,
    330-331
Interferon, alpha, 190
Intergenerational problems, 285
Interleukins, 249
Interpersonal relationships, 278-
    279, 281
Interpersonal support, 279
Interstitial therapy, 153, 156
Intestine, 167
    bacterial overgrowth in, 247
    large, 167
    small, 167, 247
"Intra-operative therapy" (see
    Radiation)
I.Q. scores, 224, 235
Iris (see Radiation)
Ischemic heart disease, risk factors
    for, 245

Jaw pain, 189
Jehovah's Witness, 223

Karnofsky scale, 242
Keratitis (see Radiation)
Kidneys, 168
Kyphoscoliosis, 229

Lacrimal gland (see Radiation)
Laminar air flow units, 90
Larynx (see Radiation)
L-asparaginase, 82, 114-115, 117
    124, 191, 195
Late effects (see Chemotherapy)
Laughter, 294
Leisure activities, 8, 289-299

Lens (see Radiation)
Leptomeningeal metastasis, 180
Leukemia
    acute lymphocytic, 16, 18, 61, 129,
        195-196, 223, 225, 227-228,
        255
    acute nonlymphocytic, 16, 130, 141,
        143, 273
Leukemogenesis, 132
Leukocyte count, 80, 82, 174
Leukocytosis, 75
Leukoencephalopathy, 191-192, 196,
    225-226, 235
Leukopenia, 75, 77, 323
Lhermitte's phenomenon, 193
Life expectancy average, 242
Liver, 120, 166
    toxicity, 120
Lorazepam, 72-74, 137, 139, 141
Lungs (see Pulmonary)
Lung volumes, changes in (see
    Pulmonary)
Lymphangiography, 34, 227
Lymphedema, 97, 173
Lymphocyte, 79, 83
    function, 248
    thymus-dependent, 248
Lymphokines, 248
Lymphopenia, 79, 83, 85, 87, 89

Magnesium depletion, 43
Maintenance fluid and electrolytes,
    46
Malabsorption (see Chemotherapy)
Malnutrition, 42, 48-52, 59, 65, 89,
    168, 261, 273
"Mantle" field (see Radiation)
Marijuana, 71
Marrow aplasia (see Chemotherapy)
Mastication (see Aging)
Melancholia, 198
Mental capacity, declining, 246

Mental competency, 265
Mental status examination, 263
Metabolic alkalosis, 65,
Metabolic encephalopathy, 185-186,
        190
Methotrexate (*see* Chemotherapy)
Methyl CCNU (*see* Chemotherapy)
Metoclopramide (*see* Chemotherapy)
Misconceptions (*see* Aging)
Misonidazole, 191
Mitomycin-C (*see* Chemotherapy)
Morphine, 28, 185, 259, 271
Mortality (*see* Aging)
Mucositis (*see* Chemotherapy)
Multifractionation (*see* Radiation)
Mutagenesis (*see* Chemotherapy)
Myelodysplastic bone marrow (*see*
        Chemotherapy)
Myeloid metaplasia, 75
Myeloma, 87-88, 131, 141, 181,
        186, 254, 269, 323
Myelopathy, 193-194, 196
Myelophthistic anemia, 75
Myelopoiesis, 79, 84
Myelosuppression, 76-77, 85, 87,
        93, 95
Myocardial infarcts, 160
Myocardium, 244

Narcotics, 184, 209-210
Nasal cavity, 152
Nasogastric tube, 159
Nausea, 2, 9, 28, 39-40, 44, 46,
        63-75, 84, 125, 139-145,
        168, 213, 246, 252-253,
        257-259, 316, 318
    chlorpromazine, 70
    haloperidol, 70, 74, 139-140,
        142, 207-208,
    metoclopramide, 70-74, 139-140,
        144, 187, 257, 259, 272
    phenothiazines, 28, 69-70, 72,

[Nausea]
        141, 144, 184, 187, 190,
        258-259
    prochlorperazine, 69-70, 74,
        137, 139-140, 143-144, 257
Neck (*see* Radiation)
Neoplastic cells, 180, 238-239
Nephrotoxicity (*see* Chemotherapy)
Neuralgia, post-herpetic, 259, 271
Neuroendocrine system, 227
Neurofibrillary tangles, 246
Neurological disturbances, 179
Neuropathies, 182-183, 188, 254,
        259
Neutropenia, 77-79, 88-89, 91-92,
        94-95, 122, 137
Nitrosourea, 85
    bischlorethylnitrosourea (BCNU)
        (*see* Chemotherapy)
Non-participation, 257
Nursing home patients, 248
Nutrient absorption, 247
Nutrition
    enteral, 63, 257, 265
    general guideline for, 59, 257,
        261
Nutritional deficiencies (*see* Aging)

Odynophagia, 158-159
Oophoropexy (*see* Gonadal)
Opportunistic organisms (*see*
        Chemotherapy)
Oral
    antibiotic, 26-27, 247
    cavity, 121, 152, 252
    diethylstilbestrol, 256
    gratification, 252
    hydration approaches, 23, 33
    poor intake, 57
    ulcers, 121
Orbit, 148
Orchiectomy, 256

Osteomyelitis, 156
Ovarian function (*see* Gonadal)
"Overcompensating smotherers", 281
Overtreatment, problem of (*see*
        Aging)
Pain, 2-3, 7-9, 15, 22, 25, 28-30,
        33, 96-97, 100-101, 103,
        114, 119-121, 181-185,
        189-191, 193, 195-196,
        201, 205, 209-210, 213,
        215-217, 246, 250-251,
        258-260, 263, 270-274,
        280, 291, 294, 302, 304,
        306, 308, 310-311, 315-
        325
Pain perception, 251, 258-260
    alterations in, 251
    control of, 258, 317-318
    decline with age, 259
    factors that influence, 260
    threshold, 258
Palliation, 1, 8-9, 20, 56, 147,
        309, 328
Palmar-plantar erythrodyses-
        thesia syndrome, 119, 141
Panic attacks, 205
Para-endocrine, 66
Paranasal sinuses (*see* Radiation)
Paraneoplastic syndromes, 47-48
Parens patriae, 221-222
Parental attitudes, 221
Parental stress, 221
Participatory self-assessment, 286
Paternalism, 265
Pearls, for more perfect practice,
        28
Peer support, 282-283, 288
Perceived support, 279
Pericardial effusion, 160
Pericardiectomy, 161
Pericarditis, acute, 160
Periodontal disease, 95-96, 260

Personality factors, 184, 208
Personnel handling antineoplastic
        agents (*see* Chemotherapy)
Personal relations, 290, 294
Phenothiazines (*see also* Nausea,
        Vomiting), 69-70, 73,
        258
Phosphorus depletion, 42
Photosensitivity reactions, 116, 119
Pigmentation (*see* Chemotherapy)
Play therapy, 220, 232-233
Pneumococcal vaccine, 262
Podophyllotoxin analogs, 259
Polyneuropathy, 188-189
"Positive cytology", 180
Post-irradiation somnolence syn-
        drome, 225
Post-thoracotomy, 259
Potassium depletion (*see* Hypok-
        alemia)
Potassium excess (*see* Hyperkalemia)
Prednisone, 71, 87, 109, 144, 254,
        259
Preleukemia, 131
Premorbid personality traits, 266
Preoperative appraisal (*see* Aging)
Preoperative irradiation, 54
Presbyesophagus, 247, 275
Prescribing, 22
Pressures, for oncologist, 20
Preventative interventions, 278,
        286
Procarbazine (*see* Chemotherapy)
Prochlorperazine, 70, 74, 257
Prognosis, discussing, 309-311, 315,
        327
Progressive muscle relaxation, 73
Prophylactic antibiotics (*see* Chemo-
        therapy, Surgery)
Prophylactic immunization (*see*
        Aging)
Psychological adaptation, 214, 231-233,

[Psychological adaptation]
    304
Psychological morbidity, related to
    side effects, 10
Psychological needs, 263, 307
Psychosis, 188, 204, 207-208
Psychosocial services, 266
Psychosocial supports, 244, 265
Psychotic distortions, 207-208
Psychotropic medication, 207, 209, 245
Pubertal development (*see* Gonadal)
Pulmonary
    changes in lung volumes, 245
    function tests, 110
    lungs, 164, 254
Pulmonary toxicity, 110, 112-114, 137-
    138

Quality of life, 20, 62, 64, 128, 203,
    252, 254-255, 260

Radiation, 61, 66, 70, 75, 77-78, 81-
    86, 94, 109, 116, 119, 122,
    131-132, 141, 144, 190-196,
    206, 237, 246, 252, 258,
    262, 270, 274, 283, 323
    auditory canal, 150
    blindness, 150
    bone necrosis, 153, 157, 173
    bowel, 167
    Caldwell-Luc, 152
    conduction system, 160
    conjunctivitis, 149
    corneal ulceration, 149
    coronary arteries, 160
    cystitis, 169
    ectropion, 149
    enteritis, 54, 168
    fetal malformations, 172
    fibrosis, 54, 149, 165, 173, 259
    hearing loss, 150
    hematologic effects, 85

[Radiation]
    hepatitis, 166-167
    hoarseness, 158
    "intra-operative therapy", 166
    iris, 149
    keratitis, 149
    lacrimal gland, 149
    larynx, 158
    lens, 149
    "mantle" field, 165
    multifractionation, 165, 168
    myocarditis, 160
    neck, 157
    nephritis, 169
    paranasal sinuses, 152
    radiation-induced tumors, 175
    pneumonitis, 164-165
    proctosigmoiditis, 170
    renal failure, chronic, 169
    retina, 149
    salivary glands, 154-155
    sarcoma, 172
    testicles, 172, 228
Radionecrosis, 192-193, 195
Radiosensitivity, 252
Receptor cells, 150
Recreation therapy, 285, 289-299
Rehabilitation programs, 2
"Rejecting avoiders", 284
Religious beliefs, 27, 286, 299-301
Renal failure, chronic (*see*
    Radiation)
Research, 18
    participation in, 28
Reserve, assessment of (*see* Aging);
        functional (*see* Aging)
Resources, financial (*see* Aging)
Retina (*see* Radiation)
Retinopathy, 133, 140
Ritual, 301, 304-305, 323
Salivary glands (*see* Radiation)
Sarcoma (*see* Radiation)

Savings (*see* Costs)
Scalp hypothermia (*see* Chemo-
    therapy)
Scalp tourniquets (*see* Chemo-
    therapy)
Screening questionnaire, 286
Secondary malignancies (*see*
    Chemotherapy)
Second opinion, 6, 38, 63
Secretion of acid, pepsin, 168
Sedation, 68, 72-73, 187, 257-
    259
  side effects of, 259
Seizures, 182, 191, 196, 225
Selection of surgical procedure, 56
Self-esteem, 202, 208, 220, 236,
    244, 281, 284, 294
Self-image, 220, 294-295, 298
Senile plaques, 246
Senile purpura, 262
Sexual dysfunction (*see*
    Gonadal)
Short stature, 227
Shunts (*see* Chemotherapy)
Sitting height, 229
Skin cleaning (*see* Surgery)
Skin toxicity, chemotherapy
    (*see* Chemotherapy)
Smell, changes in (*see* Aging)
Social control continuum,
    defined, 12
Social identity, 280
Social isolation, 289-295, 299
Social needs, 267
Social relationships, 289-294
Social support, 244, 258, 267-268,
    271, 278-280, 282, 286,
    288, 297, 299, 306-308
Sodium depletion (*see*
    Hyponatremia)
Sodium excess (*see*
    Hypernatremia)

Somnolence syndrome, 192
Sperm banking (*see* Gonadal)
Spinal cord compression, 22, 181, 193,
    195
Sphincter dysfunction, 181
Sterility (*see* Gonadal)
Steroid therapy, 37, 53, 70, 89, 164,
    262
Stomatitis (*see* Chemotherapy)
Stress buffering role, 279
Subclavian catheter, complications of
    (*see* Catheters)
Subclavian vein, thrombosis of (*see*
    Catheters)
Suicide, 198, 200-202, 215-216
Surgery, 9, 14, 19, 21, 37-60, 65-66,
    98, 140, 181, 184, 193-194,
    237, 244, 249-252, 262,
    270, 278-279, 308
  body water excess, 39-41
  electrolyte losses, 45-46, 65
  for elderly, 252
  major, risk from, 250
  prophylactic antibiotics, 54
  skin cleaning, 55
  third-space fluid losses, estimation
    of, 57
  total parenteral nutrition
    complications of, 50-51, 59
  vitamins, 46-47
Surrogate family, 284, 297
Surveillance cultures, 94-95

Tamoxifen, 133, 140, 256
Taste (*see* Aging)
Technology, use of medical, 21-22
Teleological approach, 265-266
Tension, 289, 292
Teratogenicity, 129
Terminal care (*see also* Hospice)
  expenditures on, 25-26, 309
  managerial decisions, 25

Testicles (*see* Radiation)
Tests
  ordering of, excess and prudent, 16
  types of, 18
Tetrahydrocannabinol (THC), 70-74,
    141-143, 257
Therapeutic alliance, 6, 12
Therapeutic environment (*see*
    Aging)
Third-space fluid losses, estimation
    of (*see* Surgery)
Thrombocythemia, 61, 75-77, 80-85
Thrombocytopathy, 75
Thrombocytopenia, 45, 81, 84
Thrombocytosis, 75
Thymic factors, 248
Thyroid dysfunction, 227
Tooth buds, 231
Tooth decay, 156
Total parenteral nutrition, compli-
    cations of (*see* Surgery)
Toxic fibrosis, 254
Transverse myelitis, 225
Treatment compliance, 281
Treatment protocols, selection of
    elderly for (*see* Aging)
Tremors, 261
Trismus, 157
Trust, mutual, 253
Truth-telling, 265
Tumor lysis syndrome, 125

Unconventional therapy, 222
Undertreatment, problem of,
    223-224
Urinary diversion, 170

Vein care (*see* Chemotherapy)
Ventriculostomy reservoirs (*see*
    Chemotherapy)
Vinca alkaloids (*see* Chemotherapy)
Vincristine (*see* Chemotherapy)
Visiting nurse association, 266
Vitamins, 46-47
Vitreous hemorrhages, 150
Vomiting, 2, 9, 39-40, 44, 46, 63-
    75, 84, 125, 138-145, 168,
    213, 246, 252, 257-259,
    316, 318
  chlorpromazine, 70
  haloperidol, 70, 74
  metoclopramide, 70-71, 73-74,
    257
  phenothiazines, 69-70, 258
  prochlorperazine, 70, 74, 257
Vomiting center, 68, 70

Water depletion, 40-41

Xerostomia, 121, 154

Zinc deficiency, 44
Zoster immune plasma, 94